101 Muscle Meals

101 Muscle Meals

FILL YOUR BELLY, FUEL YOUR FAT-BURNERS, AND BUILD YOUR BEST BODY EVER

Editors of *Men's Health*

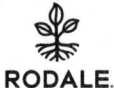
RODALE.

This book is intended as a reference volume only, not as a medical manual.
The information given here is designed to help you make informed decisions about your health.
It is not intended as a substitute for any treatment that may have been prescribed by your doctor.
If you suspect that you have a medical problem, we urge you to seek competent medical help.

Mention of specific companies, organizations, or authorities in this book
does not imply endorsement by the author or publisher, nor does mention of specific companies,
organizations, or authorities imply that they endorse this book, its author, or the publisher.

Internet addresses and telephone numbers given in this book were accurate at the time it went to press.

© 2013 by Rodale Inc.

Portions of this book have been published in *Men's Health*.

All rights reserved. No part of this publication may be reproduced or transmitted
in any form or by any means, electronic or mechanical, including photocopying, recording, or any other
information storage and retrieval system, without the written permission of the publisher.

Rodale books may be purchased for business or promotional use or for special sales.
For information, please write to:
Special Markets Department, Rodale, Inc., 733 Third Avenue, New York, NY 10017

Men's Health is a registered trademark of Rodale Inc.

Printed in the United States of America

Rodale Inc. makes every effort to use acid-free ♾, recycled paper ♻.

Book design by Mark Michaelson

Library of Congress Cataloging-in-Publication Data is on file with the publisher.

978-1-62336-284-3   hardcover

2 4 6 8 10 9 7 5 3 1   hardcover

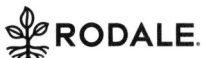

We inspire and enable people to improve their lives and the world around them.
rodalebooks.com

Special thanks to Theresa Dougherty.
Without her editorial efforts
and talent, this book would not exist.

Contents

Introduction: The Secret to Total Body Transformation...................x

Part One
The Power of Food

Chapter 1. Food, Made Simple...................3

Chapter 2. The Truth about Calories...................11

Chapter 3. The *Men's Health* Nutrition Spectrum 15

Part Two
Master Everyday Eating

Chapter 4. Rules to Eat By...................23

Chapter 5. Foods that Build Muscle...................27

Chapter 6. Fight Fat from Your Kitchen...................31

Chapter 7. The Road Warrior's Guide to Smart Eating...................43

Chapter 8. Make Eating Exciting Again...................51

Chapter 9. Think Before You Drink...................57

Part Three
Control Food, Control Yourself

Chapter 10. The Trouble with Traditional Diets **67**
Chapter 11. Crush Cravings for Good **73**
Chapter 12. Become an Expert on Portion Control **81**
Chapter 13. Why Some Foods Make You Do Bad Things **89**
Chapter 14. A Perfect Day of Eating **95**

Part Four
Fuel Your Workout

Chapter 15. Snack Smart Before You Start **105**
Chapter 16. Eat for Peak Performance **109**
Chapter 17. Recipes for Recovery **123**
Chapter 18. The All-Star Diet **131**

Part Five
Stock Up, Shape Up

Chapter 19. Master the Market **141**
Chapter 20. Pick Your Produce **149**
Chapter 21. Pantry Must-Haves **175**
Chapter 22. Shop Once, Eat for a Week **181**
Chapter 23. Best Packaged Foods for Men **187**

Part Six
Tough Nutrition Questions... Answered

Chapter 24. Is Gluten Free Worth a Shot? ... **199**

Chapter 25. Do You Need More Salt? ... **203**

Chapter 26. Should You Be Taking Probioitics? ... **209**

Chapter 27. Is Drinking Milk Risky? ... **213**

Chapter 28. How Important Are Antioxidants? ... **219**

Chapter 29. Is Sugar Toxic? ... **223**

Chapter 30. What Are the Best Supplements for Men? ... **229**

Chapter 31. Are You Getting Enough Fiber? ... **239**

Chapter 32. Do You Have a D-Ficiency? ... **243**

Chapter 33. Does Organic Really Matter? ... **249**

Chapter 34. Is Your Cooking Oil Killing You? ... **253**

Appendix
What's in Your Food?

Appendix A. Your Glossary of the Good, Bad, and Ugly in Your Food ... **259**

Appendix B. Nutritional Values of Common Foods ... **273**

Appendix C. Glycemic Loads for Selected Foods ... **287**

Index ... **291**

Recipe Index ... **301**

Introduction

The Secret to Total Body Transformation

IT'S SO SIMPLE THAT IT COMES DOWN TO ONE SHORT, SWEET WORD: EAT.

This is not a diet book. This is a book about your diet.

Big difference. Diet books, by and large, are about losing weight through calorie restriction or some specific food restriction (no carbs, for example). This book isn't about restricting foods to lose weight. It's not about finding a one-time temporary fix so you look good at your high school reunion. It's about feeding your body so you can look good at every single high school reunion for the rest of your days.

Not a bad promise, right?

See, there's a fine line between eating to lose weight and eating to build your best body, and it's easy for guys to confuse the two. Traditional diet programs that require you to restrict calories or food groups may leave you so tired, hungry, and unmotivated that you can barely make it through the day let alone a hard-core workout. You need to *eat*.

But eating too much to compensate for calories you think you're burning through exercise can be just as hazardous to your lean-body goals, not to mention your overall health. Consider this statistic from the International Food Information Council Foundation: Only 12 percent of Americans correctly estimate the amount of calories they need on a daily basis. No wonder nearly 70 percent of the same survey takers said they're concerned about their weight.

Either way, over- or under-consuming on a regular basis can ultimately lead to a fat-to-muscle ratio that's exactly the opposite of what you want it to be: too much flab and not enough muscle. And more muscle is crucial when it comes to maintaining a healthy weight, protecting your body from injury, keeping your metabolism high, and helping you look and feel your very best. Understand the numbers: One pound of muscle can burn about 6 calories per day. A pound of fat, on the other hand, burns only 2 calories per day.

It's simple. If you want to build your best body, you must eat. Eat with purpose. Eat with intelligence. Eat with the knowledge that food is the secret ingredient to total body transformation (not just "weight loss"). *Men's Health*'s *101 Muscle Meals* is designed to help you unlock this power—it's an authoritative guide on what to eat, when to eat, and how your overall health will be better for it.

We know that you may not have a lot of time to devote to narrowing down the healthiest options available, especially when you're bombarded with tons of nutrition information that can be confusing or contradictory. So we pored through the latest research to come up with the best foods for your body, at any stage of your life, no matter what your goal may be—to lose weight, build muscle, power through your next half-marathon, or just look good with your shirt off. We've also included simple tweaks, delicious recipes, and even weekly meal plans that you can easily add to your schedule as is or adapt to fit your own needs. No matter which option you choose, in no time you'll be on your way to your leanest, sexiest, most powerful body ever.

101
Muscle
Meals

The Power of Food

Part One

You know that food has the power to make you fat. You also know that controlling your food intake, on some level, can help you lose or maintain weight. But you need to go further than that. Much further. You need to understand the true power of food, its nature, and how it really works in your body. Once you learn a few basic things, detailed in this section, you'll be primed to take advantage of the rest of the information in this book—primed to begin a total body transformation, properly fueled by some of the most delicious foods known to humankind.

Food, Made Simple

UNDERSTAND HOW YOUR BODY WORKS WITH FOOD AND ELIMINATE DUMB EATING MISTAKES.

No carb. Low carb. Low fat. No fat. Caveman. Mediterranean. Gluten free. You could make a rap about all the wildly successful diets that have swept society in the past few years. And here's a little secret: They all work. Well, of course they do. If you restrict your food intake to certain kinds of foods in certain amounts, you'll lose weight.

But do you want to lose weight, or do you want to forge your best body ever? And keep that body forever? Then you have to shake off the static you hear from everyone you know about what they've been eating for the past 4 weeks (which will change in the next 4 weeks when something new comes along).

Nope, you need some food truth, because you want more than a quick fix. You need to know how food really works with your body so you can fuel that body properly. Everything comes back to food. You want to build muscle and burn fat? Eat. You want to perform in sports? Eat. You want to stay sharp all day at the office? Eat. You want to raise your bedroom game? Eat. Eating right is everything. According to *Food & Mood* author Elizabeth Somer, RD, your ability to excel is directly linked to the contents of your shopping cart. "When life is overflowing with stress, deadlines, or competitive events, it's crucial to go into these challenging situations fueled by foods that allow you to perform at your best."

But how do you know which foods are going to help increase your chances of getting the results you're gunning for? Let's start with the basics. The food that fuels you is made up of macronutrients, which are compounds that your body needs in large quantities to provide it with the energy it uses to function or to flourish. There are three types of macronutrients: fat, carbohydrates, and protein. Your body uses each in a different way. That's why it's important to eat a diet balanced in all three and why skimping on just one—by going on an extreme low-carb plan, for example—can sabotage your fitness efforts in the long run.

To best harness the power in the food you eat, it helps to grasp the fundamentals about each macronutrient.

Fat

Dietary fat is one nutrient with a serious image problem. "Our bodies need certain fats," says Bonnie Taub-Dix, RD, author of *Read It Before You Eat It*. Getting the right amounts from the right sources will not only ensure your food doesn't taste like cardboard, but also can help you lose stubborn pounds (yes, you read that correctly).

The main reason fat gets a bad rap is that much of the type we eat comes in less-than-healthy packages like doughnuts and cheese fries. The fact that we're wired to crave the flavor fat provides makes it even easier to overeat. That's because, back when mammoth was still a menu item, calories were hard to come by. Humans evolved to seek out the most concentrated supply of them, and fat, with 9 calories per gram (versus 4 calories per gram in carbs and proteins), was our best food source for survival.

Though we no longer need that primitive urge to keep us alive, fat still plays a critical role: It delivers key nutrients to your body. "Vitamins such as A, D, E, and K are called fat soluble because they need to bind to fat to be absorbed," says Taub-Dix. "If fat isn't available, the vitamins can't be absorbed properly." Top your salad with low-fat dressing and you could miss out on a lot of the benefits in those leafy greens—which can also leave you jonesing for a snack later. "Part of losing weight is being satisfied so you aren't grazing all day on other foods," says Taub-Dix. "And studies have found that foods with healthy fats, like avocado and nuts, take longer to digest and therefore help keep you fuller longer."

THE LOW-FAT LIE

Approaching fat the way you do the limbo—how low can you go?—won't send the numbers on the scale plummeting. Data from the Centers for Disease Control and Prevention (CDC) shows that while Americans consumed a lower percentage of calories from fat in 2000 than they did in 1971, the total number of calories they consumed per day increased. This is likely the result of manufacturers replacing the fat in foods with sugar. "The 'low-fat' message was interpreted as an invitation to indulge without keeping calories in mind," says Taub-Dix.

Cutting all fat from your diet means you'll also miss out on good fats that can help you in your quest to get that lean look you're after. A study in the journal *Diabetes Care* found that a diet rich in monounsaturated fats (such as almonds) may prevent the accumulation of abdominal fat. "Fat is all about the source it comes from," says Lauren Blaue, RD, a nutrition coach at Life Time Athletic Club in Minneapolis. Combining fats and carbs in the same meal will keep your blood sugar stable and help you avoid hunger-inducing spikes and dips.

This isn't license to gorge on a huge cinnamon roll, though. Calories still count (you'll read more about them later), and you're better off getting your fill of healthy, naturally occurring fats rather than gooey processed ones. For the best results, spread your fat-carb combos throughout the day: natural nut butter on whole-grain toast in the a.m., olive oil drizzled on your salad at lunch, guac with veggies for a snack.

HOW MUCH FAT SHOULD YOU EAT?

Expert guidelines suggest that 20 to 30 percent of your daily calories should come from fats, and no more than 10 percent from the saturated variety. Based on a diet of 2,000 calories a day, that's between 40 and 60 grams of fat daily. Follow these suggestions to keep your portions in control.

Saturated Fats

Many of us know saturated fats as "bad" fats, but new research has led experts to question whether they are linked to heart disease, as previously thought. And one study even found that certain saturated fats can be metabolized by your body faster than others, which means they are rarely stored as flab. If a fat is solid at room temperature (think butter or Crisco), it's probably saturated.

GET YOUR FILL:

1 tablespoon butter (salted)
(12 g fat, 102 cal)

1 tablespoon coconut oil
(14 g fat, 117 cal)

8 ounces 1% milk
(5 g fat, 122 cal)

3 ounces cooked ground beef, 85 percent lean
(13 g fat, 212 cal)

Polyunsaturated Fatty Acids (PUFAs)

These fats tend to be liquid at room temperature, like oils, and are often in plant-based foods. PUFAs can help reduce the risk for type 2 diabetes and heart disease by helping improve cholesterol.

GET YOUR FILL:

1 tablespoon safflower, corn, sunflower, soy, cottonseed, peanut, or other vegetable or nut oil
(14 g fat, approximately 120 cal)

1 ounce dry-roasted sunflower seeds
(14 g fat, 165 cal)

Monounsaturated Fatty Acids (MUFAs)

Eating this form of unsaturated fat can help improve cholesterol levels and steady blood sugar.

GET YOUR FILL:

¼ avocado
(7 g fat, 80 cal)

10 large green olives
(4 g fat, 40 cal)

1 tablespoon peanut butter
(8 g fat, 94 cal)

Omega-3 Fatty Acids

These may fight body inflammation and protect against cardiovascular disease. "Getting sufficient omega-3s is tough," says Blaue. You'd have to eat salmon three times a week to get 500 milligrams per day of omega-3s, the amount needed to reap the heart benefits.

GET YOUR FILL:

3 ounces cooked salmon
(4 g fat, 114 cal)

1 can sardines (3.75 ounces) in oil
(11 g fat, 191 cal)

1 ounce walnuts (about 14 halves)
(18 g fat, 185 cal)

Omega-6 Fatty Acids

Omega-6s can help you absorb more vitamins from food. To help decrease the risk of dying from coronary disease, "people should get a 1-to-1 ratio of omega-6 fats to omega-3s," says Blaue. Otherwise, our bodies can metabolize omega-6s in a harmful way. "Most American diets," she says, "have a 20-to-1 ratio of omega-6s to omega-3s."

GET YOUR FILL:

1 tablespoon margarine
(11 g fat, 101 cal)

2 tablespoons Caesar salad dressing
(17 g fat, 163 cal)

1 tablespoon almond butter
(9 g fat, 98 cal)

ONE TO AVOID

For all the friendly types of fat, there is one you should keep as an enemy: man-made trans fats, which have been shown to raise bad (LDL) cholesterol and lower good (HDL) cholesterol. Unlike other unsaturated fats, which tend to have health benefits, these have been chemically altered through a process called hydrogenation to make the product they are in easier to sell (for example, some packaged cookies contain hydrogenated or partially hydrogenated fats to make them last longer on store shelves).

Unfortunately, you may not even be aware they're in a product, thanks to tricky labeling laws that allow manufacturers to list zero gram of trans fats as long as a serving contains less than 0.5 gram. To avoid them, stay away from food whose ingredients panel lists hydrogenated or partially hydrogenated oils.

Finally, always remember to watch your portions, even with good fats. Fat in any form packs more than twice the amount of calories as protein and carbs. "Often, people eat the right foods but too much of them," says Taub-Dix. Follow the "Get Your Fill" guidelines above for healthy fat serving sizes. Bottom line: In small doses, fat is one of your best food friends.

Carbohydrates

Like fats, carbohydrates have been accused of a laundry list of crimes against humanity, including multiple counts of conspiracy to make us pack on the pounds. This is partly because too many of us fill our bellies with the wrong kinds—breads, chips, crackers, and pastas made from refined flour that's been processed to within an inch of its nutritional life. People have also gotten confusing messages about carbs thanks to trends like the protein-centric, grain-shunning Paleo Diet and from advocates of going gluten free. All this has many of us retreating from an essential fuel source that makes us faster, fitter, and smarter. But harnessing the power of the carbohydrate is not as simple as stocking a pantry full of bagels and filling your bottles with sports drinks. To understand why, you first need to consider some facts.

Your body uses carbohydrates to make glucose, or blood sugar, the fuel that keeps your body functioning and drives athletic performance. "All systems and tissues in your body use carbohydrates in some capacity," says Stacy T. Sims, PhD, a Stanford research exercise physiologist and nutrition scientist. Carbs fuel your immune system, enhance fluid absorption so you stay hydrated, and are even critical for muscle recovery. In fact, if you fail to feed your body the carbs it needs, it will generate them by breaking down muscle tissue. You also need carbs just to think: The brain gobbles glucose exclusively, says Michigan-based sports dietitian Donna Marlor, BSN, RD, CSSD. And maybe most surprising, especially to those of us who have been conditioned by the low-carbs-for-weight-loss craze, carbs prime the furnace for fat burning. The process of digesting them stimulates the hormones your body needs to fully break down and use fat.

BEFRIEND THE DREADED CARB

Carbohydrates fall into two categories, simple and complex. Simple carbs are made from one or two sugars, like fructose or glucose. They're found in sweeteners such as cane sugar, corn syrup, maple syrup, brown sugar, and honey. Because your body digests them quickly, they trigger a quick surge in insulin, the hormone that ushers glucose from your bloodstream into your cells to fuel activity. Refined and processed foods like white bread, white pasta, cakes, and pastries also fall into this category because they're stripped of fiber and other compounds that slow digestion and the insulin response. Simple carbs get a bad rap because sudden spikes and falls in blood sugar have been linked to overeating and, subsequently, to increased fat storage.

Complex carbohydrates are made from more than two sugar molecules and take longer to break down in your body, so you have a more measured blood sugar and insulin response. Complex carbs tend to contain fiber, which also slows digestion. About 50 percent of your total calorie intake should come from carbs, primarily the complex variety, says Marlor. Carbs like fruits, vegetables, legumes, and whole grains are lower in calories, digest more slowly, and contain vitamins, minerals, and immunity-boosting phytonutrients.

When it comes to the carbs you need to train longer and harder, your body stores carbs for fuel (in the form of glycogen), but only in a limited supply. When you exercise at an intense level, you're going to go through your stores faster. And if your body perceives that you're getting low, it will start shutting you down before you hit empty. Which means, if you don't replace some of those stores mid-workout, you could lose steam before you reach the finish line. This is where simple carbs have a place: before and during workouts when you need quick energy. Muscle contraction stimulates a special protein that transports glucose directly into your cells without insulin's help, says Marlor.

IS GLUTEN-FREE THE ANSWER? MAYBE NOT.

Some days it seems like more and more people are buying into the gluten-free or Paleo trend, but these are not necessarily the best options if you're eating with a certain athletic goal in mind or looking to shed excess weight.

There are certainly legitimate reasons to give up gluten, and you'll learn more about these in Chapter 24. Some people have celiac disease, an inability to digest the protein, which leads to gastrointestinal distress; others may have wheat allergies. A doctor can test you for both conditions. Some experts say you may simply have a gluten sensitivity, which may hamper digestion without causing more overt symptoms. The only way to test for that is to stop eating gluten and see how you feel. "Be sure to substitute in unprocessed grains like amaranth and quinoa, not just 'gluten-free' processed foods," says Sims.

But athletes who have no discernible symptoms likely won't see performance gains from giving up gluten and will miss out on the slow-burning carbs and nutrients in wheat, especially the whole-grain variety. As Marlor says, "It's an important part of an athlete's diet."

The Paleo Diet, for example, takes your everyday diet back to the Stone Age so you subsist on lean meats, fruits, and vegetables (no grains, legumes, or dairy) for most meals. The fact is, you cannot perform at a high level without the fast-acting carbohydrates that high-carb foods provide. Even the diet's creators recognize this. In their book *The Paleo Diet for Athletes*, authors Loren Cordain and Joe Friel concede that endurance athletes, like runners or cyclists, need to "bend the rules" and eat "nonoptimal foods" such as bread, pasta, bagels, rice, corn, and other items rich in glucose to fuel their efforts and promote full recovery before, during, and after exercise. As with most of these diets, you'll still wind up eating less processed crap. "If you eat 'clean' and low on the food chain," says Sims, "your body is going to respond well."

HOW MANY CARBS SHOULD YOU EAT?

Just as you wouldn't buy a bunch of perishable food before leaving on a vacation, you don't need to consume hundreds of grams of carbs if you're doing nothing more strenuous than tapping on a keyboard. Sims recommends these guidelines for matching your overall daily carb intake to how much activity you do. Each gram of carbohydrate provides 4 calories of energy.

Exercise Level	Recommended Daily Carbohydrate *
Low/easy (less than 1 hour a day)	205 to 275 g
Moderate (about 1 hour a day)	275 to 340 g
Very Active (1 to 3 hours a day)	410 to 475 g
Extremely Active (4 to 5 hours a day or more)	545 to 580 g

*Amounts based on a 150-pound person

Protein

If you think that you're currently eating enough protein, you're probably wrong. That's because nearly every part of your body needs it to function. Your skin, bones, hair, and nails are composed mostly of protein. Not to mention that it helps fuel the muscle-growing process called protein synthesis. That's why Rocky chugged eggs before his morning runs.

"At any given moment, even at rest, your body is breaking down and building protein," says Jeffrey Volek, PhD, RD, a nutrition and exercise researcher at the University of Connecticut. And every time you eat at least 30 grams of protein, says Donald Layman, PhD, professor emeritus of nutrition at the University of Illinois, you trigger a burst of protein synthesis that lasts about 3 hours.

But think about it: When do you eat most of your protein? At dinner, right? That means you could be fueling muscle growth for only a few hours a day, and breaking down muscle the rest of the time, says Layman.

What's more, your body can process only so much protein in a single sitting. A study from the University of Texas found that consuming 90 grams of protein at one meal provides the same benefit as eating 30 grams. It's like a gas tank, says study author Douglas Paddon-Jones, PhD: "There's only so much you can put in to maximize performance. The rest is spillover."

The best plan of action then is to spread out your protein intake. Eating protein at all three of your main meals—plus snacking two or three times a day on proteins such as cheese, jerky, and milk—will help you eat less overall. And people who start the day with a protein-rich breakfast consume 200 fewer calories a day than those who chow down on a carb-heavy breakfast, like a jam-smeared bagel. Ending the day with a steak dinner doesn't have the same appetite-quenching effect, Layman says.

Many foods, including nuts and beans, can provide a good dose of protein. But the best sources are dairy products, eggs, meat, and fish, Layman says. Animal protein is complete—it contains the right proportions of the essential amino acids your body can't synthesize on its own.

However, if you don't eat meat or are allergic to dairy, it's possible to build complete protein from plant-based foods by combining legumes, nuts, and grains at one meal or over the course of a day. But you'll need to consume 20 to 25 percent more plant-based protein to reap the benefits that animal-derived sources provide, says Mark Tarnopolsky, MD, PhD, who studies exercise and nutrition at McMaster University in Hamilton, Ontario.

So if protein can help keep weight off, is a chicken wing dipped in blue-cheese dressing a diet secret? Not quite: As with fats, total calories still count. Instead, try to make room on your plate for lean protein: eggs, low-fat milk, yogurt, lean meat, and fish.

PROTEIN IN THE GYM

Every guy in the gym knows he should consume some protein after a workout. But how much and when? "When you work out, your muscles are primed to respond to protein," Volek says, "and you have a window of opportunity to promote muscle growth."

When you perform a resistance exercise, it breaks down muscle. This requires a fresh infusion of amino acids to repair and build it. "If you're lifting weights and you don't consume protein, it's almost counterproductive," says Volek. Protein also helps build enzymes that allow your body to adapt to endurance sports like running and biking.

Volek recommends splitting your dose of protein, eating half 30 minutes before the workout and the other half 30 minutes after. A total of 10 to 20 grams of protein is ideal, he says. And wrap a piece of bread around that turkey, because carbs can raise insulin. This slows protein breakdown, which speeds muscle growth after your workout. Moreover, you won't use your stored protein for energy; you'll rely instead on the carbs to replenish you.

Everyone—not just muscle heads—can benefit from the quick hit of amino acids provided by a protein supplement, bar, or shake. Your best bet is a fast-absorbing, high-quality kind like whey protein powder (derived from milk). "It appears in your bloodstream 15 minutes after you consume it," Volek says.

Whey protein is also the best source of leucine, an amino acid that behaves more like a hormone in your body. "It's more than a building block of protein—it actually activates protein synthesis," Volek says. Whey contains 10 percent leucine while other animal-based proteins have as little as 5 percent.

Casein, another milk protein sold in supplement form, provides a slower-absorbing but more sustained source of amino acids, making it a great choice for a snack before you hit the sack. "Casein should help you maintain a positive protein balance during the night," says Volek. Building muscle while you sleep? Thanks to protein, anything's possible.

HOW MUCH PROTEIN SHOULD YOU EAT?

Most adults would benefit from eating more than the recommended daily intake of 56 grams, says Layman. The benefit goes beyond muscles and appetite control, he says, since protein can help prevent obesity, diabetes, and heart disease.

How much do you need? Step on a scale and be honest with yourself about your workout regimen. According to Tarnopolsky, highly trained athletes thrive on 0.77 gram of daily protein per pound of body weight. That's 116 grams for a 150-pound man.

Men who work out 5 or more days a week for an hour or longer need 0.55 gram per pound. And men who work out 3 to 5 days a week for 45 minutes to an hour need 0.45 gram per pound. So a 150-pound guy who works out regularly needs about 70 to 75 grams of protein a day.

Now, if you're trying to lose weight, protein is still crucial. The fewer calories you consume, the more calories should come from protein, says Layman. You need to boost your protein intake to between 0.45 and 0.68 gram per pound to preserve calorie-burning muscle mass.

And no, that extra protein won't wreck your kidneys, as some high-protein critics have said. "Taking in more than the recommended dose won't confer more benefit. It won't hurt you, but you'll just burn it off as extra energy," Tarnopolsky says.

GET YOUR FILL:

3 oz chicken, turkey, or tuna
(14–22 g protein, 66–100 cal)

3 eggs
(19 g protein, 232 cal)

16 oz chocolate 2% milk
(about 17 g protein, 333 cal)

30 g scoop whey powder
(24 g protein, 110 cal)

5.3 oz container Greek yogurt
(15 g protein, 80 cal)

The Truth about Calories

LOOK BEYOND THE CLASSIC WEIGHT LOSS CLICHÉ OF "CALORIES IN = CALORIES OUT."

These days you can't go anywhere without being confronted by calories. Restaurants now print calorie counts on menus. You go to the supermarket and there they are, stamped on every box and bottle. You hop on the treadmill and watch your "calories burned" click upward.

The standard school of thought dictates that the more calories we take in, the more flab we add—and if we cut back on them, then flab starts to recede, right? After all, at face value, calories seem to be the factor by which all foods should be judged. But if that were true, 500 calories of spinach would equal 500 calories of chocolate chip cookies.

Unfortunately for all of us, that's not the whole truth. But if you learn the distinctions, you can ultimately lose the lard. We've assembled some of the most common questions you may have about calories, how they work, and how you can use them to your advantage.

WHAT'S A CALORIE?

A calorie is simply a unit of measurement for heat. In the early 19th century, it was used to explain the theory of heat conservation and steam engines. The term entered the food world around 1890, when the USDA appropriated it for a report on nutrition. Specifically, a calorie was defined as the unit of heat required to raise 1 gram of water 1 degree Celsius.

To apply this concept to foods like sandwiches, scientists used to set food on fire (really!) and then gauge how well the flaming sample warmed a water bath. The warmer the water, the more calories the food contained. (Today, a food's calorie count is estimated from its carbohydrate, protein, and fat content.) In the calorie's leap to nutrition, its definition changed. The calorie we now see cited on nutrition labels is the amount of heat required to raise 1 kilogram of water by 1 degree Celsius.

Here's the problem: Your body isn't a steam engine. Instead of heat, it runs on chemical energy, fueled by the oxidation of carbohydrates, fat, and protein that occurs in your cells' mitochondria. "You could say mitochondria are like small power plants," says Maciej Buchowski, PhD, a research professor of medicine at Vanderbilt University Medical Center. "Instead of one central plant, you have several billion, so it's more efficient."

ALL CALORIES ARE *NOT* CREATED EQUAL

As you read earlier, the fuel your body needs to function properly—to keep your heart beating, your lungs breathing, or your leg muscles pushing through that tough hill workout—comes from three sources: protein, carbohydrates, and fat. "They're handled by the body differently," says Alan Aragon, MS, a *Men's Health* nutrition advisor. So that old "calories in, calories out" formula can be misleading, he says. "Carbohydrates, protein, and fat have different effects on the equation."

Here's an example: For every 100 carbohydrate calories you consume, your body expends 5 to 10 in digestion. With fats, you expend slightly less (although thin people seem to break down more fat than heavy people do). The calorie-burn champion is protein: For every 100 protein calories you consume, your body needs 20 to 30 for digestion, Buchowski says. Carbohydrates and fat give up their calories easily: They're built to supply quick energy. In effect, carbs and fat yield more usable energy than protein does.

WHEN YOU CONSUME CALORIES...

When you eat a food, it passes through your stomach and then reaches your small intestine, which slurps up all the nutrients it can through its spongy walls. But 5 to 10 percent of calories slide through unabsorbed. Fat digestion is relatively efficient—fat easily enters your intestinal walls. As for protein, animal sources are more digestible than plant sources, so a top sirloin's protein will be better absorbed than tofu's.

Different carbs are processed at different rates, too: Glucose and starch are rapidly absorbed, while fiber dawdles in the digestive tract. In fact, the insoluble fiber in some complex carbs, such as that in vegetables and whole grains, tends to block the absorption of other calories. "With a very high-fiber diet, say 60 grams a day, you might lose as much as 20 percent of the calories you consume," says Wanda Howell, PhD, a professor of nutritional sciences at the University of Arizona.

So a useful measure of calories is difficult. A lab technician might find that a piece of rock candy and a piece of broccoli have the same number of calories. But in action, the broccoli's fiber ensures that the vegetable contributes less energy. A study in the *Journal of Nutrition* found that a high-fiber diet leaves roughly twice as many calories undigested as a low-fiber diet does. And fewer calories means less flab.

WHERE DO THE CALORIES GO?

After a meal, your body begins to apportion calories to nutrient-hungry organs and growing muscles. But how, exactly, is that fuel distributed? Michael Jensen, MD, a professor of medicine in the division of endocrinology, diabetes, and metabolism at the Mayo Clinic, details what goes where (note that these numbers are estimates and that each person can process food differently, thus the total isn't exactly "100 percent"):

- Approximately 25 percent to muscles
- Approximately 23 percent to the liver, pancreas, kidneys, spleen, and adrenal glands
- Approximately 10 percent to the kidneys
- Approximately 10 percent to the brain
- Approximately 10 percent to breaking down the food you just ate
- Approximately 5 to 10 percent to the heart
- Approximately 2 to 3 percent to fat cells

THE MYTH OF "LOW-CAL" FOODS

Processed low-calorie foods can be weak allies in the weight loss war. Take sugar-free foods. Omitting sugar is perhaps the easiest way to cut calories. But food manufacturers generally replace those sugars with calorie-free sweeteners, such as sucralose or aspartame. And artificial sweeteners can backfire. One University of Texas study found that consuming as few as three diet sodas a week increases a person's risk of obesity by more than 40 percent. And in a 2008 Purdue study, rats that ate artificially sweetened yogurt took in more calories at subsequent meals, resulting in more flab. The theory is that the promise of sugar—without the caloric payoff—may actually lead to overeating.

"Too many people are counting calories instead of focusing on the content of food," says Brandon Alderman, PhD, director of the exercise psychophysiology lab at Rutgers University. "This just misses the boat."

RAISE YOUR DAILY CALORIE BURN

Most of your calories burn at a constant simmer, fueling the automated processes that keep you alive. This is your basal metabolism, says Warren Willey, DO, author of *Better Than Steroids*. On the other hand, even the most fanatical fitness nuts burn no more than 30 percent of their daily calories at the gym. So if you want to burn fuel, you need to hit the gas in your everyday activities.

"Some 60 to 70 percent of our total caloric expenditure goes toward normal bodily functions," says Howell. This includes replacing old tissue, transporting oxygen, mending minor shaving wounds, and so on. For men, these processes require about 11 calories per pound of body weight a day, so a 150-pound man will incinerate 1,650 calories a day—even if he sat in front of the TV all day.

And then there are the calories you lose to NEAT, or non-exercise activity thermogenesis. NEAT consists of the countless daily motions you make outside the gym—the calories you burn while making breakfast, playing Nerf football in the office, or chasing the bus. Emerging evidence suggests that "a conscious effort to spend more time on your feet might net a greater calorie burn than 30 minutes of daily exercise," says Alderman.

Chapter 3

The *Men's Health* Nutrition Spectrum

MAP OUT WHAT TYPES OF FOODS YOU SHOULD BE EATING AND HOW MUCH OF EACH TO CONSUME.

Eating right doesn't have to be complicated. "The best diet known to man—a diet that can help you lose weight, build muscle, and live longer—is simple," says Alan Aragon, MS, a *Men's Health* nutrition advisor. "Eat mostly whole and minimally processed foods, and start cooking at home more often." But just how much of these foods should you eat? Hit the goals shown here and you'll accelerate your path to optimal health.

1 to 2 Servings per Day

HEALTHY FATS

1 serving = 2 tbsp oil, ½ small avocado, 2 g fish oil, or 1 pat butter

WHAT THEY DO

- Improve blood cholesterol levels
- Lower blood pressure
- Fight cancer

QUICK IDEAS

Grapeseed oil: Use it for high-heat cooking (such as stir-frying) or as your go-to oil for grilling.

Avocado: Halve an avocado, fill the pit area with canned crabmeat, and dig in with a spoon.

Butter: Mix softened butter with minced fresh herbs and garlic, and use it to top grilled steak.

NUTS

1 serving = ¼ cup nuts or seeds or 2 tbsp nut butter

WHAT THEY DO

- Improve blood cholesterol levels
- Lower blood pressure
- Fight cancer

QUICK IDEAS

Any variety: Bag up an assortment of nuts for a tasty trail mix, and stash some in your gym bag or desk drawer.

Walnuts: Toss a few into your pancake batter or a salad for a healthy dose of omega-3s.

Almonds: Throw a handful into yogurt or oatmeal to add a boost of protein and a satisfying crunch.

EGGS

1 serving = 1 egg

WHAT THEY DO

- Aid muscle functioning
- Build muscle
- Improve blood pressure

QUICK IDEAS

Hard-boiled: Cook up a dozen at the beginning of the week to use in salads or to eat as snacks.

Omelets: There's no better way to add variety to your breakfast. Up the nutrient quota by filling them with vegetables, meat, or cheese.

POULTRY & PORK

1 serving = 3 oz

WHAT THEY DO

- Promote satiety
- Aid muscle functioning
- Build muscle

QUICK IDEAS

Skinless chicken breast: During the last few minutes of grilling, cover the chicken with the sauce from a can of chipotle peppers in adobo.

Pork chop: Grill until done and serve with grilled apples and peaches.

Turkey: Roast a turkey breast and eat the meat in sandwiches, wraps, and salads.

SEAFOOD

1 serving = 3 oz

WHAT IT DOES

- Helps your heart
- Fights cancer
- Boosts brain function
- Prevents eye damage as well as age-related macular degeneration
- Aids muscle functioning
- Builds muscle

QUICK IDEAS

Salmon: Grill it until done, then flake it into pasta drizzled with extra-virgin olive oil and sprinkled with freshly ground pepper and fresh herbs.

Sardines: Buy them canned and eat with hearty bread or with mustard and whole-grain crackers.

Shrimp: Keep shells on, brush with olive oil, and grill until pink. Peel and eat.

BEEF & GAME MEATS

1 serving = 3 oz

WHAT THEY DO

- Promote healthy blood cells
- Promote satiety
- Aid muscle functioning
- Build muscle

QUICK IDEAS

Skirt steak: Season with rosemary, cumin, or smoked paprika, and grill.

Lamb: Marinate kebabs in a mixture of plain yogurt, lemon juice, a little ground cinnamon, chopped fresh parsley, and a few cloves of minced garlic.

Venison: Try adding ground venison to chili for a robust flavor upgrade.

2 to 3 Servings per Day

FRUITS

1 serving = 1 baseball-size fruit, 2 egg-size fruits, 1 cup fresh fruit, or ¼ cup dried fruit

WHAT THEY DO

- Promote satiety
- Prevent diabetes
- May prevent cancer
- Aid weight loss
- Lower blood pressure

QUICK IDEAS

Apple: Chop and add to ½ cup uncooked rolled oats, along with slivered almonds and milk. Cook the oats as usual.

Strawberries: Slice and add to a spinach salad, along with balsamic vinegar and crumbled goat cheese.

Banana: For breakfast, top whole-wheat bread with peanut butter, raisins, cinnamon, and banana slices.

WHOLE GRAINS

1 serving = 1 cup cold cereal, ½ cup hot cereal, 2 bread slices, or ½ cup rice

WHAT THEY DO

- Promote satiety
- Improve blood pressure
- Reduce risk of coronary heart disease
- Fight cancer

QUICK IDEAS

Brown rice: For an Asian rice bowl, layer grilled salmon, scallions, and sautéed shiitakes over steamed brown rice. Drizzle with soy sauce and sriracha.

Popcorn: Season unflavored popcorn with Parmesan cheese and freshly ground black pepper.

Quinoa: Toss cooked quinoa with roasted peppers, chopped fresh basil, and cubed mozzarella cheese.

DAIRY

1 serving = 1 cup milk, 1 cup yogurt, or 1 oz cheese

WHAT IT DOES

- Promotes satiety
- Builds muscle
- Strengthens bones
- Aids weight loss

QUICK IDEAS

Chocolate milk: Add it to your protein shake to make it taste better and serve yourself a glass after a tough workout.

Blue cheese: Pair it with walnuts and dried apricots for an easy cheese plate.

Sour cream: For an awesome taco topping, flavor sour cream with lime juice and sriracha.

STARCHY VEGETABLES AND LEGUMES

1 serving = 1 cup cooked or 1 baseball-size portion of yams or potatoes

WHAT THEY DO

- Promote satiety
- Aid weight loss
- Lower blood pressure
- Reduce cardiovascular-disease risk

QUICK IDEAS

Black beans: For salsa, mix them with chopped fresh cilantro, chopped scallions, minced jalapeño and garlic, and lime juice. Season with salt and freshly ground black pepper.

Green peas: Toss cooked peas with a drizzle of extra-virgin olive oil and season with sea salt.

Sweet potatoes: Bake whole sweet potatoes until tender, then drizzle with maple syrup.

3 to 4 Servings per Day

NON-STARCHY VEGETABLES

1 serving = 1 cup raw or ½ cup cooked

WHAT THEY DO

- Promote satiety
- Lower diabetes risk
- Reduce cardiovascular-disease risk
- May prevent cancer
- Aid weight loss
- Lower blood pressure

QUICK IDEAS

Arugula: Try it in salads and on sandwiches to add bite.

Bok choy: Steam until tender, then toss with hoisin sauce and sesame oil. Garnish with sesame seeds.

Cabbage: For instant coleslaw, mix thinly sliced cabbage with red onions, carrots, rice wine vinegar, crushed red-pepper flakes, and a little sugar.

Optional Beverages

COFFEE
0 to 3 servings/day
1 serving = 8 oz

WHAT IT DOES

- May reduce risk of Parkinson's, Alzheimer's, and dementia
- Improves short-term memory

GREEN TEA
0 to 3 servings/day
1 serving = 8 oz

WHAT IT DOES

- Promotes satiety
- May fight cancer
- Prevents tooth decay and gum disease

WINE, BEER, SPIRITS
0 to 2 servings/day
1 serving = 5 oz wine, 12 oz beer, or 1.5 oz hard liquor

WHAT THEY DO

- May prevent diabetes
- Fight cancer
- Lower blood pressure
- Fight cavities

Master Everyday Eating

In order to maximize your muscle-building potential, you need to feed your body right all day long. That doesn't mean that you can't ever slip up or enjoy the occasional treat—you can (and we all do). But building the hard body you want is much easier when you start with a solid foundation. That's what this section is all about: How will you approach eating day in, day out? Simply employ a few smart strategies throughout the day and you can train your body to perform better— not only in the gym, but everywhere else, from the boardroom to the bedroom.

Rules to Eat By

WE'VE IDENTIFIED THE TOP 10 HEALTHY HABITS THAT WILL HELP YOU SHED FAT AND GET STRONG. IT'S NOT COMPLICATED—JUST SMART, EASY-TO-FOLLOW ADVICE.

Food used to be simple. You ate what you grew on the land or bought from nearby farmers. Processed food was nothing more than canned, frozen, or cured. Today, food is much more complicated—and we're both better and worse off for it. We can eat a greater variety of healthy foods than our ancestors did (think fresh berries in winter), but we also can eat a lot more highly processed, chemical-laden ones. And that fare seems to be winning the day, if our epidemics of obesity and diabetes are any indication.

But an increasing trend toward clean eating—with its emphasis on whole, fresh, traditional fare—could mark a turning point in our sometimes dysfunctional relationship with food and help us achieve good health, culinary satisfaction, and optimal fitness.

To help you clean up your own diet and reap the benefits (weight loss and possible decreased risk of diabetes, heart disease, and cancer), these rules will have you eating less junk and fewer hidden calories, so you can slim down and stay healthy naturally.

RULE #1:
DUMP A FEW HEAVILY PROCESSED STAPLES

Instead of overhauling your pantry all at once, start by eliminating corn oil and soda—both highly processed, says Nina Planck, author of *Real Food: What to Eat and Why*. "That alone," she says, "is a huge first step."

Also focus on eliminating added sugars from your diet. According to a USDA survey, the average American eats about 20 teaspoons of added sugar daily, or 317 empty calories. The researchers report that 82 percent of that added sugar can be attributed to soda, baked goods, breakfast cereals, candy, and fruit drinks. What's not on the list? Meat, vegetables, whole fruit, and eggs, along with unsweetened whole-grain and dairy products. Eat accordingly.

RULE #2:
MAKE VEGGIES THE CENTERPIECE

Heart disease, cancer, diabetes, and even Alzheimer's are far less common in Mediterranean countries such as Greece, Italy, France, and Spain. Eating well is easy for them because "Mediterranean eaters place an emphasis on fresh, quality ingredients," says Cynthia Sass, RD, CSSD, coauthor of *Flat Belly Diet* and *The Flat Belly Diet for Men*. Mediterranean meals typically consist of about 75 percent plant matter, from fruits, vegetables, whole grains, and beans. "Meat is considered a condiment and is eaten infrequently," says Sass. Greeks, for example, eat little red meat but consume an average of nine daily servings of fruits and vegetables. These proportions offer a broad spectrum of vitamins, minerals, and antioxidants, which stave off disease and fuel athletic performance.

To reap the same benefits at home, pick a vegetable or fruit and design the meal around it. Pair berries with oatmeal; mix broccoli into a pasta sauce. Fresh, in-season fruits and veggies deliver the highest nutrient content, and you can save them for other times of the year as well. "Freezing tends to lock in nutrients and preserve them, so many frozen foods are just as nutritious as when they are fresh," says Sass.

RULE #3:
SHOP THE PERIMETER OF THE SUPERMARKET

Most whole, natural foods are on the outside aisles of grocery stores—that's where the produce, dairy, and meat sections usually are. As you go deeper into the center of the store, you encounter more processed and packaged foods. "Find the stuff that spoils," suggests nutritionist Jonny Bowden, PhD, author of *The Most Effective Ways to Live Longer*. Also, turn to Chapter 19 for an in-depth look at how to navigate each aisle successfully.

RULE #4:
READ LABELS

It's the easiest way to distinguish a "clean" food from a highly processed one. Think about it: A head of lettuce has no label (totally natural), while a bag of ranch-flavored corn chips has a dozen or more ingredients (highly processed). Instead of eliminating all processed foods, study the labels on the packaging and choose those with fewer and simpler ingredients. Avoid hydrogenated oils, artificial flavors and colors, stabilizers, preservatives, excessive amounts of fat and sodium, and added refined sugar.

RULE #5:
THINK NUTRIENTS PER SERVING

Consider the amount of nutrients in a product rather than focusing solely on price.

Ask yourself if the price of the food is worth the nutrients (or lack thereof). You can make this assessment on every item by comparing the protein, fiber, minerals, and vitamins against fat, sodium, sugars, and chemical additives.

An organization called the Ecological Food Manufacturers Association (EFMA) is pushing for an easier way to make a healthy selection. "A consumer should be able to pick up a product and, by looking at one little score, instantly know how safe, planet friendly, and nutritious it is," says EFMA founder and CEO Winston Riley. NuVal (a food rating system designed by *Men's Health* weight loss advisor David Katz, MD, MPH, and other medical experts that gives points to foods based on their nutritional content) is available in more than 500 supermarkets nationwide. The higher the score, the more nutritious the food. Or use your smartphone (iPhone or Android) to access GoodGuide, a free application that offers health, environment, and social responsibility information, plus ratings, on more than 50,000 products. It's also available at goodguide.com.

RULE #6:
COOK MORE MEALS AT HOME

This is an easy way to shift more of your resources toward whole food and potentially save money. Plus, many restaurants rely on highly processed food to create their meals. To make home cooking easier, master a few one-pot or one-pan dishes with simple ingredients that you can whip up quickly and that will feed you or your family for days. Cooking helps you appreciate and enjoy your food more, especially if you share the process with others, says Michael Pollan, author of *The Omnivore's Dilemma* and *In Defense of Food*. He recommends involving your kids, spouse, or dinner guests by giving them a job (wash, chop, stir, set the table, etc.). As a bonus, he notes that people who cook tend to eat more healthfully and weigh less than those who don't.

RULE #7:
ADJUST YOUR TASTEBUDS

If you're accustomed to eating food with lots of salt, sugar, fat, and other additives, you'll need to retrain your tastebuds to appreciate the more subtle flavors of whole foods. For instance, if you don't immediately like the taste of brown rice, mix it with white (in decreasing amounts) until you adapt. (You can do the same thing with whole-grain pasta.) It works for salty and fatty foods, too. Instead of switching immediately to, say, reduced-sodium soups, mix a regular can with a reduced-sodium version and adjust the ratio toward less sodium as you get used to the flavor. It can take up to 12 weeks to adjust, says Richard Mattes, PhD, MPH, a professor of foods and nutrition at Purdue University. If you're still looking for more zest in your food, try adding antioxidant-rich herbs and spices such as oregano, cinnamon, or dill to entrées. Place lemon slices over fish and beans to make a zingy dish. If you're really ambitious, grow a windowsill herb garden for a supply of flavor-packed seasonings.

RULE #8:
SNACK WISELY

When you're trying to drop pounds, snacks are often the first things you cut from your diet. But that's not a smart move. In fact, it could lead you to eat more. One reason you're likely to stuff yourself at your main meals is that you're allowing too much time to pass between meals. A healthy snack can help you avoid this pitfall by breaking up the time you're not eating into smaller chunks, helping you to avoid sharp blood-sugar crashes and the cravings that ultimately accompany them. But remember, snacks should be, well, snack-size, meaning you should keep them to significantly smaller sizes than your regular meals.

RULE #9: FOLLOW AN 80-20 STRATEGY

Eating plans go bad (and are eventually abandoned) when they turn obsessive. To avoid that trap, take an 80-20 approach. That is, try to eat natural, healthy food 80 percent of the time, with a 20 percent buffer for when you're traveling or socializing or simply want to indulge.

RULE #10: FEEL THE LOVE

For Mary Ellen Camire, PhD, a professor of food science and nutrition at the University of Maine, eating is all about the pleasures of food. She remembers some advice that celebrity chef Alton Brown of the Food Network delivered at an Institute of Food Technologists conference a few years ago. "I'll never forget it," she says. "He said, 'You know, as long as it's made with love …' That really stuck with me because it goes back to the whole French paradox thing: While the French are talking with family, drinking wine, and turning eating into a celebration, we're scarfing down handheld food in our cars. His message was to think about where your food is coming from, who's preparing it, and especially how you're eating it."

In other words, be mindful. It's a word that comes up repeatedly in discussions of eating for your health. Be more mindful of how you shop, how you cook, and how you eat.

"I choose to eat this way for many reasons, and one of the biggest is enjoyment," says Pollan. "There doesn't have to be a trade-off between pleasure and health. If you eat this way, you can have both. It's not rocket science. In fact, it's not even science; it's just common sense."

Chapter 5

Foods that Build Muscle

CHOOSE THE BEST ITEMS TO ADD TO YOUR MEALS AND SET YOURSELF UP TO BE STRONGER, FASTER, AND LEANER.

So many diets center on all of the foods that you shouldn't eat. When it comes down to it, what you consume is the fuel your body uses to function on a daily basis. The foods that we've highlighted in this section are shining examples of what you should be eating every day.

MACADAMIA NUTS

Australian scientists found that men with high cholesterol who ate 12 to 16 macadamia nuts a day raised their HDL (good) cholesterol levels by 8 percent. "Because macadamia nuts contain the highest amount of monounsaturated fat of all nuts, this degree of HDL-raising effect may be unique to them," says Manohar Garg, PhD, the study's author. Macadamia nuts are also a good source of zinc, which is important for sexual health.

EGGS

A large egg contains a powerful 6.3 grams of high-quality protein and only about 75 calories. A study published in the International Journal of Obesity found that people who replaced carbs with eggs for breakfast lost 65 percent more weight than those who didn't eat eggs. And while the old school of thought was that you should eat egg whites rather than whole eggs, studies have proved that the fat in the yolk is important to keep you satiated and is packed with vital nutrients. Researchers in Michigan found that egg eaters were about half as likely to be deficient in vitamin B_{12}, nearly 24 percent less likely to be deficient in vitamin A, and 36 percent less likely to be deficient in vitamin E than those who ate few or no eggs. If you're worried about cholesterol, don't be. The same study found that those who ate at least four eggs a week had significantly lower cholesterol levels than those who ate fewer than one. Turns out the dietary cholesterol in the yolk has little impact on your serum cholesterol.

OLIVE OIL

Of all the oils out there, olive oil contains the best combination of high monounsaturated fatty acids and good ratio of omega-3 to omega-6 fatty acids (13:1). An abundant intake of omega-6 fats relative to omega-3 fats increases inflammation (a 1:1 ratio in your overall diet is best), which may ultimately increase your risk of developing heart disease, diabetes, and cancer, according to the results of a 2008 review of studies conducted by the Center for Genetics, Nutrition, and Health. Extra-virgin olive oil has a robust flavor and is best when saved to use to dress salads, vegetables, and cooked dishes. For cooking, regular or light olive oil is fine. But remember, in this case, "light" refers to color, not fat or calorie content.

MACKEREL

Fish may be the healthiest food on the planet, and omega-3 fatty acids are the key to their nutritional power. Those who eat two servings of fish a week live longer and have lower rates of cardiovascular disease, greater mental capacity, and less abdominal fat than those who avoid seafood. Mackerel is a fish superstar—it provides omega-3 fatty acids, zinc, and vitamin D. Consider this: You'd have to eat two salmon fillets to get the omega-3 power in one serving of mackerel.

PORK TENDERLOIN

Ounce for ounce, pork tenderloin has less fat than a chicken breast. And food scientists are finding ways to make it leaner every year. This cut is an excellent source of zinc and iron. And it cooks up great on a grill.

GRASS-FED BEEF STRIP STEAK

All cows are raised on grass for the first year or so of their lives, after which, if they're headed to a conventional slaughterhouse, they'll eat an unlimited supply of corn to fatten them quickly. A cow raised solely on grass, however, yields a completely different type of meat—in taste as well as in chemistry—because it's practically a wild animal. Grass-fed beef has 16 percent fewer calories than conventional beef, 27 percent less fat, 10 percent more protein, and a healthier balance of omega-3 to omega-6 fatty acids. Grass-fed beef strip steak is the best combination of vitamin B_{12} and iron that you'll find in the beef and game meats family. Strip steak delivers 24 grams of protein per 4 ounces. It also has the least fat of any loin cut (17 grams, compared with 20 or 21 grams in other loin cuts).

RASPBERRIES

These berries are a must-eat food, dense with antioxidants and other powerful nutrients that defend against such conditions as cancer and memory loss. They also contain anthocyanins, which protect against diabetes by increasing insulin production and lowering blood-sugar levels.

OATS

Oats reduce your risk of heart disease, high blood pressure, and type 2 diabetes and deliver muscle-building protein. And of all the whole grains, oats offer the best combination of fiber, folate, and magnesium. Some oat options include rolled (old-fashioned and instant) and steel-cut. Old-fashioned oats are groats (the hulled grain) rolled into flakes; they cook in about 5 minutes. Instant oats are rolled oats cut up to cook faster (but beware of the sugar in "flavored" instant oatmeal). Steel-cut oats are groats that are cut up but not rolled. They're nutty and toothsome but take a half hour to cook unless you soak them overnight. Still, they are worth the extra time and effort. "The enzymes in your gastrointestinal tract take a longer time to penetrate the unrolled groats in steel-cut oatmeal," says David Jenkins, MD, PhD, a nutrition and metabolism researcher at the University of Toronto. "This results in a slower uptake of glucose, and that makes steel-cut oatmeal better, especially for people who are at risk of diabetes."

1% MILK

Drinking two to three glasses of milk a day lowers the likelihood of both heart attack and stroke—a finding confirmed by British scientists. Also, because milk contains bone-strengthening calcium and muscle-building protein, it's worthy to add to your daily calorie allotment. The USDA recommends that adults ages 19 to 50 get at least 1,000 milligrams of calcium a day, and teens and those over 50 should get at least 1,300. The less fat in your milk, the more calcium you'll receive (1% milk has 290 milligrams per cup). Lower-fat milk varieties are also your best option if you want to cut calories—1% offers the best balance of high protein with low calories.

NAVY BEANS

Perfect little fiber bombs, white beans are one of the more versatile beans. They also pack a great combination of magnesium, potassium, and vitamin C. Surveys reveal that men consume only about 80 percent of the recommended 400 mg of magnesium a day, which is a serious shame because this lightweight mineral is a multitasker: It's involved in more than 300 bodily processes, including muscle function. A study published in the *Journal of the American College of Nutrition* found that low levels of magnesium may increase your blood levels of C-reactive protein, a key marker of heart disease. "Without enough magnesium, every cell in your body has to struggle to generate energy," explains Dana King, MD, a professor of family medicine at the Medical University of South Carolina.

SPINACH

Spinach is a great muscle builder. In one study, researchers discovered a hormone in spinach that allows muscle tissue to repair itself faster. Spinach also contains abundant amounts of the nutrients vitamin K, calcium, phosphorus, potassium, zinc, and selenium, which may help protect the liver and ward off Alzheimer's. A study in the *Journal of Nutrition* suggests that the carotenoid neoxanthin in spinach can kill prostate cancer cells. Spinach reigns supreme over other green vegetables because it contains the powerful combination of folate, vitamin A, and potassium.

COFFEE

A deluge of studies confirms that java delivers a major health jolt, thanks to its rich source of nutrients that lower cholesterol, improve insulin sensitivity, and destroy damaged cells. Caffeine is protective, so don't opt for decaf unless you suffer from insomnia, headaches, or high blood pressure. The results speak for themselves: A review of research found that compared with people who drink the least, drinking at least 1 cup of coffee lowers your risk of early death from all causes by 37 percent, while at least 2 cups per day reduces your risk of death from heart disease by 25 percent, 3 cups per day slashes your risk of dementia and Alzheimer's by 65 percent, and 4 or more cups per day makes you 56 percent less likely to develop type 2 diabetes.

GREEN TEA

Literally thousands of studies have been carried out to document the health benefits of catechins, the group of antioxidants concentrated in the leaves of tea plants. Among the most startling results came from a study published by the American Medical Association in 2006. The study followed more than 40,000 Japanese adults for a decade, and at the 7-year follow-up, those who had been drinking five or more cups of tea per day were 26 percent less likely to die of any cause compared with those who averaged less than a cup. Looking for more immediate results? Another Japanese study broke participants into two groups, only one of which was put on a catechin-rich green tea diet. At the end of 12 weeks, the green tea group had achieved significantly smaller body weights and waistlines than those in the control group. Why? Researchers believe that catechins are effective at boosting metabolism.

RED WINE

Oxidative stress plays a major role in aging, and an antioxidant in red wine called resveratrol may help extend life by neutralizing disease-causing free radicals. And polyphenols found in grape skins are potent weapons against heart disease. That doesn't mean you have permission to go crazy: Canadian researchers found that by dilating blood vessels, a single drink of wine allows your heart to work less, but the second drink may increase heart rate and bloodflow without additional dilation. The researchers warn that repeated high consumption can lead to higher risk of heart attack.

Chapter 6

Fight Fat from Your Kitchen

IT'S TIME TO MAKE YOUR COOKING SKILLS YOUR BIGGEST ASSET IN YOUR QUEST FOR A BETTER BODY, AND THESE EASY RECIPES—AND 5-DAY MEAL PLAN— CAN HELP YOU DO JUST THAT.

Eating more of the foods we've highlighted is a perfect way to increase your intake of essential nutrients on a daily basis. Not only will these superfoods help you lose weight and help your body perform at its peak level, but they'll also save you from downing foods that are high in calories, fat, and preservatives. Start with this 5-day menu.

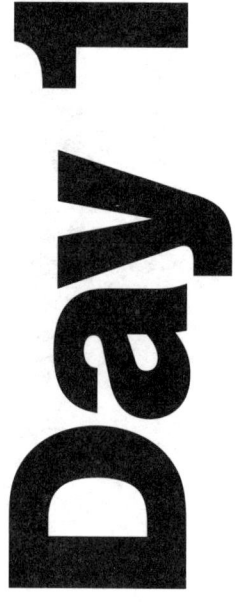

BREAKFAST

1 cup Greek yogurt with strawberries, blackberries, and 1 tsp flaxseeds

MIDMORNING SNACK

Raw veggies with hummus

LUNCH

VIETNAMESE PORK SALAD

- 12 oz pork tenderloin
- ¼ tsp salt
- 3 Tbsp lime juice
- 3 Tbsp sugar
- 1 clove garlic, minced
- 2 Tbsp fish sauce
- 6 cups shredded coleslaw mix
- ¾ cup chopped fresh cilantro
- 1¼ thinly sliced scallions
- ½ cup lightly salted chopped peanuts

1. Preheat oven to 400°F.

2. Place pork on a foil-lined baking sheet. Sprinkle with ⅛ tsp of the salt and cook until thermometer registers 160°F, 20 to 24 minutes. Let meat rest 10 minutes. Cut meat crosswise into 4 sections and shred.

3. Place lime juice, sugar, and garlic in a microwaveable bowl. Cover with microwaveable plastic wrap and microwave on high until sugar melts, 20 to 30 seconds. Let cool. Stir in fish sauce and remaining ⅛ tsp salt.

4. In large bowl, gently toss coleslaw mix, cilantro, and scallions. Pour lime mixture over veggies, add pork, and toss gently. Divide evenly into 4 salad bowls. Top salad with nuts before serving.

MAKES 4 SERVINGS.

Per serving: 362 calories, 27 g protein, 25.5 g carbohydrates (6 g fiber), 19 g fat (4 g sat), 1,137 mg sodium

DINNER

ITALIAN-STYLE CHICKEN AND MUSHROOMS

- 1 Tbsp unsalted butter
- 4 tsp olive oil
- ½ lb sliced mushrooms, such as cremini or stemmed shiitake
- 1 small onion, chopped
- ¼ cup all-purpose flour
  Salt and freshly ground black pepper
- 1 lb chicken breast cutlets (¼" thick), halved crosswise
- 1 cup Marsala or dry red wine
- 1¼ cups reduced-sodium chicken broth
- 2 Tbsp chopped parsley

1. Heat butter and 2 tsp of the oil in large nonstick skillet over medium-high heat. Add mushrooms and cook until golden, 5 minutes. Transfer to bowl. Cook onion in skillet until tender, 4 minutes. Add to bowl. Reserve skillet.

2. Put flour on plate and season with salt and pepper. Coat chicken with flour mixture, shaking off excess. Reserve 1½ Tbsp of the flour mixture. Heat remaining 2 tsp oil in skillet over medium-high heat. Add chicken and brown, turning, about 3 minutes. Transfer to plate and keep warm. Add wine to skillet. Simmer, scraping up browned bits, until reduced by half, about 3 minutes.

3. Add broth and bring to a simmer. Remove ¼ cup liquid and whisk in reserved flour. Whisk back into skillet. Bring to a boil. Add chicken and mushroom mixture and simmer until chicken is cooked through and sauce is slightly thickened, about 5 minutes. Serve sprinkled with parsley.

MAKES 4 SERVINGS.

Per serving: 281 calories, 26.5 g protein, 9 g carbohydrates (1 g fiber), 10.5 g fat (3 g sat), 426 mg sodium

EVENING SNACK

BUTTERSCOTCH CHIP MACADAMIA COOKIES

- 1 cup plus 2 Tbsp all-purpose flour
- ½ tsp baking soda
  Pinch of salt
- ½ cup trans-fat free spread
- ½ cup brown sugar
- 1 egg yolk
- 1 tsp vanilla extract
- ½ cup (3 oz) butterscotch chips
- ¼ cup macadamia nuts, finely chopped

1. Preheat oven to 350°F.

2. In medium bowl, stir together flour, baking soda, and salt with a fork.

3. In mixing bowl, beat spread with a wooden spoon until smooth. Add sugar and beat until smooth. Add egg yolk and vanilla and beat until smooth. Stir in dry ingredients. Add butterscotch chips and nuts and stir to mix.

4. Roll dough into 24 equal balls. Place dough balls, 1" apart, on nonstick baking sheet. Bake until puffed and golden on the bottom, 10 minutes.

5. Allow to cool on sheet before removing to rack.

MAKES 24 SERVINGS.

Per serving (1 cookie): 93 calories, 1 g protein, 10 g carbohydrates (<1 g fiber), 5 g fat (2 g sat), 66 mg sodium

Day 2

BREAKFAST

BREAKFAST STUFFINS

- 1 bakery loaf whole-wheat or whole-grain bread
- 1 jar (12 oz) roasted red peppers, rinsed and drained
- 1 cup chopped onion
- 5 oz baby spinach, coarsely chopped
- 3 large eggs
- 3 large egg whites
- 1½ cups 2% milk
- 1 Tbsp Dijon mustard (optional)
- Salt and freshly ground black pepper
- ¾ cup shredded reduced-fat Cheddar cheese

1. Heat oven to 350°F. Coat standard 12-cup muffin pan with baking spray.

2. Remove crust from bread and cut into ½" cubes to get 3¾ cups. Set aside. Reserve remaining bread for another use. Pat roasted peppers dry, remove any seeds, and dice. Set aside.

3. Coat medium skillet with olive oil spray and heat over medium-high heat. Add onion and cook until golden, about 4 minutes. Add spinach and cook, stirring, until wilted, about 1 minute. Let cool.

4. In large bowl, whisk together eggs, egg whites, milk, mustard (if using), and salt and pepper. Stir in cheese, reserved peppers, and spinach mixture. Gently fold in bread cubes and let stand 15 minutes.

5. Divide mixture evenly among prepared muffin cups. Bake until puffed and set, 20 to 25 minutes. Let stand 5 minutes before removing.

MAKES 12 SERVINGS.

Per serving (1 stuffin): 118 calories, 7 g protein, 14 g carbohydrates (2 g fiber), 4 g fat (2 g sat), 235.5 mg sodium

LUNCH

HEARTY MINESTRONE SOUP

- 2 Tbsp extra-virgin olive oil
- 1 onion, chopped (about 1 cup)
- 4 cloves garlic, minced
- 1½ tsp dried basil
- 1 sweet potato (8 oz), peeled and cut into ½" pieces
- 1 zucchini (8 oz), cut into ½" pieces
- 1 yellow squash (8 oz), cut into ½" pieces
- 1 fennel bulb (8 oz), cut into ½" pieces
- 5 cups reduced-sodium fat-free chicken broth
- 1 can (14.5 oz) diced tomatoes
- 1 bag (5 oz) baby spinach
- 1 can (15 oz) red kidney beans, rinsed and drained
- ¼ tsp freshly ground black pepper
- ¼ cup grated Parmesan cheese

1. Heat oil in large saucepan over medium-high heat. Add onion, garlic, and basil. Cook, stirring occasionally, until starting to soften, 2 to 3 minutes. Add sweet potato and cook 1 minute. Stir in zucchini, yellow squash, and fennel and cook until just starting to soften, 2 to 3 minutes.

2. Add broth and tomatoes. Bring to a boil, reduce heat to medium, and simmer, uncovered, until vegetables are crisp-tender, about 25 minutes.

3. Stir in spinach and cook until wilted, 5 minutes. Add beans and pepper and cook until hot, 3 minutes.

4. Remove from heat and stir in cheese.

MAKES 8 SERVINGS.

Per serving: 177 calories, 8 g protein, 27 g carbohydrates (9 g fiber), 5 g fat (1 g sat), 502 mg sodium

MIDAFTERNOON SNACK

THAI ICED COFFEE POP

- ¼ cup sugar
- ¼ cup water
- ¼ tsp almond extract
- 1 cup strongly brewed coffee, cooled (prepared with ½ tsp ground cardamom added to coffee grounds)
- 2 Tbsp half-and-half

1. In saucepan, boil sugar and water, stirring until sugar is dissolved. Remove from heat and add almond extract. Stir to combine, then stir in coffee and half-and-half.

2. Distribute into 4 ice-pop molds, add sticks, and freeze for 8 hours.

MAKES 4 SERVINGS.

Per serving (1 pop): 65 calories, <1 g protein, 14 g carbohydrates (<1 g fiber), 1 g fat (<1 g sat), 12 g sodium

DINNER

PERFECT GRILLED MACKEREL

- ½ cup olive oil
- 1 Tbsp Dijon mustard
- Juice of 2 lemons
- 1 handful fresh parsley
- 2 mackerel fillets
- Salt and freshly ground pepper

1. Whisk together olive oil, mustard, lemon juice, and parsley.

2. Season mackerel with salt and pepper and a spoonful of olive oil mixture. Cook over medium heat on clean, oiled grill until lightly charred and firm to the touch, 3 to 4 minutes per side.

3. Drizzle on remaining olive oil mixture before serving.

MAKES 2 SERVINGS.

Per serving: 347 calories, 25.5 g protein, 33 g carbohydrates (8 g fiber), 14 g fat (4.5 g sat), 161 mg sodium

EVENING SNACK

Raspberries and a few squares of dark chocolate

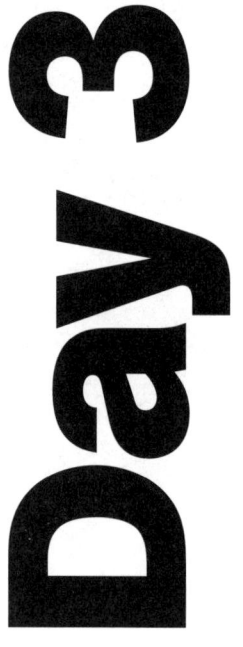

BREAKFAST

MAPLE-BACON OATMEAL

- 2 slices natural turkey bacon
- ¼ cup rolled oats
- 2 Tbsp maple syrup

1. Cook natural turkey bacon.

2. Cook oats according to package directions. Mix in maple syrup, then crumble bacon on top.

MAKES 1 SERVING.

Per serving: 361 calories, 11 g protein, 61 g carbohydrates (5 g fiber), 8 g fat (2 g sat), 404 mg sodium

MIDMORNING SNACK

1 cup green tea with a handful of pistachios

LUNCH

ESCAROLE SOUP WITH FENNEL, NAVY BEANS, AND MINI MEATBALLS

Meatballs
- 8 oz mild Italian pork sausage in bulk (otherwise, remove from casings)
- 1 Tbsp extra-virgin olive oil

Soup
- ½ yellow onion, chopped
- 1 bulb fennel, chopped
- 3 cloves garlic, minced
- 8 cups (packed) chopped escarole

- 1 can (15 oz) navy beans, rinsed and drained
- 4 cups reduced-sodium chicken broth
- ½ tsp freshly ground black pepper
- 1 cup water
- 6 tsp olive oil

1. To make meatballs: Form sausage into 30 teaspoon-size balls. In soup pot, heat oil and brown meatballs over medium-high heat, 5 minutes. Remove to a plate.

2. To make soup: In same soup pot, sauté onion and fennel in drippings over medium-low heat, 10 minutes. Add garlic and sauté 1 minute. Add escarole, reserving a handful. Increase heat to medium-high and toss until leaves wilt, 2 minutes.

3. Return meatballs to soup pot. Add beans, broth, pepper, and water. Bring to a boil. Reduce heat, cover, and simmer until meatballs are cooked through, about 5 minutes.

4. Stir in reserved escarole. Divide among bowls and drizzle each with oil.

MAKES 6 SERVINGS.

Per serving: 268 calories, 13 g protein, 20 g carbohydrates (6 g fiber), 15.5 g fat (4 g sat), 700 mg sodium

DINNER

Grilled salmon with pineapple and asparagus

EVENING SNACK

RICH CHOCOLATE PUDDING

- ⅓ cup packed brown sugar
- ¼ cup unsweetened cocoa powder
- 3 Tbsp cornstarch
- 1 tsp instant espresso powder (optional)
- ⅛ tsp ground cinnamon
- Pinch of salt
- 2 cups 1% milk
- 1 large egg
- 2 oz bittersweet chocolate bits (about ⅓ cup)
- 1½ tsp vanilla extract

1. In medium saucepan, whisk together sugar, cocoa, cornstarch, espresso powder (if using), cinnamon, salt, and ½ cup of the milk. Slowly pour remaining 1½ cups milk into mixture while whisking.

2. Bring to a simmer over medium-low heat. Simmer, whisking constantly, until slightly thickened, about 2 to 3 minutes.

3. Beat egg lightly in small bowl. Whisk in 1 cup of the hot milk mixture. Pour egg mixture back into saucepan. Cook over medium-low heat, stirring, 2 minutes.

4. Remove from heat. Add chocolate and whisk until mixture is smooth. Stir in vanilla extract.

5. Pour mixture into 4 serving dishes. Chill, covered, 2 hours or overnight.

MAKES 4 SERVINGS.

Per serving: 250 calories, 8 g protein, 40 g carbohydrates (3 g fiber), 9 g fat (5 g sat), 114.5 mg sodium

Day 4

BREAKFAST

Ham, mushroom, onion, and bell pepper omelet made with 2 eggs and 2 egg whites

MIDMORNING SNACK

RASPBERRY JAVA SMOOTHIE

- 2 pitted dates
- ¾ cup 1% milk
- ½ cup frozen raspberries
- 1 cup coffee ice cubes (about ¾ cup brewed and frozen)

1. Soak dates in water up to 1 hour.

2. In blender, combine dates, milk, and raspberries. Blend on high speed 1 minute. Add coffee ice cubes and blend until smooth.

MAKES 1 SERVING.

Per serving: 291 calories, 8 g protein, 66.5 g carbohydrates (12 g fiber), 2 g fat (1 g sat), 89 mg sodium

LUNCH

STEAK QUESADILLAS

- 1 tsp olive oil
- 8 oz grass-fed strip steak
- 4 100-calorie tortillas
- ½ avocado, sliced
- 1 small red onion, sliced
- ¼ cup salsa
- ¼ cup black beans
- ¼ cup Monterey Jack cheese

1. Heat oil in skillet and cook strip steak to desired level of doneness. Slice and divide among tortillas.

2. Top with avocado, onion, salsa, black beans, and cheese. Heat quesadillas in skillet until cheese is melted.

MAKES 4 SERVINGS.

Per serving: 405 calories, 26 g protein, 39 g carbohydrates (8 g fiber), 20 g fat (8 g sat), 1,011 mg sodium

MIDAFTERNOON SNACK

Spinach Dip with 1 cup baby carrots

SPINACH DIP

- 1 package (9–10 oz) frozen chopped spinach, thawed
- 1 container (16 oz) plain 0% Greek yogurt
- 2 oz crumbled feta or goat cheese or finely grated Parmesan cheese
- 2 Tbsp store-bought basil or cilantro pesto

1. Squeeze spinach dry with hands to extract as much liquid as possible.

2. Place spinach, yogurt, cheese, and pesto in food processor. Pulse until just combined. Season to taste with salt and pepper. Transfer to serving bowl.

MAKES 8 SERVINGS.

Per serving (1/3 cup): 81 calories, 8 g protein, 4 g carbohydrates (1 g fiber), 4 g fat (1 g sat), 119 mg sodium

DINNER

BAKED EGGPLANT WITH TOMATO CHUTNEY

- 1 medium eggplant
- 2 Tbsp olive oil
- 1/4 tsp salt
- 1/4 tsp freshly ground black pepper
- 1 onion, chopped
- 1 clove garlic, chopped
- 1/4 cup balsamic vinegar
- 1 Tbsp chopped fresh basil or 1 tsp dried
- 1 can (14.5 oz) diced tomatoes
- 1/4 cup pine nuts

1. Preheat oven to 425°F. Coat 13" × 9" baking dish with cooking spray.

2. Cut eggplant into 1/2" slices and brush with 1 tsp of the oil. Sprinkle each side with salt and pepper and lay slices in baking dish. Bake for 30 minutes, or until eggplant is tender.

3. Heat remaining oil in nonstick saucepan over medium-high heat. Cook onion and garlic, stirring, until softened, 3 minutes. Add vinegar and basil and cook, stirring, 1 minute. Add tomatoes and simmer 5 minutes.

4. Remove from heat and stir in pine nuts. Spoon over eggplant and bake 10 minutes.

MAKES 4 SERVINGS.

Per serving: 99 calories, 2 g protein, 10 g carbohydrates (3 g fiber), 6 g fat (1 g sat), 158 mg sodium

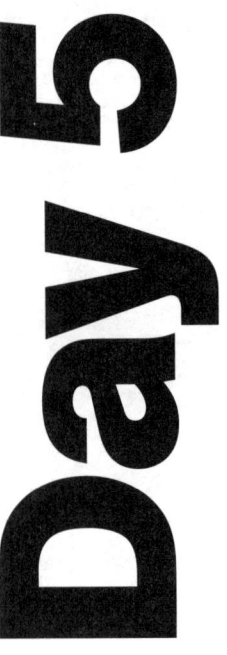

BREAKFAST

GREEN TEA FRENCH TOAST

- 1 tsp matcha (green tea) powder
- 1 cup 1% milk
- ½ tsp vanilla extract
- 1 egg
- ½ tsp ground cinnamon
- ½ tsp cardamom
- ⅛ tsp ground cloves
- 8 slices whole-wheat bread
  Mandarin preserves (optional)

1. In medium bowl, whisk matcha powder, milk, vanilla, egg, cinnamon, cardamom, and cloves.

2. Dip bread into mixture. Heat a large nonstick skillet and fry until golden brown, 3 to 4 minutes per side.

3. Serve with warm mandarin preserves.

MAKES 8 SERVINGS.

Per serving: 237 calories, 11 g protein, 37 g carbohydrates (4 g fiber), 5 g fat (2 g sat), 387 mg sodium

MIDMORNING SNACK

Banana with 1 cup chocolate milk (made with 1% milk)

LUNCH

BABY SPINACH SALAD WITH GOAT CHEESE AND TOASTED PISTACHIOS

- 1 Tbsp sherry or balsamic vinegar
- ¼ cup extra-virgin olive oil
- Salt and freshly ground black pepper
- 4 cups loosely packed baby spinach
- 4 oz crumbled goat cheese
- ¼ cup shelled pistachios, toasted

1. Place sherry in medium bowl. Slowly drizzle in oil, whisking continuously. Season to taste with salt and pepper.

2. Toss spinach in vinaigrette, using tongs to coat spinach evenly.

3. Divide spinach between 2 plates and top with cheese and pistachios.

MAKES 2 SERVINGS.

Per serving: 573 calories, 17 g protein, 11 g carbohydrates (4 g fiber), 52 g fat (16 g sat), 447 mg sodium

DINNER

ROAST COD WITH POMEGRANATE-WALNUT SAUCE

- 1 cup black or regular quinoa
- 1 Tbsp olive oil
- 1 shallot, finely chopped (about ¼ cup)
- ⅓ cup ground walnuts
- 3 cloves garlic, minced
- ⅓ cup dry red wine
- ¼ cup reduced-sodium chicken broth
- 1½ Tbsp pomegranate molasses or frozen cranberry juice concentrate
- 1 Tbsp honey
- 4 cod fillets (6 oz each)
- ¼ cup chopped fresh parsley
- ¼ cup broken walnut halves

1. Prepare quinoa according to package directions.

2. Meanwhile, heat oil in medium nonstick skillet over medium heat. Add shallot and cook, stirring, until softened, 2 minutes. Add ground walnuts and garlic and cook, stirring, until walnuts are golden brown, about 4 minutes. Remove from heat and add wine, broth, molasses, and honey. Return to heat and simmer, stirring occasionally, until thickened, about 4 minutes. Transfer sauce to gravy boat.

3. Heat broiler. Line a sheet pan with nonstick foil. Arrange fish in single layer on pan and season with salt and pepper. Broil until cooked through, about 6 minutes.

4. Toss quinoa with parsley and broken walnuts. Spoon onto 4 plates and top with fish and sauce.

MAKES 4 SERVINGS.

Per serving: 481 calories, 39 g protein, 43 g carbohydrates (5 g fiber), 16 g fat (1.5 g sat), 136.5 mg sodium

EVENING SNACK

1 cup frozen grapes

The Road Warrior's Guide to Smart Eating

USE THESE TIPS TO SIDESTEP DIET DISASTERS ON THE ROAD, IN THE AIRPORT, AND ANY OTHER TIME YOU EAT AWAY FROM HOME.

How many times have you left for a vacation, business trip, or family visit only to return feeling seven or eight meals heavier? It's no coincidence that when you spend time on the road or away from home, your diet takes a nosedive. It's a combination of factors: travel stress, unhealthy convenience foods, and a sense that, once you leave the confines of your normal day-to-day home life, anything goes. "There seems to be an assumption that when you travel, you can't eat healthfully, so you don't even make an attempt," says exercise physiologist Monika Woolsey, RD.

Fueling up is even more important when you're on the move. The right foods can help prevent jet lag, ward off road rage, and give you the energy to deal with your family or business clients when you finally get where you're going. The pickings may be slim (in a not-so-good way) at some common travel pit stops, but dietary salvation is still entirely achievable—as long as you think ahead.

Chapter 7

And it's not just when you're miles away that you face situations that have the potential to derail your healthy eating habits. Anytime you've stepped out of your kitchen—whether you're at the corner deli or your favorite sports bar—you face temptation over what you put in your mouth. Try the following strategies to avoid diet disasters the next time you're away from home.

On the Road

LOOK FOR LEAN PROTEIN AT BREAKFAST

Tempted to hit a drive-thru? Keep in mind that many menus still lack calorie counts, and those that are listed may not be accurate, according to a study published in *The Journal of the American Medical Association*. But a study published in the journal *Obesity* found that a protein-rich breakfast can help increase feelings of fullness and reduce cravings later in the day. Some solid choices:

Ham and Egg on an English Muffin or Whole-Grain Bread

"A lot of high-protein options on menus also tend to be pretty high in fat," says Woolsey. Eggs are an exception. Don't go the egg-whites-only route just because it sounds healthier. The yolk actually contains most of an egg's nutrients, including cancer-battling choline and antioxidants that keep your eyes sharp. Make this sandwich a slim one by opting for ham over sausage or bacon (both are much higher in artery-clogging saturated fat) and choosing an English muffin or bread, both of which have a fraction of the calories packed into bagels and croissants.

Breakfast Burrito

Wraps have a decent protein-to-carb ratio, which means you won't feel ravenous a few hours later, and they may even include veggies like tomatoes and peppers. Avoid any burrito larger than an iPhone or that has words like *loaded*, *meaty*, or *cheesy* in its name or description. Top it off with the hottest sauce you can stand; you could get an extra metabolism-boosting kick from the capsaicin.

Smoothie

The mistake most people make is drinking a smoothie with their meal instead of drinking it *as* their meal, says Charles Platkin, PhD,

MPH, author of *The Diet Detective's All-American Diet*. Research shows that, unlike many other liquid calories, a smoothie can satisfy hunger. Just be sure to pick one that's made with protein-rich low-fat yogurt instead of ice cream. Other ingredients to avoid: apple juice, fruit syrups, and sorbet. These additions can all send the calorie count in a concoction (not to mention your blood sugar) skyrocketing.

Skip this: Fruit and Granola Parfait
Despite its health-food reputation, granola packs more than 500 calories and nearly 30 grams of fat per cup! Plus, it's often loaded with added sweeteners and high-cal items like dried fruit.

AVOID SNACKS THAT ARE HIGH IN SUGAR AND FAT
When the needle on the gas gauge is edging toward E—and so is your stomach—make sure you choose premium fuel at the gas station. Inside the mini-mart, bypass the high-profit (and high-sugar) impulse buys at the counter and be on the lookout for these healthy choices:

Low-Fat Yogurt
Besides being a great source of creamy, satisfying protein in a portion-controlled cup, yogurt contains probiotics. These healthful, naturally occurring bacteria can help settle your stomach on a long car ride.

Banana
If you're prone to migraines while riding in a car, one of these may help. Bananas are rich in magnesium; a deficiency in this mineral can result in headaches and fatigue. Plus, a medium banana has only about 100 calories.

Nuts
Yes, they're high in calories, but their combo of healthy fat and protein can help keep you fuller longer and reduce your total calorie intake for the day. "It pays to get the most nutritional value for your calories," says Platkin. "That way, you won't be hungry again for a while." If traffic jangles your nerves, opt for walnuts. Research in the *Journal of the American College of Nutrition* found that their polyunsaturated fats may help buffer the body's natural reaction to stress. Whatever nut you go for, unsalted is best.

Skip this: Protein Bar
Unless you can find a brand you know and trust, you might end up with a bar that's closer to candy than a healthy snack. Some manufacturers jam their bars with sugar and artificial ingredients. Look for bars that have fewer than 30 grams of carbohydrates and at least 20 grams of protein.

In the Airport

EAT BEFORE YOU FLY

By the time you've lugged your overstuffed carry-on through security and to your gate, you're probably famished—and most planes don't even serve pretzels anymore. Before you leave for the airport, it's smart to fill up on a healthy entrée. If you can't, sharpen your eye for healthier options at the terminal's chain restaurants. Here are three options that will get you from takeoff to baggage claim—and help you avoid the siren call of the warm cinnamon roll at the kiosk next to your departure gate.

Black Bean Soup

Soups in general are filling options, and this one has the bonus of fiber and protein. But even better, black beans are a top source of immunity-enhancing antioxidants, which are always a smart idea when you fly. "Planes tend to have very low humidity, so you can get pretty dried out, and dehydration can put you at risk for germs and colds," says Susan Levin, RD, director of nutrition education for the Physicians Committee for Responsible Medicine (PCRM), in Washington, DC, a group that has studied airport food for the past 10 years.

Vegetarian Wrap

As long as they're not loaded with cheese, meat-free meals tend to be low in saturated fat. And veggie dishes also tend to be high in water content, fiber, and other nutrients that help keep you hydrated and full but not feeling overstuffed, says Levin. Plus, they're increasingly easy to find at airports: PCRM's 2010 report found that 82 percent of airport restaurants now offer at least one low-fat, high-fiber, cholesterol-free vegetarian entrée.

Sushi Roll

Choose one with avocado, which contains vitamin B6, a nutrient that helps your body produce the calming chemical serotonin (good news for nervous fliers).

Skip this: Salad

Prepared salads are often a sneaky source of hidden calories, and the majority of dressings are loaded with bloat-inducing sodium, which is bound to make you feel uncomfortable in an already-cramped airline seat.

PACK LIGHT

We know that you probably don't have a lot of extra room in your carry-on, but who wants to pay $5 for a tiny bag of peanuts when you could have a few smart, healthy options always at the ready. Here are four healthy, travel-friendly snacks to stow in your bag.

Cereal, sans Milk

It's satisfyingly crunchy but way better for you than chips or pretzels. Look for boxes with no more than 120 calories per cup and a decent amount of fiber to tide you over.

Turkey Jerky

This practically fat-free protein source is chewy enough to keep your mouth busy as the miles roll by.

Fruit Snacks

Go for the most durable fresh picks (such as apples and oranges) or stash a few no-sugar-added dried fruits in your bag for a fiber-filled way to satisfy a sweet tooth. Skip sugary dried fruit or the neon-colored, faux-fruity snacks you remember from childhood.

Nut Butter

Some brands make single-serve packs (200 calories or fewer). Eat the nut butter straight from the container or spread it onto celery sticks, apple slices, or whole-grain crackers to make them extra filling.

At a Hotel

CONSIDER STAYING AT A BED-AND-BREAKFAST

Per the name, B and Bs typically offer a convenient, home-cooked breakfast, unlike motel chains, which usually provide a serve-yourself selection of cold cereals and pastries. At a B and B, you'll have access to plenty of low-carb menu items. (Omelet, anyone?) For a nationwide directory of more than 6,000 B and Bs, go to bedandbreakfast.com.

MANAGE TEMPTATION

When reserving a room at a major hotel, ask for your mini-fridge to be stocked for someone who has diabetes. "This is a frequent request, and most hotels oblige by swapping out high-sugar junk foods for milk, cheese, vegetables, diet soda, and fruit," says Cynthia Finley, RD, a clinical dietician at the Johns Hopkins Weight Management Center. The downside? Don't expect a break from the normal in-room price-gouging.

KEEP YOUR LAPTOP ON THE DESK

"If you work in bed, you associate the bed with wakefulness and activity, not with sleep and relaxation," says Mark Rosekind, PhD, the president of Alertness Solutions and a former sleep scientist at NASA. Why is that so important? Because men average 2 to 3 fewer hours of sleep when they are traveling for business. This disturbance in your internal clock decreases your levels of leptin (a hormone that delivers feelings of satiety), and increases levels of ghrelin (a hormone that sparks hunger). "The net effect is that your appetite increases by 23 percent," says Rosekind.

At a Restaurant

DETERMINE YOUR ORDER BEFORE YOU EVEN SEE THE OPTIONS

"Most people choose with their eyes and not with their heads," says Christopher Mohr, PhD, RD, a personal nutrition consultant in Louisville, Kentucky. At dinner, for example, you should decide that you're ordering a salad as your appetizer (eat it instead of the bread), and steak, chicken, or fish with the vegetable of the day as your entrée. Another reason to avoid quality time studying the menu: A study in the *Journal of Consumer Research* found that large, vivid images increase the probability that you'll impulsively order that food. And where the photo is placed also matters: The most profitable items get prime real estate, which in the menu world is the upper corners and the center of the page—hot spots where your eyes naturally travel. "The more attention we can bring to an item, the more likely you are to order it," says Gregg Rapp, a menu engineer consultant in Palm Springs, California.

READ BETWEEN THE LINES

Ordering up a dessert called German Black Forest Indulgence sounds a lot better than plain ol' chocolate cake, doesn't it? Sexed-up monikers can boost food sales by up to 27 percent, according to industry research. "Enticing descriptions create a positive emotion about how something will taste," says Sybil Yang, a researcher and menu psychologist at Cornell University. That's why saying something is "hand-battered" or "crispy" can be a home run: It triggers a craving and draws your attention away from the harsh reality that the food is fried.

SIMPLIFY YOUR VEGETABLES

The presence of veggies—even if they're carb-coated, deep-fried, and cheese-slathered—

convinces you that you're making the right food choices. Don't fall for it. "A seemingly healthy addition to a less-than-wholesome dish sounds like a smart compromise," Yang says. But in reality, these "veggie" delights can often be worse for you than more notorious diet killers like pizza and hamburgers.

SIDESTEP THE SAMPLER

Instead of ordering a few appetizers, you get the sampler, thinking you'll try just a wee bit of everything offered. But research from the University of Pennsylvania reveals that when you're given a wide selection, you'll eat 10 percent more than you would have if there had been only one option. That's because having more variety makes you feel as if you're not eating as much. In other words, when you're given a couple of mozzarella sticks as opposed to the usual six, you feel entitled to gobble those up and then move on to the chicken wings, the potato skins, the poppers, and so on.

INVITE SOMEONE NEW TO DINNER

In a study, researchers at the State University of New York at Buffalo observed that men consumed 35 percent fewer calories when eating with strangers than when breaking bread with friends.

BE YOUR OWN MAN

When ordering dinner with a group, don't follow the overeating crowd. An added bonus? If you're dining with colleagues, it could benefit your career. "If your boss and colleagues see you eating healthfully, you're going to look like an outcome-driven leader," says behavioral therapist Robinson Welch, PhD, former clinical director of Washington University's weight management program. "It sends a message that you want to be successful, that you'll take care of business the same way you take care of yourself—effectively."

Beware of Calorie Deception

More and more restaurants are putting calorie counts next to food items on their menus. You may think it's a smart idea to glance at those numbers before making your final meal choice (1,000 calories in a turkey burger?!), but take those numbers with a grain of salt. They're hit or miss. When USDA researchers tested food samples from 42 chains, they found that some restaurants played by the rules while others broke them. In general, the calorie data at fast-food joints tended to be more accurate, while data from sit-down restaurants varied—sometimes by a lot. About one in five samples had at least 100 more calories than stated, and one in 10 had more than 275 extra calories.

"Fast-food workers usually just field food shipments and then reheat and serve them, while restaurant employees have to assemble dishes," says study author Susan Roberts, PhD, a professor of nutrition at Tufts University and coauthor of The "I" Diet. "By adding more dressing or sauce, a chef can skew the calorie count." A safe bet: Use the nutrition numbers at a chain restaurant as a guide, not gospel, and be especially careful with salads and soups—their calorie counts were underreported most often, the USDA study found.

At the Deli

SELECT THE RIGHT CUT

Sliced whole roasted ham, turkey, and pot roast are known in deli-speak as "whole cuts." Far more common, though, are processed meats, which tend to be fattier and are made by adding preservatives (mostly salt) and sometimes fillers (anything from meat by-products to corn syrup) to ground meat. You can usually recognize processed meats by their unnaturally uniform shape—the better to fit on a bun, says Jan Novakofski, PhD, associate vice chancellor for research and former professor of nutritional science in the meat science laboratory at the University of Illinois at Urbana-Champaign. The best way to make sure you're getting a whole cut is to ask for it.

CONSIDER FOOD SAFETY FIRST

If you're worried about Listeria, relax. This invisible foodborne bacteria isn't common, and even if it is ingested, it's rarely deadly unless your immune system is already compromised. If you're iffy about an order, try this trick from Mindy Brashears, PhD, director of the International Center for Food Industry Excellence at Texas Tech University: "When you get home, microwave the meat until it's steaming (a temperature of about 165°F) before putting it away in the refrigerator."

KNOW YOUR NITRATES

A study in the journal *Circulation* found that a daily dose of 50 grams (about two slices) of processed red meats such as bologna and salami increases heart disease risk by 42 percent and diabetes risk by 19 percent. Processed red meats typically contain nitrates, chemicals that are added for flavor and color (cured meats, including smoked turkey, may also have them). The study findings suggest that high amounts of nitrates (and sodium) may explain the higher risk of heart attacks and diabetes, says lead study author Renata Micha, PhD, RD. Worse, researchers have discovered that when sodium and nitrates combine with the digestive juices in the stomach, they can turn into carcinogenic compounds and have been linked to several types of cancer.

This doesn't mean you can never have another pastrami on rye—just make sure it's loaded with greens. "Some studies show that the antioxidants in vegetables may prevent nitrates from converting into cancer-causing compounds," says Rebecca Scritchfield, a registered dietitian in Washington, DC. "Stuff your sandwich with lots of veggies, not just lettuce. Spinach, alfalfa, and tomatoes are all high in antioxidants and nutrients and low in calories."

STACK YOUR SANDWICH WITH FLAVOR, NOT SALT

Surprise! Some sandwiches can pack 150 percent of your RDA of sodium. Usually, they're the ones stuffed with processed red meats such as salami and pepperoni; they have an average of four times the sodium of whole cuts. Low-sodium meats and cheeses slash salt by anywhere from 30 to 85 percent. When going low sodium, pick a meat or cheese you don't normally eat, says Marjorie Nolan Cohn, a registered dietitian in New York. That way, your tastebuds won't be expecting the same flavor. And choose a variety with herbs or spices, like chipotle chicken or peppered roast beef, so you don't miss the salt.

Build a Slimmer Sandwich

Making your own sammie saves you at least 85 calories compared with deli-made subs—and that's just between the bread. "Deli sandwiches often have enough meat for two lunches," says Keri Gans, RD, author of *The Small Change Diet*. Here are three more ways to save.

Flavor Up: Honey- and maple-spiked meats have about 15 more calories per serving, so pair them with low-calorie condiments.

Don't Overdo It: Three slices of meat or one slice of cheese is one serving.

Be a Softie: Sub a slice of American with an ounce of goat cheese or feta, and you'll save 17 calories and 1 gram of fat.

The Road Warrior's Guide to Smart Eating

CHOOSE YOUR CHEESE WISELY

Swiss has 83 percent less sodium than American cheese and more calcium—about 25 percent of the recommended daily value, says Keri Gans, RD, author of *The Small Change Diet*. And although no regular cheese can claim to be low fat, mozzarella is the best one for your bod, with about 6 grams of fat per ounce. Ask for your order to be sliced thin. Not only will you save calories, but thin cheese slices are a better choice for hot sandwiches. "Their lower density helps them melt better," says Cathy Strange, global cheese buyer for Whole Foods Market.

AVOID SHINY SIDES

When the veggies in deli salads are slick and glistening, it's usually a good sign that they've been bathed in high-calorie oil. Instead, go for a cucumber salad or mayo-free coleslaw, says Gans. And don't eat straight from the deli dish: "A container is not necessarily a serving size," she says. "It can be tightly packed, and what looks like a quarter pound may actually be half a pound."

Chapter 8

Make Eating Exciting Again

BREAK OUT OF A FOOD RUT BY SWAPPING IN A FEW OF THESE GOOD-FOR-YOU ALTERNATIVES FOR YOUR USUAL BORING STAPLES.

Salmon? So over. Sure, it's delicious. Sure, it's incredibly good for you. But it's just so . . . done. It has perched atop the "healthiest entrée" throne long enough, and now any way you slice, sauté, steam, stir-fry, or glaze it, you've had your fill. After years of salmon consumption in the name of good health, the urge to pound several double bacon cheeseburgers just for the sake of variety is understandable.

Rediscover your will to eat well with these 10 foods—each just as healthy and delicious as the standbys. Make one of our recipes tonight and give your tried-and-true (and tried again) fallbacks a rest.

INSTEAD OF BROWN RICE ... TRY QUINOA

The ancient Inca believed quinoa (pronounced "KEEN-wah") gave their armies a fighting edge. While it may not help you conquer any empires, it will give your diet a boost. "Unlike other grains, quinoa is considered a complete vegetarian protein on par with dairy," says Marjorie Livingston, R.D., an associate professor at the Culinary Institute of America. (Your body can't use most vegetarian proteins unless you pair them with another, different protein—like peanut butter and whole-wheat bread, or rice and beans. But you can eat quinoa solo.) That's not all this light and nutty grain can do. "Quinoa is an excellent source of fiber, vitamins, and minerals often insufficient in women's diets, like vitamin E, iron, zinc, copper, and magnesium," Livingston says. Since it contains no gluten, even the wheat intolerant can enjoy.

Make It Tonight

Give uncooked quinoa a good rinse to remove any bitter coating. To deepen its flavor, toast it in a skillet in oil over low heat before cooking, says Carol Fenster, PhD, president of Savory Palate, a cookbook company. "For a wonderful flavor twist, add a stick of cinnamon to the boiling water," she suggests.

QUINOA SALAD WITH BLACK BEANS AND SWEET POTATOES

- ½ cup quinoa
- 1 Tbsp olive oil
- 1 medium sweet potato, peeled and diced
- 1 scallion, thinly sliced
- ¼ tsp dried red-pepper flakes
- 1 cup water
- ½ tsp salt
- ¾ cup canned black beans, drained and thoroughly rinsed
- Juice of 1 lime
- 2 Tbsp chopped fresh cilantro

1. Place quinoa in small-mesh sieve and rinse thoroughly. Heat oil over medium-high heat in medium skillet with tight-fitting lid. Add sweet potato, scallion, and pepper flakes and sauté until fragrant, about 2 minutes.

2. Add quinoa and toast 2 minutes. Add water and salt. Bring to a boil, reduce heat to medium low, and cover. Simmer until quinoa and sweet potato are tender, about 10 to 12 minutes. If liquid remains unabsorbed in pan, raise heat to high and cook until it boils off, 2 minutes.

3. Stir in black beans and lime juice. Serve warm or chilled, sprinkled with cilantro.

MAKES 2 SIDE-DISH SERVINGS.

Per serving: 350 calories, 11 g protein, 62 g carbohydrates (10 g fiber), 10 g fat (1 g sat), 1,090 mg sodium

INSTEAD OF SALMON ... TRY ARCTIC CHAR

You've already heard our beef with salmon. For a more interesting substitute that has a mild, light, salmonlike flavor, but less of a fishy taste, look no further than arctic char. Traditionally a protein staple of the Inuit, arctic char swims in the waters off northern Alaska and other icy depths. Like salmon, it's a fatty cold-water fish, which means it's chock-full of heart-healthy omega-3 fats, with fewer dangerous PCBs—heavy metals that are found in salmon feed.

Make It Tonight

Once hard to find outside specialty stores, arctic char is now widely available at well-stocked fish markets. You can also buy it online at shop.legalseafoods.com. You can use it in any recipe that calls for salmon, and it lends itself to just about any cooking method. "Marinades work very nicely with arctic char," Fenster says. Italian salad dressing or teriyaki sauce both work in a pinch.

SEARED ARCTIC CHAR WITH CITRUS-FENNEL SALSA

- 1 small fennel bulb with some fronds attached
- 1 small pink grapefruit
- 1 orange
- ½ cup black olives, roughly chopped
- 2 tsp extra-virgin olive oil
- Coarse kosher salt
- Freshly ground black pepper
- 2 arctic char fillets (4 oz each)

1. Remove stalks from fennel bulb and finely chop 1 Tbsp of the feathery leaves. Remove outer layer from bulb and dice the rest. Set aside.

2. Cut grapefruit in half crosswise. Using small serrated knife, cut around segments of each half to release from membrane. Pop out into bowl. Repeat with orange. Add olives, chopped fennel bulb, fennel leaves, and olive oil to bowl. Season salsa with salt and pepper and stir gently.

3. Heat medium nonstick skillet on high until hot but not smoking. Sprinkle pan with 1 tsp salt. Season fillets with pepper and lay in pan, skin side down. Cook until skin is crispy brown, about 3 minutes. Turn over and cook 1 to 2 minutes more. Let rest 1 minute. Top with salsa.

MAKES 2 SERVINGS.

Per serving: 340 calories, 26 g protein, 26 g carbohydrates (7 g fiber), 16 g fat (1 g sat), 380 mg sodium

INSTEAD OF BROCCOLI... TRY BROCCOLI SPROUTS

Despite their small size and mild taste, tiny broccoli sprouts are a stronger cancer fighter than their grown-up counterparts. "Broccoli sprouts can have 50 times more sulforaphane than mature broccoli," says Paul Talalay, MD, professor of pharmacology at Johns Hopkins Medical School. Sulforaphane, one of the many antioxidants found in the sprouts, has the ability to increase so-called phase two enzymes, which neutralize cancer-causing chemicals before they wreak havoc. "It's chemoprotection through food," Talalay says.

Make It Tonight
Look for the Brocco-Sprouts brand. Brocco-Sprouts are produced under license from Johns Hopkins, which guarantees that each batch has high sulforaphane levels. They're available in most supermarkets.

SHRIMP AND SPROUT LETTUCE WRAPS

- 2 Tbsp reduced-sodium soy sauce
- 2 Tbsp lime juice
- 1 tsp freshly grated ginger
- ¼ tsp sugar
- 1 head Bibb or Boston lettuce
- 1 cup broccoli sprouts
- 4 oz cooked medium shrimp, tails removed
- 1 medium carrot, grated
- 1 daikon root, grated
- Mint or cilantro leaves

1. In small bowl, stir together soy sauce, lime juice, ginger, and sugar.

2. Choose 4 large lettuce leaves without any bruises or holes. Lay them flat. Arrange one-quarter of the broccoli sprouts down the center of 1 leaf. Top with 2 or 3 shrimp. Sprinkle with carrot and daikon, and add a few mint or cilantro leaves. Repeat with remaining lettuce leaves.

4. Loosely roll in sides of lettuce leaves, leaving ends open. Serve with soy-lime dipping sauce.

MAKES 2 APPETIZER SERVINGS.

Per serving: 106 calories, 13 g protein, 10 g carbohydrates (3 g fiber), less than 1 g fat (0 g sat), 1,230 mg sodium

INSTEAD OF PEANUT BUTTER... TRY ALMOND BUTTER

Okay, you're probably not sick of peanut butter. But that's no reason not to swap it out once in a while, as almond butter is higher in calcium, magnesium, and phosphorus. "These three minerals work together to improve bone strength," says Anne VanBeber, PhD, RD, nutrition professor at Texas Christian University in Fort Worth. It's not just your bones that benefit. A study in the *Journal of the American College of Nutrition* found that when participants included almond butter in their diets for 4 weeks, their LDL "bad" cholesterol levels fell. "Almond butter has also been spared the trans fat and sugars that plague many processed peanut butters," VanBeber says.

Make It Tonight

Anywhere peanut butter goes—from cookies to sauces—this can, too. "Just make sure you stir in the oil at the top to prevent it from going dry," Fenster says.

BANANA-ALMOND SMOOTHIE

- ½ cup fat-free plain yogurt
- 1 medium banana
- 1 Tbsp almond butter
- ¾ cup orange juice
- Dash of ground cinnamon

In blender, combine yogurt, banana, almond butter, and orange juice. Blend until smooth. Sprinkle with cinnamon.

MAKES 1 SERVING.

Per serving: 280 calories, 8 g protein, 59 g carbohydrates (5 g fiber), 3.5 g fat (0 g sat), 95 mg sodium

INSTEAD OF BEEF... TRY BUFFALO

Love red meat but hate the fat? Enter buffalo. The cuts are the same, but the health benefits are much different. "Buffalo gets a green light from the American Heart Association because it's low in fat and high in nutrients such as protein, zinc, and vitamin B_{12}," says Martin Marchello, PhD, a professor of animal and range sciences at North Dakota University. "Buffalo also has fewer fats that can raise your cholesterol." Throwing a buffalo burger on the grill is a great way to meet iron requirements, too, since buffalo often contains more of the mineral than other meats do. The taste? Almost indistinguishable from beef, though a bit sweeter and more tender.

Make It Tonight

You don't have to live on the range to get buffalo, though it may set you back a dollar more a pound than beef. Many specialty meat shops and natural food stores stock it. Or buy it at exoticmeatsandmore.com. You can use buffalo in recipes calling for beef, but make sure you prepare it carefully. "Because it's low in fat, you need to employ quick cooking methods or you'll end up eating a hockey puck," VanBeber says.

BUFFALO BURGERS IN PITA WITH MINT-YOGURT DRESSING

- ½ cup reduced-fat plain yogurt
- ¼ cup fresh mint leaves, chopped
- 1 tsp white wine vinegar
- 1 clove garlic, minced
- Salt and freshly ground black pepper
- 8 oz ground buffalo meat
- ½ tsp cumin
- ½ tsp coriander
- 2 whole-wheat pitas
- ½ medium cucumber, thinly sliced

1. In small bowl, stir together yogurt, mint, vinegar, and garlic. Season to taste with salt and pepper.

2. In medium bowl, combine meat, cumin, coriander, and ½ tsp salt until thoroughly mixed. Season with pepper. Shape mixture into 2 patties about ½" thick.

3. Heat large skillet over medium heat. Coat with cooking spray and cook burgers to medium rare, turning once, about 5 to 6 minutes total (be careful not to overcook).

4. Cut tops off pita pockets. Stuff each pita with 1 burger and several slices of cucumber. Drizzle with mint-yogurt dressing and serve.

MAKES 2 SERVINGS.

Per serving: 260 calories, 31 g protein, 22 g carbohydrates (3 g fiber), 6 g fat (2 g sat), 900 mg sodium

INSTEAD OF CARROTS... TRY PARSNIPS

This cousin of the carrot has a more complex, sweet, nutty flavor. And 1 cup packs a whopping 7 grams of fiber (double that of carrots), which fends off hunger pangs. Other perks: a stellar amount of vitamin C and folate, plus almost 40 percent of your daily requirement of vitamin K, a hard-to-get nutrient that researchers are realizing may improve bone health and control blood sugar.

Make Them Tonight
Toss parsnips into salads and stir-fries as you would carrots, or make parsnip cakes by combining 1 pound peeled and grated parsnips, ¾ cup whole-wheat flour, 1 teaspoon baking powder, 3 eggs, and ¼ cup fat-free milk. Season to taste with salt, freshly ground black pepper, and nutmeg, and spoon onto a skillet lightly coated with vegetable oil. Brown on both sides.

INSTEAD OF PLUMS... TRY FIGS

You get the sweetness of plums without all the drippy juice. "Fresh figs have a deliciously sweet pulp and are a good source of potassium, dietary fiber, calcium, and manganese," says Elizabeth Pivonka, PhD, RD, president and CEO of the Produce for Better Health Foundation.

Make Them Tonight
Remove the stems, then cut an X into one end without slicing all the way through. Pinch to open the flesh and fill with a small dollop of low-fat ricotta cheese, ½ teaspoon maple syrup, and a dusting of cinnamon.

INSTEAD OF LETTUCE... TRY BOK CHOY

The stalks of this Asian leafy green are crunchy and mild, and the leaves are more like cabbage. Bok choy is among the top cancer-fighting picks in the produce aisle, thanks to its high levels of the antioxidants glucosinolate and indole.

Make It Tonight
Stir-fry sliced bok choy in a few drops of sesame oil with onion and vegetables. Add chopped toasted peanuts, soy sauce, and a splash of balsamic vinegar.

INSTEAD OF POTATOES... TRY SUNCHOKES

With its mellow taste and flaky texture, the sunchoke (aka Jerusalem artichoke) is easy to pair with any main dish. The tuber is also brimming with 5 grams of energy-boosting iron per serving (massive for a veggie that isn't a bean) and inulin, a soluble fiber that may help lower blood cholesterol and stabilize blood glucose levels.

Make Them Tonight
Slice sunchokes into matchsticks, toss with vegetable oil, rosemary, cayenne, salt, and pepper, and bake at 350°F for 15 minutes.

INSTEAD OF SPINACH . . . TRY SWISS CHARD

A vitamin powerhouse with a more intense flavor than spinach, Swiss chard adds zing to any dish. Chard has huge amounts of vitamins A and K and more of the vision-protecting antioxidants lutein and zeaxanthin than spinach. More great news: A 2009 study in *The American Journal of Clinical Nutrition* found that boosting your intake of nutrient-dense greens such as chard will also help you dodge heart disease.

Make It Tonight
Sauté torn Swiss chard in a little olive oil, garlic, and salt and serve as a bed for fish. Or steam and toss with pasta along with shrimp, olive oil, sun-dried tomatoes, and lemon juice. Stalks can be sliced raw and served with hummus for a standout snack.

Chapter 9

Think Before You Drink

ONE OF THE EASIEST WAYS TO REVAMP YOUR DIET? RECONSIDER YOUR LIQUID INTAKE.

America has a serious drinking problem. But it's not the dirty martinis and shots of Patrón that we're hooked on. It's the soft stuff—regular soda, juice, and, yes, the beloved grande mocha— that fuels this addiction. In fact, a study in *The American Journal of Clinical Nutrition* showed that around 37 percent of our total daily liquid calories come from sugar-sweetened drinks. And here's the really crazy part: Guzzling those beverages can have a bigger impact on your waistlines than anything else you eat.

"Our evolution over hundreds of thousands of years didn't prepare us to process liquid calories," says Barry Popkin, PhD, a distinguished professor of nutrition at the University of North Carolina. After all, he says, we drank only water for most of human history. For reference, you can figure that's a duration of, say, 200,000 years. "High-sugar drinks didn't even exist until 150 years ago, and they weren't consumed in significant amounts until the past 50 years. This is just a blip on our evolutionary timeline," says Popkin.

The problem, it seems, is that beverages don't make us feel full. Popkin hypothesizes that humans developed this way so that satisfying our thirst with water wouldn't also blunt our hunger for food. Unfortunately, our bodies weren't reprogrammed for the 21st century, a time when more than 20 percent of our total calorie intake comes from beverages.

Perhaps all of this explains why our appetite for sugary drinks is seemingly insatiable: The drinks taste great but aren't filling.

When Purdue University researchers had people consume 450 calories a day from either jelly beans or soft drinks for 4 weeks, the candy eaters consumed no more total calories than usual. The soda swiggers, however, downed 17 percent more calories each day. So on a 2,500-calorie diet, for example, the pop drinkers would have taken in an extra 425 daily calories. "People simply don't reduce their food intake when they drink their calories from soda and other beverages," says Popkin. Not surprisingly, the group that consumed the liquid calories gained weight during the study.

Now consider that the average person consumes 459 calories, in the beverages he or she drinks each day. So by cutting back or even eliminating the kinds of drinks that contribute to those empty calories, you'll instantly kick-start weight loss. Where to begin? Start by slashing your consumption of soda and focus on chugging more H_2O. Then use this guide to fill out the rest of your drink list.

Drink Freely

UNSWEETENED TEA

After water, tea is the world's most popular beverage. But in the United States, regular soda rules. That's a shame, because not only does tea contain antioxidants that may help protect against heart disease and fight cancer, it's also calorie-free. And studies have found that compounds in green tea known as catechins rev your metabolism for up to 24 hours—meaning it actually helps you burn more calories.

But when you load this naturally good beverage with sugar, you detract from those health benefits. So order unsweetened when you can, and check labels: You want beverages that provide little or no sugar. To make your own comparisons, remember that every 4 grams of the sweet stuff is the same as eating one sugar packet or sugar cube.

But what if the product label doesn't list nutrition information? That's good news, since it's an indicator that the calorie content is negligible. For instance, you typically won't find a nutrition label on tea bags, because they contain less than 1 gram of carbohydrates per serving, and thus, virtually no calories.

While green, black, and oolong bag teas are all great choices, there are many other types of tea that come in a variety of different flavors. Check out the ones listed below and experiment with as many as you can. You'll no doubt find several you enjoy, and you won't miss the sugar at all.

Genmaicha
Best for: An afternoon pick-me-up. This Japanese green tea is mixed with roasted rice kernels. It has a savory smell, almost like popcorn.

Matcha
Best for: An antioxidant boost. Leaves are ground into a fine powder, which you can whisk into water for tea. Since you consume

the actual leaves, which gives it a strong, grassy flavor, you get more antioxidants than from other green teas. As an alternative to sipping, stir 1 teaspoon of powder into a smoothie or dust it over vanilla ice cream or a bar of dark chocolate. The tea's earthiness is a pleasant contrast to the food's sweetness.

Sur le Nil
Best for: After-dinner relaxing. Its flavor is more delicate than that of many green teas. Think of it as chamomile-plus, with hints of lemon and spice.

Dragon Well
Best for: Sipping on a chilly afternoon. This yellowish-green flat leaf tea is one of the most popular drinking teas in China, and its soft chestnut notes give it a comforting, toasty flavor. Give your dinner a lift by chopping the tea leaves, combining them with spices, and using them to coat chicken or steak before cooking.

High Mountain Oolong
Best for: Relaxing after work. It's made with thick tea leaves, which give it a full floral flavor with an earthy finish—a good balance for before dinner.

Wood Dragon Oolong
Best for: Guys who've quit coffee. Because it contains more stem than leaf, this strong, woodsy brew has significantly less caffeine than other oolong teas.

Honey Phoenix Oolong
Best for: Wintertime defrosting. It's a robust tea, with a flavor almost like a cherry pit. That makes it sweet, with a tinge of bitterness.

Hojicha
Best for: When you want less of a jolt. It's made from leaves that are roasted until they're dark brown, which gives it a toasty, nutty flavor. Because it's picked at the end of the season and processed at a higher heat than other teas, hojicha contains lower levels of caffeine. For a tasty autumn meal, ladle a cup of steeped hojicha tea over a mixture of brown rice and roasted fall veggies, like squash. Garnish with a sprinkle of chestnuts.

Vanilla Rooibos
Best for: Dessert—and not just because it's free of caffeine. You'll taste a light sweetness followed by a creamy finish.

Sencha
Best for: Green tea beginners. The most popular green tea in Japan, sencha leaves are steamed, producing a bright green color, then rolled into needle form. It's sweet and mellow, without the bitter bite of some other green brews. Sip it with sushi or dessert. Or, after mixing the dough or batter for cookies, muffins, or scones, fold 2 tablespoons of dried sencha tea leaves directly into it, then bake as usual.

Cassis
Best for: Snapping awake on a cold morning. This black tea is rich and powerful. You'll taste black currants, with a sweet, dry finish.

Pu-Erh Tuocha
Best for: Coffee drinkers. It's strong and earthy, and has a kick of caffeine. The black tea comes pressed into nuggets, which break apart when you boil them.

Kukicha
Best for: When you want a lighter flavor. Called twig tea, kukicha is derived from thinly cut stalks of sencha and gyokuro leaves. Its light flavor is balanced with smooth, woody notes. It's also a perfect flavor balance for sweeter varieties of fish or shellfish, like scallops or halibut. Add a few tablespoons to a marinade.

COFFEE
Studies show that coffee can help ward off mental decline, certain cancers, Parkinson's disease, high blood pressure, and even extra

pounds (yes, really!). A study published in the *Archives of Internal Medicine* found that each time you refill your cup of java (caffeinated or decaf) in a day, you slash your diabetes risk by 7 percent; in another study, drinking two to three cups of coffee each day was associated with a 21 percent lower risk of heart disease.

Want to reap all these benefits without the jitters or coffee breath? Give your next meal a shot of espresso.

"Coffee can give both sweet and savory dishes a rich, earthy element," says chef David Guas, owner of Bayou Bakery Coffee Bar & Eatery in Arlington, Virginia. "It works particularly well in recipes that star chocolate, cherries, blueberries, lemon, and stronger-tasting nuts such as pecans and walnuts."

To let a bold coffee flavor come through in a finished recipe, Guas says it's best to brew a dark roast with half as much water as you would normally use (let the coffee cool to room temperature if you're adding it to a batter). Or use coffee grounds as a rub for poultry, pork, or steak.

In terms of drinking the brew, it's best to do it in moderation, despite the body benefits. "Coffee is a natural stimulant, and high intake can bring on headaches, increased heart rate, or insomnia," says Nyree Dardarian, RD, an adjunct faculty member at Drexel University College of Nursing and Health Professions in Philadelphia. She recommends capping your daily fix at four 6-ounce cups and finishing the last one at least 4 hours before turning in for the night.

Become a Coffee Connoisseur

Now that you know coffee is good for you, how do you reap all the benefits of a java jolt? Stay informed. Pour yourself a second cup and read on, because we've compiled everything you've ever wanted to know about your morning brew.

The Bean

Out of the nearly 100 different varieties of coffee beans, only two make their way to the cup. Arabica, known for its deep, complex flavor, accounts for about 75 percent of the beans sold throughout the world. Robusta, a cheaper bean usually considered a filler, is often found lurking in the canisters you buy in the supermarket.

The Roast

Roasting can be done anywhere, from a factory to your home oven. Bringing out the richness in a raw bean without destroying its inherent flavor is a delicate art. "A medium roast of a good coffee is like a nice table wine—really bright, with that pleasant acidity," says Kenneth Davids, a cofounder of CoffeeReview.com and the author of *Coffee: A Guide to Buying, Brewing, and Enjoying*. "The darker the roast, the fewer characteristics of the bean you taste." Most single-origin coffees, such as Colombian, Sumatra, and other coffees named after countries, are lightly roasted to preserve the beans' natural flavor. Blends are typically roasted for a desired flavor. The three main roasting categories are:

Medium. These coffees are roasted for 9 to 11 minutes, like most grocery-store varieties. Also called Breakfast Roast.
Dark. In this common European method, batches are roasted for 12 to 13 minutes until the oils reach the surface of the beans. Also called French Roast.
Extra dark. Roasted for at least 14 minutes, these oily beans taste so smoky that it's nearly impossible to identify where they were grown. You drink it for the deep roast, not the nuance of the bean. Also called Italian or Espresso Roast.

Beware of flavored beans. These are usually cheap Robusta beans roasted to oblivion and flavored artificially. If you need a hazelnut or vanilla fix, buy a bottle of flavored oil and mix a teaspoon into a cup of the good stuff.

The Region

All good coffee is grown between the Tropic of Cancer and the Tropic of Capricorn, where the climate is ideal for producing rich, full-flavored beans. Each of the three major coffee-growing regions produces a distinct flavor. Known for their lighter coffees, the Americas produce more joe than any other region. "Latin American coffee's crisp, bright acidity comes as a direct result of its climate and the volcanic soils the beans grow in," says Andy Fouché, a former certified coffee specialist with Starbucks Coffee. Africa/Arabia, the region where coffee was born 1,200 years ago, produces a smoother, less acidic cup than the Americas. The Asia/Pacific region produces the boldest of coffees, often with a heavy, earthy taste.

The Preparation

Good coffee is about proper flavor extraction from the bean, and each brewing method demands a different grind. French presses and percolators use the coarsest grind (about 5 to 10 seconds in your grinder), automatic-drip machines need a medium grind (10 to 15 seconds), and espresso machines require the finest grind (25 seconds).

The Brew

Even the most carefully roasted beans can be ruined by sloppy brewing. Start by buying your coffee fresh in small batches every 2 weeks. Skip the preground stuff and the oversize supermarket grinder, and buy your beans whole instead; grinding them just before you brew will make the best cup. For a standard automatic-drip machine, use filtered water and 1 to 2 tablespoons of ground beans for every 6 ounces of brewed coffee. When it comes to storing your beans, keep them out of the freezer—it destroys the essential oils that make coffee delicious. Keep coffee in your cupboard in a dark, airtight container.

The Effect

Within about 15 minutes of your first sip, the caffeine starts the release of dopamine in your brain's prefrontal cortex. This effect, which increases wakefulness and mental focus, among other things, peaks in about 30 minutes.

Give Espresso a Shot

"Espresso is all about the crema," says Matt Riddle, a designer for Intelligentsia Coffee and the 2006 winner of the United States Barista Championship. "Think of a Guinness when it's poured. That's how the shot should look—a nice dark body, but with a reddish-brown top." Achieve crema perfection and espresso ecstasy in five steps:

Step 1: Find the "Roasted On" or "Best Before" date, and make sure the coffee's less than 2 weeks out of the roaster. "Coffee is a food. It can spoil like anything else in your cupboard," says Riddle.

Step 2: Use a burr grinder to make sure the beans are ground evenly. Setting the grinder on the finest setting should make the grounds about the size of table salt.

Step 3: Fill your basket until there's a quarter inch of room at the top. Now press down with your tamper, using about 30 pounds of pressure. "Use a normal bathroom scale to see how much force you need," says Riddle. Then tightly place the basket in the machine.

Step 4: Make sure the temperature is between 198° and 204°F and the pressure is around 8 or 9 bars. The 2-ounce shot should take between 20 and 30 seconds to pour.

Step 5: Keeping your equipment clean is the most important part. "Whether it's a $50 machine or a $5,000 machine, simply wiping down the parts with a dry paper towel once a week will keep oily buildup from forming," says Riddle.

The Flavor Boost

Like tea, unsweetened coffee is filled with healthful compounds and almost no calories. But when was the last time you drank unsweetened coffee? Gourmet-coffee drinkers consume, on average, 206 more calories a day than people who sip regular joe. Not ready to break up with your barista? Try an Americano (espresso plus water) or a café au lait with skim milk. If you can't skip cream and sugar, be stingy with them or use low-cal or fat-free versions. Cream and sugar add needless calories and may delay the uptake of antioxidants into your blood, says a study in the *Journal of Nutrition*. Instead, flavor your grinds with these spices, then brew as usual.

Cardamom: Remove the seeds from three pods, and crush using a mortar and pestle or the flat side of a knife.

Fresh orange zest: Grate in ½ teaspoon.

Star anise: Add one whole dried star-shaped fruit for a spicy-sweet licorice flavor.

Cinnamon: Grate 1 teaspoon from a stick or sprinkle the same amount of ground cinnamon.

Nutmeg: Use a spice grater to shave in ¼ teaspoon.

Go Easier on These

MILK

Like soda, milk doesn't make you feel full, says Popkin. However, other researchers disagree. And because milk contains bone-strengthening calcium and muscle-building protein, it's a worthy beverage to work into your daily calorie allotment. (Of course, you can also derive the same nutrients from solid dairy foods, such as cheese and yogurt.)

Still, some studies show that milk drinkers are leaner than those who skip the beverage—so unless you're downing it by the gallon, it's not likely to be the reason for your love handles. If you're trying to manage your weight, make it a policy to cap your intake at two glasses a day. Just make sure you opt for the unsweetened kind—flavored milk is loaded with added sugar. Interestingly, in an analysis of vending-machine sales in schools, flavored milk, such as chocolate and strawberry, outsold the regular kind nine to one. That just goes to show that our taste for sweet drinks isn't limited to sodas, coffee, and tea—and it probably starts at a young age. For even more information on milk, turn to Chapter 27.

JUICE

It's time to dispel a popular myth: All juice is healthful because it comes from fruit. This has led many people to take a more-is-better approach to these beverages. The trouble is, many juices contain not only the natural sugar from the fruit, but also copious amounts of added sugars, so that they aren't as tart. Cranberry juice, in fact, is too sour to drink when it hasn't been sweetened.

Keep in mind, though, that a medium orange contains just 62 calories and 12 grams of sugar, and it has 3 grams of belly-filling fiber. An 8-ounce glass of Minute Maid OJ has 110 calories, 24 grams of sugar, and no fiber.

So the best approach is to eat the whole fruit, which also ensures that you get all the beneficial nutrients. (The skin of an apple is loaded with antioxidants.) And if you want juice, take it in smaller doses—2 to 3 ounces is a good rule of thumb. Another option: Go ahead and have the juice, but make sure you're monitoring your total calorie intake.

DIET SODA

No-cal pop may not pile on the pounds directly, but research from Purdue University suggests that drinking these artificially sweetened beverages can screw with the brain's ability to measure caloric intake. Also, emerging research suggests that consuming sugary-tasting beverages—even if they're artificially sweetened—may lead to a high preference for sweetness overall. And that might best explain why nobody takes their coffee black anymore. Plus, if you swig diet drinks all day, you're taking in fewer healthy liquids, such as tea. Get your carbonation fix with zero-calorie seltzer instead, or make your own with a home soda maker that carbonates your drink of choice.

ALCOHOL

Happy hour is good for plenty of things, but weight loss isn't one of them. Savoring a drink every now and then does have its perks, including reducing your risk of heart disease, but alcohol packs a lot of calories into a small glass, and it may even stimulate your appetite. And unlike the calories in fat, carbohydrates, and protein, those in alcohol can't be stored in your body, so they have to be used immediately. As a result, your body stops burning fat until the alcohol is processed—that's roughly an hour for every drink. Most wines ring in between 100 and 120 calories a glass, but you can stretch it out by adding club soda and ice to make a spritzer. If you can't stomach that, have a Bloody Mary—a 6-ounce glass delivers around 76 calories. That's reasonable.

Control Food, Control Yourself

Part Three

Food makes us do crazy things. We get deep cravings. Some foods seem to call our very names across long distances, and we float toward them like Bugs Bunny drifting on a wave of carrot waft. It would be easy to say that willpower is the problem. But it goes deeper than that. Some food is engineered to trigger our cravings so we eat (and buy) more of it. So the problem—and this section—is less about willpower and more about how to achieve control over what you eat.

Chapter 10

The Trouble with Traditional Diets

HERE ARE THE REASONS MOST DIETS FAIL, AND HOW YOU CAN FIND WHAT WORKS FOR YOU.

If you've ever tried to slim down, you've probably amassed a menu-ful of calorie-cutting tips and tricks. So it may come as a shock to learn that many of the ones you've sworn by are actually keeping you fat. "In their quest to lose weight, many people unknowingly sabotage themselves," says Elisa Zied, RD, an American Dietetic Association spokesperson and coauthor of *Feed Your Family Right!* Here are 10 well-intentioned approaches to weight loss that can go awry, and the expert and research-proven ways to drop pounds for good.

DIET DOWNFALL #1: YOU SAVE YOUR CALORIES FOR A BIG DINNER

Yes, cutting total calories can lead to weight loss. But bank most of those calories for the end of the day and your hunger hormones will go haywire, making you eat more. Men who ate their daily number of calories in one supersize supper produced more ghrelin, a hormone that causes hunger, than when they ate the same number of calories in three square meals, researchers at the National Institute on Aging found.

Smarter Move
Front-load your calories. Overeating at night keeps you from being hungry in the morning, setting off a vicious cycle in which you're never interested in breakfast but always starving by dinner. The key is to rebalance your day so you don't set yourself up for an evening binge. To get your appetite back in the morning, cut your evening meal in half. Then eat a breakfast of about 450 calories, such as a scrambled egg with cheese on a whole-wheat English muffin with an 8-ounce glass of juice—an amount that should keep you satisfied until lunch, says George L. Blackburn, MD, PhD, associate director of the Division of Nutrition at Harvard Medical School and author of *Break Through Your Set Point*. Once your appetite adjusts, don't go more than 5 hours without another meal of roughly the same size.

DIET DOWNFALL #2: YOU GRAZE INSTEAD OF EATING REGULARLY SCHEDULED MEALS

Trouble is, eating in this manner may contribute to weight gain, according to a 2005 *American Journal of Clinical Nutrition* study. When researchers asked participants to eat at regular, fixed times or to break their usual amount of food into unscheduled meals throughout the day, they made a startling discovery: The panelists actually burned more calories in the 3 hours after eating the regular meals than they did after the unplanned meals. They produced less insulin, too, potentially lowering their odds of insulin resistance, which is linked to weight gain and obesity. What's more, grazing instead of planning ahead can set you up to eat mindlessly, says Zied. In the end, we rarely realize how many calories all those little nibbles and noshes really add up to.

Smarter Move
Figure out how many times a day you need to eat—everybody is different—and then stick to a schedule. "It's not great to feel starved, but it is okay to feel slightly hungry," says Zied. You can home in on your body's internal cues with a food diary. It's so effective that researchers at Kaiser Permanente's Center for Health Research found that dieters who kept a food journal lost twice as much weight as those who didn't record what they ate.

DIET DOWNFALL #3: YOU ASSUME HEALTHY, NATURAL FOODS ARE LOW CALORIE

People consistently underestimate the calories in nutritious items such as yogurt, fish, and baked chicken, found researchers at Bowling Green State University who quizzed students on calorie counts. "Just because a food is healthy doesn't mean you can eat big portions," says D. Milton Stokes, PhD, MPH, RD, owner of One Source Nutrition in Stamford, Connecticut. "A handful of nuts can be 200 calories or more. And if you add that without cutting back elsewhere, it could be the reason you're not losing weight."

Smarter Move

Count all calories for a few days or weeks. Once you learn that $1/2$ cup of cereal can have as much as 200 calories or that there are about 220 calories in that "single-serving" bottle of OJ, you'll be more prudent about how much you consume.

DIET DOWNFALL #4: YOU CRASH DIET FOR A MONTH BEFORE A BIG EVENT

Slashing significant calories might sound like the fast track to weight loss, but it's likely to backfire. In fact, nutrition experts recommend you don't dip below 1,200 to 1,500 calories a day. "If you crash diet for more than 2 weeks or so, your metabolism will temporarily slow down," says Blackburn. "So the same exact dieting effort results in less and less weight loss." The reason: Your body is conserving energy to keep you from losing weight too quickly. And that's not all. When you drastically cut calories, you lose muscle along with fat—especially if you haven't been exercising. Because muscle is your body's calorie-burning furnace, this can slow down your metabolism, even long after your crash diet is done.

Smarter Move

Aim to shed about a pound a week—the slow, steady weight loss ensures you lose fat, not muscle. "If you want to drop 10 pounds, get started 10 weeks before your goal, not 4," says Blackburn. "You'll have a better chance of actually taking off the weight permanently." To drop a pound a week, shave 250 calories from your diet and burn an extra 250 calories through exercise each day.

DIET DOWNFALL #5: YOU SET SHORT-TERM WEIGHT LOSS GOALS

The National Weight Control Registry (NWCR) estimates that only 20 percent of dieters successfully keep off lost weight for more than a year. That's because after we reach our goal, we let old eating habits creep back in. But people who win at weight loss consistently eat the same way even after they've slimmed down. In fact, the NWCR found that dieters who maintain their healthy eating habits every single day are 1 1/2 times more likely to maintain their weight loss in the long run than those who relax their diets on the weekends.

Smarter Move

Think of healthy eating as a work in progress, not as a "diet" with a beginning and an end. The key: making small changes you can maintain so they become long-term habits. Start by creating a list of problem areas in your diet, then tackle them one at a time. For example, if you snack on a heaping handful of cookies every night before bed, set a goal of having two instead of six, and cut back by one a day. Once you've made that a habit, pat yourself on the back and move on to your next goal.

DIET DOWNFALL #6: YOU SPLURGE ON "DIET" FOODS

Research suggests that when a food is described as a diet food, we're subconsciously primed to eat more—even if it's actually as caloric as regular food. When Cornell University researchers offered the same candies labeled either regular or low-fat to visitors at a university open house, visitors ate 28 percent more of the "low-fat" snacks. While less fat does not mean fewer calories, people make the assumption that it does, setting them up to overeat, say scientists.

Smarter Move

First, check food labels. So-called diet foods frequently don't save you calories. Take low-fat chocolate chip cookies—because they've been infused with extra carbs to add flavor, you save only 3 calories per cookie. Once you have that reality check, follow the golden rule for any food: Keep close tabs on portions. Limit yourself to two small cookies, for example, or trade in a bowl of frozen yogurt for a kid-size scoop. Measure out condiments such as low-fat sour cream or low-fat ranch dressing. And remember—if you prefer the flavor of full-fat foods, you'll still lose weight if you watch your portion sizes.

DIET DOWNFALL #7: YOU'VE GONE NO-CARB OR FAT FREE

Cutting back markedly on any one food group—say, carbs or fat—can leave you short on the nutrients you need to stay energized. One study found that dieters low in calcium and vitamin C had higher odds of putting on belly fat.

Smarter Move

The trick is a varied diet that includes healthy fats and good carbs such as fruits. After all, the biggest reason low-carb diets backfire is that, for the vast majority of people, they aren't sustainable over the long haul. It's a rare soul who can pass up birthday cake and pasta dinners for a lifetime. And as with all diets, once you quit, you regain the weight you lost and (often) more. These fluctuations can make it an even bigger challenge to lose weight next time.

DIET DOWNFALL #8: YOU AREN'T EATING ENOUGH

You may need to bump up your calories to stoke metabolism. When you dip below about 1,200 calories per day, not only are you not eating enough to get all your nutrients, but your body slows metabolism in order to hold on to precious calories, says Christine Gerbstadt, MD, RD, author of *Doctor's Detox Diet*. Also, if you skip meals to lose weight, your body could lose its ability to feel full.

Smarter Move

If you skip breakfast, the body assumes food is scarce and goes into survival mode. The best way to break this cycle? Eat breakfast. You need a morning meal to let your body know it's okay to burn calories. "Within 1 hour of waking, you should consume a 350- to 500-calorie breakfast, with 10 to 15 grams of protein and fiber to stoke the metabolic fire," says Gerbstadt.

DIET DOWNFALL #9: YOU REWARD YOURSELF WITH FOOD AFTER EXERCISE

Burning 300 calories during a workout is cause for celebration—but rewarding yourself with a high-calorie treat doesn't add up to weight loss. You're likely to overestimate how much the workout burned off and underestimate how much you ate.

Smarter Move
"Even if you're just working out for well-being, you still have to keep calories in check," says Heidi Skolnik, coauthor of *Nutrient Timing for Peak Performance*. If you want to give yourself a reward for a workout well done or when you reach a certain goal in your training, indulge in a nonedible treat, like a sports massage, new GPS watch, or an afternoon of doing an activity you enjoy.

DIET DOWNFALL #10: YOUR FRIENDS ARE FAT

Your chances of being overweight or obese increase half a percent with every friend in your network who is obese, finds a November 2010 study from Harvard. That more than adds up: Your chances of obesity double for every four obese friends you have, say researchers. Even if that friend lives thousands of miles away, your chances of gaining weight still go up, according to a 2007 *New England Journal of Medicine* study. That may be because your perception of being overweight changes—living larger seems acceptable since the heavy person is a friend. (Interestingly, having an obese neighbor that you don't know does not raise your risk.) Experts also think that a person's lifestyle and behaviors can subconsciously rub off on those in the individual's inner circle.

Smarter Move
You don't have to ditch overweight friends to lose weight. Instead, use the group mentality to get fit. If you embark together on an exercise plan, you can increase your fun and calorie burn. Research from Oxford finds that exercising with friends as a team can actually make the agony of exertion less intense. The same hormones that are released during social bonding—endorphins—also help quell pain. And once a friend starts to lose weight, you have a greater chance of losing as well (the mechanisms work both ways).

Chapter 11

Crush Cravings for Good

THEY HAPPEN TO EVERYONE AND ARRIVE WHEN YOU'RE AT YOUR WEAKEST. NEVER CAVE IN TO A CRAVING EVER AGAIN.

A craving is like a little devil, constantly encouraging you to indulge. And dieting only turns up the pressure. A study published in the *International Journal of Obesity* found that 91 percent of participants reported experiencing food cravings when they weren't on a diet; once they started restricting calories, that figure went up to 94 percent.

The good news is that these unhealthy tormentors can be fended off. The reason: Cravings are all about blood sugar. If your levels stay consistent throughout the day, your eating patterns will, too. It's when you starve yourself for hours that cravings call.

"Your blood sugar can fall too low after just 4 hours of not eating," says Valerie Berkowitz, MS, RD, nutrition director at the Center for Balanced Health in New York City. So you search the fridge, food court, or seat cushions for carbohydrates, which will provide a quick boost.

Trouble is, fast-rising blood sugar triggers your pancreas to release a flood of insulin, a hormone that not only lowers blood sugar but also signals your body to store fat. And in about half of us, insulin tends to "overshoot," which sends blood sugar crashing. "This reinforces the binge, because it makes you crave sugar and starch again," says Berkowitz.

Worse, when it comes to quelling cravings, manufacturers are often stacking the deck against us, in an effort to get us to eat—and buy—more of their products. In their natural state, whole foods may be high in fat or sugar, but they're rarely high in both. Today we have man-made snack foods with a tantalizing combination of fat and sugar rolled into one. "Foods have become so 'hyperpalatable' that they're now capable of hijacking our brains the same way that nicotine and alcohol do," says Ashley Gearhardt, the lead author of a Yale University study on food addiction. With all these forces arrayed against you, how can you resist?

The most effective way to keep blood sugar in check is to avoid foods that are made with added sugar, such as soda, some fruit juices, and baked goods. Also try the following strategies, which are designed to stop 99 percent of cravings before they start—and help you muzzle the 1 percent that never seem to shut up.

CRAVING CRUSHER #1: RAMP UP YOUR RESOLVE

One reason most diets fail is that long-term goals can be deceptively difficult. When the plan is to watch what you eat for the next 6 months, chugging one caramel latte with whipped cream seems like a minor slip. To avoid that kind of thinking, commit to eating well for a fixed amount of time that you're 100 percent confident you can manage, even if it's just a few days. "Once you make it to your goal date, start over," says Mary Vernon, MD, former chair of the board of the American Society of Bariatric Physicians. "This establishes the notion that you can be successful and gives you a chance to notice that eating better makes you feel better, reinforcing your desire to continue."

CRAVING CRUSHER #2: FIND MEANINGFUL MOTIVATION

If the main purpose of your diet is cosmetic—i.e., to look amazing shirtless—you're unlikely to stick with it for the long haul. The solution: "Arm yourself with additional motivators," says Jeffrey Volek, PhD, RD, a nutrition and exercise researcher at the University of Connecticut. He suggests keeping a daily journal in which you monitor other issues you have, like migraines, heartburn, acne, canker sores, or sleep quality in addition to body measurements and the number on the scale. "Discovering that your new diet improves the quality of your life and health is powerful motivation," Volek says.

CRAVING KNOWLEDGE

Think you're prepared to fend off the next chocolate doughnut that enters your field of vision? Find out how much you really know about your cravings.

FACT: Chewing gum can help reduce cravings.
A study presented at the 2007 annual scientific meeting of the Obesity Society found that chewing gum at one-, two-, and three-hour intervals after lunch significantly reduced the desire to eat.

FICTION: Cravings are your body's way of communicating that it needs certain nutrients.
This is probably just wishful thinking. Researchers have found no evidence of it for the vast majority of commonly craved foods.

FACT: Eating the same thing every day can increase the number of cravings you have.
According to a study published in the journal *Obesity*, eating the same foods all the time can increase your number of cravings.

FICTION: The most successful dieters never give in to their cravings.
A 2007 Tufts University study found that dieters who occasionally give in to cravings have the most weight loss success.

FACT: Chocolate is the most-craved flavor.
A study in the *Journal of the American Dietetic Association* found that while there's not yet proof that chocolate is biologically addictive, it is the most sought-after flavor in North America.

FICTION: The easiest way to kill a craving is to think about something else.
Smell or look at something else instead. Researchers at Flinders University in Australia found that visual and olfactory distractions could help.

CRAVING CRUSHER #3: RESTOCK YOUR SHELVES

How many times have you driven to the store in the middle of the night to satisfy a craving? Probably not nearly as often as you've raided the fridge. You're more likely to give in to a craving when the object you desire is close at hand. So make sure it's not: Toss the junk food and restock your cupboard and fridge with almonds and other nuts, cheese, fruits and vegetables, and canned tuna, chicken, and salmon. And do the same at work. "By eliminating snacks that don't match your diet and providing plenty that do, you're far less likely to find yourself at the doughnut shop drive-thru or the vending machine," says Christopher Mohr, PhD, RD, a personal nutrition consultant in Louisville, Kentucky.

CRAVING CRUSHER #4: ROLL OUT OF BED AND INTO THE KITCHEN

Sure, you've heard this advice from us already. But consider that if you sleep for 6 to 8 hours and then skip breakfast, your body is essentially running on fumes by the time you get to work. And that sends you desperately seeking sugar, which is usually pretty easy to find. The most convenient foods are typically packed with sugar (doughnuts, lattes) or other quickly digested carbohydrates (bagels, muffins). Which brings us to our next strategy.

CRAVING CRUSHER #5: OPTIMIZE YOUR COOKING TIME

If you're ravenous by the time you get home from the office, join the club. When you're ready for dinner—but dinner's not ready for you—it's easy to make a beeline for the fridge and inhale whatever you can get your hands on. By the time dinner's on the table, you're not hungry. But you eat a full meal anyway. In this case, "planning is key," says Patricia Bannan, MS, RD, author of *Eat Right When Time Is Tight*. Start before you get home by eating something light and healthy to tide you over so you won't be inclined to gobble up everything in sight. If you're starving while you cook, munch on some raw veggies like sugar snap peas. Next, "set yourself up for success by planning quick, healthy meals so you can get dinner on the table in a hurry," says Bannan. With bags of frozen mixed vegetables, along with a rotisserie chicken and microwavable brown rice, you can have a real meal on the table in 5 minutes flat. Can't last that long? "Many grocery stores offer healthy meals to go or even deliver them, so dinner will be ready when you walk in the door," she says.

CRAVING CRUSHER #6: SPOT HUNGER IMPOSTORS

Have a craving for sweets even though you ate just an hour ago? Imagine sitting down to a large, sizzling steak instead. "If you're truly hungry, the steak will sound good, and you should eat," says Richard Feinman, PhD, a professor of biochemistry at SUNY Downstate Medical Center in Brooklyn, New York. "If it doesn't sound good, your brain is playing tricks on you." His advice: Change your environment, which can be as easy as stretching at your desk or turning your attention to a different task.

CRAVING CRUSHER #7: OVERHAUL YOUR OFFICE

Between the office candy bowl, the break room vending machine, your coworkers' home-baked brownies, and leftover platters of bagels from the morning staff meeting, your office probably stocks more snacks than a 7-Eleven. Free food is a temptation under the best of circumstances (and because you're only nibbling, it has no calories, right?). But it's especially dangerous when you're too busy for a proper lunch, encouraging you to graze throughout the day. Avoid temptation by bringing in healthy snacks—say, tamari-roasted almonds or a few squares of dark chocolate—that you actually prefer over the junk. Knowing that these are tucked away in a desk drawer will give you the strength to resist the disastrous jelly doughnuts. And if you know ahead of time that you're not going to be able to leave your desk for lunch, brown-bag it. With a healthy lunch within arm's reach, you can eat as soon as hunger hits, and you won't need to raid your colleague's candy jar.

CRAVING CRUSHER #8: MAINTAIN CONTROL ON THE HOME FRONT

If you work at home or spend your days inside on any given weekend, you may not have the office vending machine to tempt you. But there's just you and the fridge and nobody watching. Because you have no meetings or structured activities, you can check the mail, toss in a load of laundry, play with the dog, and—while you're at it—grab a snack (or two or four). "The more breaks there are in a person's schedule, the more opportunities there are to snack," says Brian Wansink, PhD, director of the Cornell University Food and Brand Lab and author of *Mindless Eating*. Keep a log of your daily activities, including every time you get up to eat. Chances are, once you see how often you're noshing, you'll be shamed into cutting back. But if you still feel you need to snack, eat at the kitchen table without doing anything else at the same time. Without the distraction of the computer, TV, or newspaper, you'll become much more aware of how often you're eating out of habit rather than hunger.

CRAVING CRUSHER #9: FOCUS ON YOUR FAMILY

It's the diet dilemma of nearly every parent. The kids badger you into buying them sugary snacks. Then you eat them. Before you know it, you're helping with homework and munching on a Pop-Tart. And who can resist those snack-size bags of cookies that no one put away? To stop yourself from downing the last of the iced animal crackers, ditch the foods designed for kids, says Barbara Rolls, PhD, author of *The Volumetrics Eating Plan*. "Family-friendly snacks should include low-calorie foods that are high in water or fiber and aren't loaded with fat," she says. Try no-fuss fruits like grapes or berries drizzled with all-natural vanilla yogurt—or fix yourself some air-popped popcorn (it counts as a whole grain) sprinkled with a dash of Parmesan. Not only will these keep you and your clan fuller, but they also take more time to eat and chew so you can't mindlessly suck them down.

CRAVING CRUSHER #10: MOVE ON AFTER A MISTAKE

Okay, you overindulged. What's the next step? "Forget about it," says James Newman, a nutritionist at Tahlequah City Hospital, in Tahlequah, Oklahoma, who followed his own advice to shed 300 pounds. (That's right, 300.) "One meal doesn't define your diet, so don't assume that you've failed or fallen off the wagon," he says. Institute a simple rule: Follow any "cheat" meal with at least five healthy meals and snacks. That ensures you'll be eating right more than 80 percent of the time.

Chapter 12

Become an Expert on Portion Control

LEARN HOW TO SERVE UP PROPER PORTIONS—
WITHOUT THE HELP OF MEASURING CUPS, BOWLS,
OR SCALES.

You snack on fruit, check calorie counts, and squeeze in a workout on most days of the week. So when you step on that scale and the needle stays put, you wonder what the heck you're doing wrong. Even with such healthy habits, one of the biggest contributors to keeping those pounds in place is portion size. Gauging reasonable portions is easier than you think—even without complicated measuring devices. Try these simple, slight adjustments in how you eat and think to help you reach your weight loss goal.

Handy Portion Control

Eating right-size portions pays off. Researchers at Penn State University conducted a study to found out how easily big servings lead to calorie overload.

On two consecutive days in each of 3 weeks, 32 subjects chose as many food portions as they wanted. But the serving sizes changed: Regular-size portions during week 1 became 50 percent larger the second week and doubled during week 3. Compared with the first week, total daily calories jumped by 504 for men during the second week and by an astonishing 812 in the last week.

Eyeballing portion sizes is tricky, but you have the best measurement tools at your fingertips. "Using your hand to gauge portions is a simple way to judge how much you should be eating at meals," says Alan Aragon, MS, *Men's Health* nutrition advisor.

YOUR FIST
Equivalent: 1 cup
Foods: Rice or pasta; fruit; veggies
Calories: 200; 75; 40

YOUR PALM
Equivalent: 3 ounces
Foods: Meat; fish; poultry
Calories: 160; 160; 160

ONE HANDFUL
Equivalent: 1 ounce
Foods: Nuts; raisins
Calories: 170; 85

TWO HANDFULS
Equivalent: 1 ounce
Foods: Chips; popcorn; pretzels
Calories: 150; 120; 100

THE LENGTH OF YOUR THUMB
Equivalent: 1 ounce
Foods: Peanut butter; hard cheese
Calories: 170; 100

THE TIP OF YOUR THUMB
Equivalent: 1 teaspoon
Foods: Cooking oil; mayonnaise, butter; sugar
Calories: 40; 35; 15

Table-Setting Tricks

Kids are told to clean their plates at every meal, so it's no wonder they grow into adults who feel compelled to finish whatever's in front of them. Breaking that habit can be next to impossible—but switching up your plates, silverware, and utensils can help you downsize your dinners without extra hassle.

PLATES
Keep them saucer-size (about 6 inches in diameter). Yes, it might feel like you should be having tea with Alice in Wonderland, but in a Cornell University study, people who ate hamburgers off of saucers believed they were eating an average of 18 percent more calories than they really were. People who ate off of 12-inch-diameter dishes, on the other hand, had no such delusion.

BOWLS
Research shows that the bigger the bowl, the more you'll stuff into it. So stick with small ones, or use a teacup or a mug for foods you tend to gulp down, like cereal and ice cream. Save the giant bowls for salad and broth-based soups so you can fill up on fewer calories.

GLASSES
According to a study in the *Journal of Consumer Research*, adults pour about 19 percent more liquid into short, wide glasses than they do into tall tumblers. This may be because our brains tend to focus more on an object's height than its width, so short glasses don't appear quite as full.

SPOONS
Stick with teaspoons, even to load up your plate. Another Cornell study found that people who used 3-ounce serving spoons shoveled out nearly 15 percent more food than those who scooped using 2-ounce spoons.

SERVING DISHES
In studies, people ate as much as 56 percent more when they served themselves from a 1-gallon bowl than they did from a half-gallon one. You can also hedge your bets by choosing ceramic over glass: One study in the *International Journal of Obesity* found that people ate 71 percent more out of transparent containers than they did out of dishes they couldn't see through.

WALLS
Paint them blue—it's thought to be a natural appetite suppressant. In a study published in *Contract* magazine, gala attendees who dined in a blue room ate 33 percent less than those who ate in a yellow or red room. "Blue lights make food look less appealing, while warmer colors, especially yellow, have the opposite effect," says Val Jones, MD, president and CEO of Better Health. "Fast-food restaurants have known and used this fact for decades, which is why almost all of them have yellowish interiors—they want you to eat more."

Cut Calories without Counting

Whether it's Spanish tapas, Chinese dim sum, or Greek mezes, small plates have become a staple in American restaurants. And no one's walking away hungry. Why? Because big flavors can be just as filling as big portions. "Most places specializing in small plates create taste-rich sensations in microsize bites," says Brian Wansink, PhD, director of the Cornell University Food and Brand Lab and author of *Mindless Eating*. "And we've found that much of a man's eating satisfaction is derived from the flavor intensity and visual impact of a meal, not necessarily the amount served."

So forget mounds of mediocre food. Instead, eat half as much and feel twice as full, by downsizing your dinner—and your gut—with these small but hugely satisfying dishes, courtesy of some of America's top small-plate chefs.

SPICY GARLIC SHRIMP

The chef: Seamus Mullen
The restaurant: Tertalia, New York City

- ¼ cup olive oil
- 1 Tbsp red-pepper flakes
- 4 cloves garlic, thinly sliced
- 16 oz shrimp, peeled and deveined
- Salt and freshly ground black pepper
- 1 Tbsp chopped parsley

1. Heat oil in small sauté pan until it starts to shimmer (just below smoking temperature). Add pepper flakes and then garlic.

2. As garlic begins to brown, season shrimp with salt and pepper, then place shrimp in pan, swirling it gently. Sauté over medium-high heat 1 minute, then stir in parsley. Sauté another minute, remove from heat, and serve.

MAKES 4 SERVINGS.

Per serving: 249 calories, 23 g protein, 3 g carbohydrates (<1 g fiber), 16 g fat (2 g sat), 315 mg sodium

MINI BLUE-CHEESE STEAKS ON SALAD

The chef: Chris Santos
The restaurant: The Stanton Social, New York City

- 1 lb hanger or skirt steak, cut into 4 equal portions
- Salt and freshly ground black pepper
- 1 tsp cooking oil
- 2 cups toasted large, cubed pieces of baguette, crusts removed
- 1 bag mixed salad greens
- 2 pt cherry tomatoes
- 1 red onion, sliced thin
- ¼ bunch chives, chopped
- 2 Tbsp red-wine vinegar
- ½ Tbsp tomato paste
- ⅛–¼ cup olive oil
- ½ cup Cabrales or other soft blue cheese

1. Preheat oven to 500°F.

2. Rub steaks liberally with salt and pepper. Heat cooking oil in ovenproof sauté pan until it begins to smoke lightly. Add steaks and cook 1 minute. Turn steaks, then place pan in oven for 5 minutes. Remove steaks from pan and allow to rest.

3. In large bowl, toss baguette cubes, salad greens, cherry tomatoes, onion, and chives. In small bowl, mix together vinegar, tomato paste, and olive oil. Toss dressing with salad and divide among 4 plates. Slice steaks thinly and place on top of salad. Garnish with cheese.

MAKES 4 SERVINGS.

Per serving: 488 calories, 38 g protein, 22 g carbohydrates (5 g fiber), 28 g fat (10 g sat), 513 mg sodium

VIETNAMESE CHICKEN SKEWERS

The chef: Michael "Bao" Huynh
The restaurant: Mai House, New York City

- 2 cloves garlic, minced
- 1 small red onion, minced
- 1 stalk lemongrass, inner leaves only, minced
- 1 Tbsp fresh ginger, peeled and minced
- 2 jalapeño chile peppers, split, seeds removed (wear plastic gloves when handling)
- 1 Tbsp cilantro, chopped
- 1 cup fish sauce
- 2 Tbsp sugar
- Juice of 1 lime
- 2 boneless, skinless chicken breasts, cut into 1" cubes

1. In saucepan, combine garlic, onion, lemongrass, ginger, chile peppers, cilantro, fish sauce, sugar, and lime juice. Slowly bring to a boil over medium heat, then remove from stove and cool.

2. Toss chicken into mixture and let marinate 1 to 2 hours. Meanwhile, soak wooden skewers in cold water 30 minutes.

3. Skewer chicken cubes and grill until firm and lightly charred, 3 to 4 minutes per side.

MAKES 4 SERVINGS.

Per serving: 112 calories, 16 g protein, 11 g carbohydrates (<1 g fiber), less than 1 g fat (<1 g sat), 598 mg sodium

CHICKPEAS WITH CHORIZO

The chef: Ken Oringer
The restaurant: Toro, Boston

- ½ large onion, chopped
- 5 cloves garlic, minced
- 1 bay leaf
- ¼ cup extra-virgin olive oil
- 2 oz Serrano ham or prosciutto, chopped
- 4 oz ready-to-eat Spanish chorizo, sliced in ¼" rounds
- 3 Tbsp tomato paste
- ¼ cup dry white wine
- 1 cup chopped frozen spinach
- 1 cup canned chickpeas
- Salt and freshly ground black pepper
- 2 hard-boiled eggs, quartered

1. In large skillet, sauté onion, garlic, and bay leaf in oil over medium heat 10 minutes. Add ham and chorizo, and cook 5 minutes. Stir in tomato paste and wine and cook 10 minutes.

2. Once wine has evaporated, add spinach and chickpeas and their liquid. Simmer 10 minutes. Season to taste with salt and pepper, and turn off heat.

3. Remove bay leaf. Serve with eggs and a drizzle of olive oil.

MAKES 4 SERVINGS.

Per serving: 438 calories, 20 g protein, 22 g carbohydrates (5 g fiber), 29 g fat (7 g sat), 1,108 mg sodium

BRAISED SALMON WITH SOY AND GINGER

The chef: Susanna Foo
The restaurant: Susanna Foo Chinese Cuisine, Philadelphia

- 16 oz salmon fillet
- 2 Tbsp extra-virgin olive oil
- 1 Tbsp minced ginger
- ¼ cup mirin
- 2 Tbsp soy sauce
- 2 Tbsp vodka
- 1 Tbsp butter
- 2 scallions (white parts only), chopped
- 3–4 sprigs cilantro

1. Cut salmon into 1" squares.

2. Heat oil in 12" nonstick pan over medium-high heat and add salmon cubes and ginger. Sear together about 1 minute, then pour mirin, soy sauce, and vodka over salmon.

3. Reduce heat to medium and cook until fish turns pale, about 3 minutes. Add butter and turn off heat.

4. Spoon salmon onto serving plate and top with scallions and cilantro.

MAKES 4 SERVINGS.

Per serving: 359 calories, 24 g protein, 6 g carbohydrates (1 g fiber), 22 g fat (5 g sat), 668 mg sodium

Completing the Meal

For a full meal, add a salad and a small vegetable plate to your main entrée. Each option has been infused with the biggest flavors from around the globe. (Each recipe makes 4 servings.)

SALADS

Start with 4 cups loosely packed mixed greens.

For an American flavor, add:
1 ripe pear, peeled and sliced
2 Tbsp crumbled blue cheese
2 Tbsp toasted walnuts

TOSS WITH:
1 Tbsp balsamic vinegar
2 Tbsp olive oil
Pinch of salt and pepper

For an Asian flavor, add:
1 orange, peeled and sectioned
1 carrot, grated
2 scallions, chopped

TOSS WITH:
1 Tbsp rice vinegar
1 Tbsp peanut oil
2 tsp soy sauce
1 tsp minced ginger

For a Mediterranean flavor, add:
¼ cup roasted red bell peppers
½ cup marinated artichoke hearts, quartered
2 Tbsp toasted almonds

TOSS WITH:
1 Tbsp red or white wine vinegar
2 Tbsp olive oil
1 Tbsp Dijon mustard

VEGETABLES

Start with a 2-pound mix of any of the following vegetables, cut into similar-size pieces: asparagus, zucchini, carrots, onions, cherry tomatoes. Toss with one of the options below and brown in a 400°F oven for 15 minutes.

For an American flavor, add:
2 Tbsp olive oil
2 cloves garlic, roughly chopped
1 Tbsp chopped fresh thyme or 1 tsp dried

For an Asian flavor, add:
2 cloves garlic, chopped
1 Tbsp minced ginger
1 Tbsp low-sodium soy sauce
2 tsp sesame seeds

For a Mediterranean flavor, add:
2 Tbsp pesto, fresh or bottled
Squeeze of lemon

Why Some Foods Make You Do Bad Things

Chapter 13

JUST AS SOME DRUGS LEAD THE WAY TO HARDER ONES, SOME EATS CAN OPEN THE GATES TO A FLOOD OF UNHEALTHY CHOICES

In a perfect world, all you'd need to do to maintain a high standard of fitness is exercise and watch what you eat. Sounds simple, right? Or not. What if other forces were at work, trying to put pounds on your frame until you join the 58 percent of the world predicted to be overweight or obese by 2030? Many scientists now believe that it's not your stomach you should worry about—it's your brain. In the past few years, scientists have published nearly 40 studies on whether the temptation of food can veer into actual addiction.

Guess what? It's very possible, says Gary Wenk, PhD, author of *Your Brain on Food*. "Some foods are like gateway drugs," he says. "From your brain's viewpoint, there is no difference." These so-called gateway foods make you feel out of control, maybe even physically unable to stop reaching for more, in part because of their addictive effect on your mind and body, according to research. But rehab is probably easier than you think.

HOW WE BECAME JUNK FOOD JUNKIES

It may seem silly to think about being addicted to food, something we'd die without, but most of us eat for a lot more than just survival. Merely looking at or thinking about a food you love activates the reward portion of your brain, the nucleus accumbens—the same area stimulated by drugs and alcohol. This triggers the release of dopamine, a feel-good chemical that enhances your awareness of that food (so forget ignoring it!).

And once you've taken that first bite, watch out. Tasting food engages all of your senses. Your nervous system responds by secreting insulin (which drops blood glucose) and relaxing your stomach muscles, which makes you feel like you need to eat more to be satisfied, says Susan Roberts, PhD, a professor of nutrition at Tufts University and coauthor of The "I" Diet.

Still skeptical that the addiction concept is nothing more than an overeater's cop-out? Experts aren't. Researchers are currently debating whether food addiction should be included in the Diagnostic and Statistical Manual of Mental Disorders, the go-to reference for members of the American Psychiatric Association.

Scientists speculate that only some people are *truly* addicted to food. However, a far greater number of us may be vulnerable to the ways food can trick the brain into making us eat more than we want to, says Joseph Frascella, PhD, director of the National Institute on Drug Abuse's Division of Clinical Neuroscience and Behavioral Research. And with the current profusion of food-themed TV shows and an escalating fast-food arms race, it's becoming more and more difficult for our brains to resist cues to overeat.

FOOD, ON THE BRAIN

Emerging science shows that the minds of overeaters may look like those of drug addicts. The proof is in neuroimaging scans, says Gene-Jack Wang, MD, of the Brookhaven National Laboratory. When Wang's team scanned the brains of obese overeaters and meth addicts, they found that the people in both groups had fewer dopamine receptors available in their brains than healthy individuals. What's the big deal? Just as meth users need more and more of the drug to get high, obese overeaters may need more and more food to produce the same intensity of dopamine "high"—a cycle that can reinforce addictive behavior, according to Wang.

THE EVOLUTION CONNECTION

When the call for more is especially powerful, there's a reason it happens almost exclusively with fatty and sugary foods and not, say, lettuce. We exist on the planet because of fat and sugar, those valued treasures in the evolutionary struggle. Fat was survival fuel for cavemen, since it contains more calories per gram than either protein or carbs. And back in the day, sugar carbohydrates helped keep us alert to potential dangers. Today we and our deskbound brethren burn far fewer calories, yet we maintain that Cro-Magnon connection to the pleasures that high-fat, high-sugar foods bring to our brains, says Nicole M. Avena, PhD, a food addiction researcher and assistant professor of psychiatry at the University of Florida. So the food we're wired to desire isn't always the food we need.

A 2010 Scripps Research Institute study found that when rats were presented with a "cafeteria-style" diet of large amounts of high-fat food, they ate almost twice as many calories as rats given only standard laboratory chow. It's another piece of evidence that fatty, sugary foods may be more habit-forming than other foods, Avena says. Yes, humans are more evolved than rats, but who hasn't had a similar experience at an unlimited pizza-and-dessert buffet?

And when you give in to one of these primal desires, here's what happens: The saturated fats in foods like bacon and cheese impair your brain's normal ability to regulate appetite and cravings, so you don't realize you're full until you're completely stuffed, says Kelly McGonigal, PhD, a health psychologist at Stanford University and author of *The Willpower Instinct*. What's more, that effect on your appetite can last for up to 3 days, the length of time it takes to flush those fats from your system. So one unhealthy indulgence can end up triggering a major relapse.

Add sugar to the fatty food—ice cream, cake, doughnuts—and you have a double whammy. High-sugar foods increase your levels of ghrelin, a hormone that stimulates appetite and increases cravings. "So you may tell yourself, 'Just one bite,' but find yourself wanting more and more, the more you eat," says McGonigal.

Sugar also has been shown to enhance memory storage, which may explain why you want it in the first place—and so much of it on special social occasions. As a result, your brain has evolved a system of rewards that gives you a real high when you eat sugar. "The brain responds to both sugar and fat by releasing endorphins," says Wenk. Chemically, those feel-good compounds are similar to morphine and can have a biological impact similar to a shot of heroin, including causing you to jones for another fix when the initial euphoria begins to fade.

HOW YOU CAN REGAIN CONTROL

Avoiding the call of these dangerous gateway foods entirely is tough, given that they can become especially powerful when you're stressed or even just thinking about eating. But there's plenty you can do to avoid skidding down the slippery slope toward total diet disaster.

Interrupt yourself. If you're three bites into a pint of fudge ripple when you feel a pang of regret, try switching to a healthier snack. Once your senses have been engaged, your body is going to demand more food, but you can still decide what to give it. Sorbet or a piece of fruit can freshen up your palate, which can help put the brakes on thinking about the stuff you want most.

Hide your triggers. You don't need psychotherapy to stop emotional eating. You just need to reverse the reward patterns. That means hitting the pause button, says Gary Foster, PhD, director of Temple University's Center for Obesity Research and Education, who has explored the topic of emotional eating. Recognize triggers for what they are, ride out the emotions, and then praise yourself for doing so, Foster says. "It's difficult at first, but each time you reinforce the positive behavior, you drive emotional eating into extinction."

Stow your snacks. Proximity to food influences how much of it you eat, says James Painter, PhD, RD, a professor at Eastern Illinois University who studies behavioral eating. Try keeping healthy foods right where you can see them and stash unhealthy ones in a hard-to-reach drawer—or just don't keep them around at all.

Retrain your brain. "People eat for any number of reasons—they're happy, sad, stressed, bored, anxious. When the trigger occurs, like Pavlov's dog you start salivating," says Foster. The more often you use a fridge raid as a stress buster, the more your brain will come to expect that behavior. Repeating this cycle can reinforce the habit, says Foster. Instead, think of your growing belly, not your growling stomach. Mindless eating is just that—your brain shuts down as your gullet opens up. "We've found that most people focus only on the short-term rewards when it comes to foods," says Ashley Gearhardt, lead author of a Yale University study on food addiction. "But what we've found is that if you can train yourself to focus on the long-term consequences—the weight gain, the sickness—then you'll activate your prefrontal cortex, or the 'brakes' in your brain that may prevent you from overeating."

Escape the food traps. It's hard to resist the call of the 24-hour meal. "Our modern eating environment isn't like it was 10,000 years ago. Cheap, high-calorie foods are available on every corner," says Frascella. Fast-food joints pump out aromas to entice you, and "food porn" TV shows are spliced with ads for double-stuffed pizzas and towering burgers. "For people who have a tendency to overeat, these stimulating cues trigger unhealthy food behaviors," says Foster. Some tips for limiting your exposure to triggers: Ask your server for the check before the dessert menu reaches the table. Change the channel if commercials start splashing unhealthy foods across the screen. Think twice about that pizza buffet. And if there's a burger chain gassing the road with char-broiled aromas on your way to the salad place, take a detour. "The less you engage with these cues, the easier it will be to eventually stop the behavior," Foster says.

THE FOOD PORN PROBLEM

A picture is worth a thousand... calories? New research proves that the growing obsession with images of sinfully seductive dishes can make us feel hungrier and cause us to overeat. Here's how to control an obscene appetite.

"Like the sexual kind, food porn allows us to lust after taboo things," says psychologist Susan Albers, PsyD, author of *Eating Mindfully*. "And now it's on our terms: We can search for exactly what turns us on, enlarge the images, and linger for as long as we want."

Just a few short years ago, food sites were predominantly recipe driven. Now, a growing number shamelessly flaunt the fact that few people visit for the articles. FoodPornDaily.com (tagline: Click, drool, repeat) stripped away recipes altogether in favor of luscious panned-in shots. Food images are also the fastest-growing category on Pinterest. If you don't find anything that turns you on there, you can log on to Flickr's Food Porn Group. Boasting nearly 600,000 images, it's one of the most active categories on the photo-sharing site.

Problem is, that Flickr group isn't the only thing that's growing. Photos seem harmless, but they provoke a real emotional and physical hunger response that can be tough to control, says neuroscientist Laura Martin, PhD, an assistant professor at the University of Kansas Medical Center who studies how we respond to food. And straight out of the insult-meets-injury department: Those who are overweight appear to be more sensitive to the effect of viewing irresistible food. Does that mean you can never ogle your cake without eating it too? Not necessarily. There are savvy ways to curb your appetite—online and in real life.

Eating with Your Eyes

The best food porn plays on the fact that the more indulgent a photo appears, the more likely it will trigger our instinct to eat. "Food porn relies on a phenomenon called supernormal stimuli, which exaggerates qualities we're already hardwired to love," says Deirdre Barrett, PhD, an evolutionary psychologist at Harvard Medical School's Behavioral Medicine Program and author of *Waistland: The (R)Evolutionary Science behind Our Weight and Fitness Crisis*. Usually, that translates to visual cues that a food is high in calories—things like pooling oils and the sheen of sugar—which were coveted assets back in hunter-gatherer days, when calories (particularly the gooey, fatty ones) were harder to come by, says Barrett. That might explain why, according to a study from 360i, a marketing firm that studies online trends, pictures of desserts are the most likely to be shared online. Cheesy, oozy comfort foods also get favorited more frequently on sites like FoodGawker.com.

But it rarely ends there. A study in the journal *Obesity* found that simply seeing food increases levels of the hunger hormone ghrelin, even after eating a regular meal. And maybe worst of all, the part of your brain that governs self-control fails to kick in with food porn the way it does with actual food.

Dieters, unsurprisingly, are among the most susceptible to this seduction. A study published in the journal *Appetite* found that nondieters ate the same amount of candy whether food was featured in the television programming they were viewing or not; dieters consumed 60 more calories when they came across a food image.

"Food was never meant to be experienced from just a visual perspective," says Amy Sousa, PhD, an anthropologist at the Hartman Group, a research consulting firm that tracks food culture. "When we see food, we need to fill in the blanks of what it will taste like. Merely looking makes for an unsatisfying experience."

The Food Porn Diet

Cutting back doesn't mean blocking every friend who Instagrams an amazing meal. But you can start by seeking out healthier foods in your online searches. After all, if photos can make you crave nachos and chicken wings, a good enough shot might turn you on to Brussels sprouts (that's part of the point of us including in this book a section of photos based on healthy recipes).

The Munchie Shot

What makes some food photos particularly drool-inducing? Barrett, who also wrote *Supernormal Stimuli*, deconstructs the gut-tricking details in one of the most-liked savory shots on FoodPornDaily.com.

- **It's larger than life.** This extreme close-up (you can practically see the holes in the bread crumbs!) is no accident. Zooming in on food makes you feel as though you're having an intimate experience with it. The result: You end up eating more.
- **Every calorie counts.** Even if the portion itself isn't huge, showing a hyperconcentration of salt, fat, and refined carbs in every bite makes you want to dig in.
- **Oooh, shiny!** Your body craves fat, so you seek out the slickness of oils and refractive shine—found, in this case, cradling the pasta in an orgy of butter, three different cheeses, and bacon grease.
- **Imaginary mouthfeel.** Blistering at the dome suggests texture. Can't you just imagine piercing through the crust?

And although food porn temporarily disables your willpower, certain activities have been shown to weaken your brain's response to food. A study in the *Journal of Applied Physiology* found that after men biked for an hour, their brain's food-reward response barely registered. Researchers believe the vigorous activity dampened the desire to seek out food (and, they theorize, regular intense exercise could keep this effect intact long-term).

On the flip side, not getting enough sleep leaves you wide open to food porn's seduction. A study in the *Journal of Clinical Endocrinology & Metabolism* showed the brain's hunger- and appetite-regulating center is more likely to be stimulated by images of food when you're sleep deprived. Yet another reason to get those 8 hours of shut-eye—or, at the very least, to not prowl the Internet when you don't.

But the most effective technique is probably the same whether you're using it in the bedroom or the kitchen: Turn your online fantasies into inspiration to get busy at home. Research shows that we consume fewer calories when we cook, because we control portions and ingredients. Also, a growing number of sites are serving up food porn with nutritional information (like Edamam.com) or ones like Foodily.com that allow you to search for a dish without certain ingredients (say, carrot cake without raisins). And the benefits go beyond the scale. "Consumers who cook tend to have a healthier relationship with food and are more likely to be satisfied by what they eat," says Sousa. "They may peruse these images online, but they are less inclined to eat mindlessly as a result of it, because they're actually experiencing all the sensual pleasure that comes with food."

Chapter 14

A Perfect Day of Eating

OPTIMIZE YOUR FAT-BURNING POTENTIAL WITH THESE SUGGESTIONS, WHICH WILL KEEP YOU GOING STRONG FROM DAWN 'TIL DUSK.

You're probably thinking, *If I want to slash fat and drop pounds, shouldn't I eat less food and spend more time in the gym, not the other way around?* But you can accomplish both of these goals in your own kitchen simply by choosing foods that increase calorie burn and fuel muscle building—like the ones in this chapter.

This plan isn't about depriving yourself of your favorite foods or spending hours in the gym. Instead it's about finding the right (and did we mention delicious?) foods to eat and learning the best times to eat them so you'll not only see the results you're looking for, but also do it without going hungry.

7:00 A.M. BREAKFAST

After a full 7 or 8 hours without food, your body craves a healthy dose of high-quality protein. Start your day right with at least 30 grams, along with plenty of slow-digesting carbs. Because your carbohydrate stores are low after an overnight fast, there's no better time to fill your tank. Just make sure your carbs come primarily from fruit and 100 percent whole-grain sources.

PROTEIN-PACKED OATMEAL

Prepare:

- 1 package instant oatmeal with flax

Mix in:

- 1 scoop strawberry whey protein powder (choose a product that's 100 percent whey protein)
- 3 Tbsp 1% milk

Have on the side:

- 1 medium pear
- 1 cup green tea or coffee

MAKES 1 SERVING.

Per serving: 472 calories, 32 g protein, 76 g carbohydrates (9 g fiber), 8 g fat (1 g sat)

OPTION 2: SPICY OMELET

Make with:

- 1 cup egg substitute
- 1 medium egg
- ½ cup fresh spinach
- 2 mushrooms, sliced
- 2 Tbsp shredded light Cheddar cheese
- ½ cup salsa

Have on the side:

- 1 slice 100% whole-wheat bread with 1 Tbsp low-sugar jelly
- 1 cup vegetable juice

MAKES 1 SERVING.

Per serving: 421 calories, 37 g protein, 40 g carbohydrates (5 g fiber), 11 g fat (4 g sat)

OPTION 3: STRAWBERRY-AND-BANANA WORKOUT SHAKE

If you work out first thing in the morning, choose this option, drinking half of the shake right before your session and half immediately afterward.

Blend together:

- 2 scoops vanilla whey protein powder
- 6 oz fat-free strawberry yogurt
- 8 frozen strawberries
- 1 large banana
- Plenty of ice

MAKES 1 SERVING.

Per serving: 491 calories, 52 g protein, 61 g carbohydrates (5 g fiber), 6 g fat (1 g sat)

10:00 A.M. MIDMORNING SNACK

Eating protein- and fiber-rich meals or snacks every 2 to 3 hours helps keep your blood-sugar levels normal. This not only improves your body's ability to burn fat, but also reduces risk factors for heart disease by lowering cholesterol and triglycerides. Frequent eating also prevents afternoon binges on useless calories, like the leftover Krispy Kremes from your morning staff meeting.

GRAPES, CHEESE, AND HAM

Eat together:

- 1½ cups seedless grapes
- 2 slices fat-free American cheese singles
- 4 oz low-sodium ham slices

MAKES 1 SERVING.

Per serving: 352 calories, 28 g protein, 51 g carbohydrates (2 g fiber), 4 g fat (1 g sat)

OPTION 2: MEXI-TUNA

Mix together:

- 1 can or packet (3 oz) light tuna in water
- ¾ cup canned black beans
- ½ cup salsa
- ½ cup canned green beans

MAKES 1 SERVING.

Per serving: 335 calories, 45 g protein, 41 g carbohydrates, 15 g fiber, 1 g fat (0 g sat)

OPTION 3: CHILI

Microwave:

- ½ can reduced-sodium chili with beans

MAKES 1 SERVING.

Per serving: 340 calories, 18 g protein, 30 g carbohydrates (9 g fiber), 17 g fat (7 g sat)

NOON LUNCH

These lunches not only are high in protein and healthy fat, but also score low on the glycemic index. So, like the midmorning snack, they contain carbohydrates that have little impact on your blood sugar. This keeps your fat-burning furnace stoked and helps prevent the dreaded midday lull.

TUNA SANDWICH

Make with:

- 2 slices 100% whole-wheat bread
- 1 can or packet (3 oz) light tuna in water
- 1 Tbsp reduced-fat mayonnaise
- 1 Tbsp mustard
- 1 lettuce leaf
- 2 slices tomato
- 1 tsp chopped onion
- 1 Tbsp chopped celery

Have on the side:

- 1 oz mixed nuts

MAKES 1 SERVING.

Per serving: 506 calories, 45 g protein, 41 g carbohydrates (7 g fiber), 17 g fat (2 g sat)

OPTION 2: CHEF'S SALAD

Combine:

- 2 cups chopped romaine lettuce
- 1 large hard-boiled egg
- 2 oz turkey breast
- 2 oz ham
- 1 oz sliced light Cheddar cheese
- 1 oz sliced light American cheese
- 6 cherry tomatoes
- ½ oz sliced almonds
- 2 Tbsp reduced-fat ranch dressing (Or, for a different flavor, try dressing your salad with olive oil and vinegar, which has zero gram of sugar.)

MAKES 1 SERVING.

Per serving: 493 calories, 54 g protein, 20 g carbohydrates (4 g fiber), 22 g fat (6 g sat)

3:00 P.M. MIDAFTERNOON SNACK

As the day goes on, your ability to utilize carbohydrates for energy decreases, boosting the likelihood that they'll be stored as fat. So late afternoon is a good time to start downsizing your carb intake and increasing the amount of healthy fat you consume. This also leads to fewer total carbohydrates in your daily diet, which speeds fat loss, according to multiple studies over the past 5 years.

CHEESE STICKS AND NUTS

- 2 sticks light string cheese
- 1 oz walnuts

MAKES 1 SERVING.

Per serving: 307 calories, 24 g protein, 5 g carbohydrates (2 g fiber), 24 g fat (6 g sat)

OPTION 2: BEEF JERKY AND CELERY WITH PEANUT BUTTER

- 2 oz beef jerky
- 1 celery stalk
- 1 Tbsp natural creamy peanut butter

MAKES 1 SERVING.

Per serving: 277 calories, 33 g protein, 14 g carbohydrates (3 g fiber), 10 g fat (2 g sat)

OPTION 3: LOW-CARB PROTEIN BAR

Look for one that contains fewer than 30 g carbohydrates and 20 g or more protein.

6:00 P.M. DINNER

Your sense of satiety, or feeling of fullness, is less sensitive in the evening than in the morning, which may help explain why you crave foods like ice cream at night. It's also another reason it makes sense to eat a dinner that's high in protein and healthy fat, both of which keep you full longer than carbohydrates do.

PAN-FRIED SALMON WITH BROCCOLI AND BEANS

Pan-fry:

- 1 salmon fillet (5½ oz) in 2 Tbsp olive oil, preheated in a nonstick skillet, over medium-high heat for 4 minutes. Turn and fry for another 5 minutes. Season with lemon juice and dill.

Have on the side:

- 2 cups steamed broccoli (measured raw)
- ½ can dark-red kidney beans (wash thoroughly, then serve without cooking)

MAKES 1 SERVING.

Per serving: 516 calories, 56 g protein, 36 g carbohydrates (18 g fiber), 19 g fat (3 g sat)

OPTION 2: MEAT LOAF WITH GREEN BEANS

Combine:

- 1 lb extra-lean ground beef
- ½ cup oats
- ½ cup organic ketchup
- 1 large egg
- ½ tsp salt
- ½ tsp freshly ground black pepper
- 2 Tbsp dried onion flakes
- 1 tsp dried mustard
- 1 tsp Worcestershire sauce

In a baking pan, mix and form the ingredients into a loaf with your hands, then place into a preheated 350°F oven. Cook for 15 to 20 minutes.

MAKES 2 SERVINGS.

Have on the side:

- 1 cup cooked green beans

MAKES 1 SERVING.

Per serving: 530 calories, 52 g protein, 28 g carbohydrates (5 g fiber), 20 g fat (9 g sat)

9:00 P.M. EVENING SNACK

Slow-absorbing proteins such as casein—the type of protein found in dairy products—deliver a steady supply of amino acids to muscle cells while you sleep, protecting your hard-earned muscle.

PROTEIN PUDDING

Mix together, then chill for 1 hour:

- 1 scoop chocolate whey protein powder
- 6 oz 1% milk
- 1 tsp sugar-free pudding mix

MAKES 1 SERVING.

Per serving: 239 calories, 33 g protein, 17 g carbohydrates (1 g fiber), 4 g fat (1 g sat)

OPTION 2: COTTAGE CHEESE AND STRAWBERRIES

Mix together:

- 1 cup 2% cottage cheese
- ¾ cup sliced strawberries

MAKES 1 SERVING.

Per serving: 198 calories, 29 g protein, 14 g carbohydrates (3 g fiber), 3 g fat (0.5 g sat)

Fuel Your Workout

Part Four

Food can help ensure that you perform at the peak of your abilities. It's not just about, "Oh, I had an epic workout today, felt great, must be the food." Of course you want to feel great and fully fueled while you work out. You'll find plenty of info on that very thing in this section. But what about eating before your workout? Or after? What should you eat depending on your fitness goal? Should a guy training for a triathlon eat the same as a guy trying to bulk up with muscle? You need to personalize your eating to fit your life. All the answers are in here.

Snack Smart Before You Start

TO GET THE MOST BANG FOR YOUR WORKOUT BUCK, FIND OUT HOW MUCH YOU NEED TO EAT TO STAY FUELED WITHOUT BEING WEIGHED DOWN.

Many people think snacks mean junk—and they probably do if they come from a cookie jar or candy bowl. But snacking is a valid nutrition strategy, especially if you're active. It helps you fuel up for workouts, get a variety of nutrients, and spread calories evenly throughout the day. Snacks also sustain blood-sugar levels (which reduces cravings) and keep your metabolism high, warding off weight gain. "Without a snack to take the edge off, people eat faster, eat more, and choose higher-calorie foods because they're overly hungry," says Suzanne Farrell, RD, a former spokesperson for the American Dietetic Association.

The key is to keep portions small—around 200 to 300 calories—and choose healthy, nutrient-dense foods, says Kelli Montgomery, a coach and nutrition consultant in Connecticut. By going for fruits, vegetables, whole grains, and healthy fats, you can get nutrients you may have missed at meals. But it's important to know what to choose and when, since some foods offer the most benefit at particular times. Here's how to snack smart to get the fuel your body needs.

PREWORKOUT SNACK

If you're like many people, your workout often takes place hours after your last meal. Morning exercisers haven't eaten since last night's dinner, and late-afternoon sweat sessions take place long after lunch. To curb preworkout hunger, 30 to 60 minutes before hitting the gym, eat high-carb, low-fiber foods that are easy to digest and provide fast energy. You can eat some protein and fat to steady your blood sugar during a long workout, but include them sparingly, says Montgomery: Fats and protein break down slowly and, like fiber, can lead to an upset stomach.

Pick This
Piece of fruit and cottage cheese. Other options: fig cookies; half a bagel with nut butter and jam; an energy bar; sports drink.

POSTWORKOUT SNACK

Even if you eat a meal before exercising, you may be hungry afterward—especially if you trained long and hard and your muscles need fuel. Choose a more substantial snack combining a 4:1 ratio of carbs to protein. The mix speeds muscle recovery, especially if eaten right away since foods consumed within 30 minutes of your workout provide the maximum recovery benefit. Not hungry? "It's okay to skip a snack after shorter, easier runs," says Montgomery. If a tough workout leaves you feeling queasy, try chocolate milk—it provides that 4:1 ratio and helps you rehydrate but won't strain your stomach.

Pick This
Save half of your turkey sandwich at lunch for later as a snack with juice. Or, try a fruit-and-yogurt smoothie.

AFTERNOON SNACK

Lunch at 1 p.m. and dinner at 7 p.m. means 6 hours without food. "That's longer than people should go," says Farrell, who suggests eating every 4 hours. To stave off hunger without tons of calories, go for fiber and protein—both are slowly digested and feel satisfying. Work in an extra serving of veggies, which are less appealing before or after a workout or run because of their fiber content. Crave pretzels or carb-rich snacks? Measure out a portion. A 2008 study found that people who eat 100-calorie snack packages consume about 120 fewer calories a day than those who snack from a regular-size bag.

Pick This
A cup of vegetable soup; salad with egg whites; yogurt with berries and almonds.

EVENING SNACK

Sometimes the urge to snack after dinner isn't hunger but a craving for comfort food. "Evening is a big time for emotional eating, especially after a stressful day," says Farrell. Try to avoid overdoing sugary foods, which can cause a spike in blood sugar and interfere with sleep. Go for protein and high-fiber carbs (which top off energy stores while you sleep), or snack on high-fiber cereal. One study found that people who eat a serving of cereal 90 minutes after dinner consume fewer calories daily than those who don't have cereal.

Pick This
Need a sweet? Try a portion-controlled dessert like a frozen yogurt pop.

ANYTIME OPTIONS

Popcorn. High in fiber and low in calories, popcorn is also a heart-healthy food. In a study presented at the 2009 American Chemical Society national meeting, University of Scranton researchers tested a wide range of whole grains for polyphenol count. Polyphenols are antioxidant plant chemicals that may protect your body from cell and tissue damage linked to heart disease and certain cancers. Researchers found that among snack foods, popcorn has the highest polyphenol level.

Dark chocolate. Juggling family, work, and training is challenging, and too much stress may raise your heart disease risk. According to a study, dark chocolate may help. Researchers gave participants 1.4 ounces of dark chocolate (the size of a matchbook) daily for 2 weeks. The chocolate reduced stress-hormone levels in anxious participants. There's also evidence that dark chocolate may help lower blood pressure—another key to reducing heart disease risk, says sports nutritionist Deborah Shulman, PhD. But keep an eye on calories. "It's like red wine," says Pamela M. Nisevich Bede, MS, RD, a nutrition consultant for Swim, Bike, Run, Eat!. "It can provide health benefits but should be consumed in moderation."

Roasted peanuts. A study published in the journal *Food Chemistry* discovered that the longer peanuts are roasted, the higher their levels of antioxidants. The extra-long roasting preserves more manganese and vitamin E (which helps protect your bones and red blood cells, respectively) than lightly roasted or even raw nuts. Peanuts are rich in protein, fiber, and healthy unsaturated fats—three nutrients that help keep you feeling full. Store small bags of peanuts in your desk drawer, or make your own trail mix with peanuts, dried fruits, cereal, and pretzels, says Nisevich Bede.

Cereal and milk. Turns out the breakfast of champions can help speed recovery after a tough workout. In a study published in 2009 in the *Journal of the International Society of Sports Nutrition*, cyclists rode for 2 hours and then ate whole-grain cereal with fat-free milk or drank a carbohydrate sports drink. Several days later they repeated the test. Researchers found the pantry staple replenishes energy stores equally as well as sports drinks. Milk also provides quality protein, which is ideal for muscle recovery, says Shulman—making this less-expensive (and less-processed) option a smart snack.

Chapter 16

Eat for Peak Performance

THE FOODS IN THIS CHAPTER WILL HELP YOU
GO LONGER, HARDER, AND FARTHER.

To get the most from your workouts, you have to give your body the right fuel. That means eating nutritious meals filled with plenty of lean protein, fiber, and healthy fats. And good news: The same foods that pump up your energy can help shrink your waistline, and often come hand-in-hand with other body-boosting benefits, like immune-system-supporting vitamin C. To power your next workout—and your overall health—whip up these tasty recipes.

Apple-Sausage Sauté

BODY BENEFIT: Apples pack a wallop of vitamin C and cancer-fighting antioxidants, as well as 18 percent of your daily fiber requirement—more than a bowl of bran cereal—for less than 100 calories each.

- 4 tsp olive oil
- 1 lb cooked chicken or pork sausages, cut into ½" diagonal slices
- 4 medium tart apples (such as Granny Smith or Idared), peeled, quartered, and cut into ½" wedges
- ¼ tsp freshly ground black pepper
- ¼ tsp dried thyme
- 2 Tbsp maple syrup

1. Heat 2 tsp of the oil in large nonstick skillet over medium heat. Add sausages and cook, turning often, until lightly browned, about 6 minutes. Remove from skillet.

2. Add remaining 2 tsp oil to skillet. Add apples, pepper, and thyme and drizzle with syrup. Cook, tossing often, until tender, 12 to 14 minutes.

3. Return sausages to skillet and toss with apples to heat through.

MAKES 4 SERVINGS.

Per serving:
375 calories, 19 g protein,
45 g carbohydrates (4 g fiber),
14 g fat (3 g sat), 643 mg sodium

Cran-Almond Muffins

BODY BENEFIT: Cranberries help maintain urinary tract health and are a good source of vitamin C and fiber.

- 1 cup all-purpose flour
- ½ cup whole-wheat flour
- ¾ cup plus 2 tsp sugar
- 1½ tsp baking powder
- ¼ tsp salt
- 1 large egg
- ½ cup 1% milk
- 4 Tbsp butter, melted
- 1 tsp almond extract
- 1⅔ cups whole cranberries
- 1 Tbsp butter, cut in 12 cubes
- ¼ tsp ground cinnamon
- ½ cup sliced almonds (optional)

1. Heat oven to 375°F. Line muffin pan with 12 baking cups.

2. In large bowl, mix together flours, ¾ cup sugar, baking powder, and salt.

3. In medium bowl, whisk together egg, milk, melted butter, and almond extract. Fold into flour mixture. Stir in cranberries.

4. Pour batter into baking cups. Top each with butter cube. Sprinkle the muffins with 2 tsp sugar, cinnamon, and almonds (if using). Bake until wooden pick comes out clean, about 22 minutes.

MAKES 12 SERVINGS.

Per serving:
169 calories, 3 g protein,
27 g carbohydrates (2 g fiber),
6 g fat (3 g sat), 143 mg sodium

Linguine with Walnut-Tomato Pesto

BODY BENEFIT: Walnuts score highest of all nuts in the omega-3s that protect against heart disease. And their stores of fiber and unsaturated fat can help you lower "bad" LDL cholesterol naturally.

- 1 cup fresh basil leaves
- ¼ cup walnut pieces
- 2 cloves garlic
- 6 oil-packed sun-dried tomatoes
- 2 Tbsp grated Parmesan cheese
- ½ tsp salt
- ¼ tsp red-pepper flakes
- 6 Tbsp olive oil
- 12 oz linguine

1. In food processor, combine basil, walnuts, and garlic and chop. Add tomatoes, cheese, salt, and pepper flakes. Pulse to combine, scraping down sides.

2. Drizzle in oil with machine running. Process to a coarse paste.

3. Cook pasta according to package directions. Add 1 cup of cooking water to processor and pulse until smooth. Toss pesto with drained pasta in warm pot.

MAKES 4 SERVINGS.

Per serving:
563 calories, 14 g protein,
66 g carbohydrates (4 g fiber),
27 g fat (4 g sat), 346 mg sodium

Smoky Paprika Kale Chips

BODY BENEFIT: Kale is rich in vitamins A, C, and K and is a great source of calcium. What's more, eating cruciferous veggies like kale may lower your cancer risk.

- 1 large bunch kale
- ¼ cup olive oil
- 1 Tbsp smoked paprika
- ½ tsp sea salt

1. Preheat oven to 400°F.

2. Remove stems from kale and tear leaves into large pieces. In large bowl, toss kale pieces with oil and paprika.

3. Line baking sheet with parchment paper. Scatter kale on sheet and roast until greens are dry and crispy, about 30 minutes. Toss with salt and serve.

MAKES 6 SERVINGS.

Per serving:
150 calories, 5 g protein,
14 g carbohydrates (3 g fiber),
10 g fat (1.5 g sat)

Lentil Quinoa Burgers

BODY BENEFIT: Just ¼ cup of these tiny legumes is crammed with 13 grams of protein, 11 grams of belly-filling fiber, and 5 milligrams of fatigue-fighting iron—all for only 161 calories. And some research suggests that because lentils keep blood sugar steady, they may even cut back on hunger, boosting weight loss.

- ½ cup quinoa
- 1 cup water
- ½ cup plain bread crumbs
- 1 egg, lightly beaten
- 2 cloves garlic, chopped
- 2 tsp cumin powder
- ⅓ cup cilantro
- Juice of ½ lemon
- 1 can (19 oz) lentils, rinsed
- Salt and freshly ground black pepper
- ½ cup walnut pieces
- 1 Tbsp butter
- ½ lb crimini mushrooms, sliced
- ¼ cup dry red wine
- 2 tsp vegetable oil
- 6 100% whole-grain buns

1. In saucepan, combine quinoa and water. Bring to a boil and simmer about 10 minutes. Let quinoa cool.

2. In a bowl, combine bread crumbs, egg, garlic, cumin, cilantro, lemon juice, cooked quinoa, half the lentils, and salt and pepper to taste. Place in food processor or blender and process or blend until well combined. Add remaining lentils and walnuts and pulse until incorporated. Form into 6 patties. Preheat grill to medium.

3. Meanwhile, melt butter in skillet over medium heat. Add mushrooms and sauté, stirring regularly, 5 minutes. Stir in wine and cook another 5 minutes.

4. Brush burgers with oil and grill 4 minutes per side. Toast buns 2 minutes. Serve burgers on buns and top with sautéed mushrooms.

MAKES 6 SERVINGS.

Per serving:
436 calories, 19 g protein,
60 g carbohydrates (13 g fiber),
15 g fat (3 g sat), 304 mg sodium

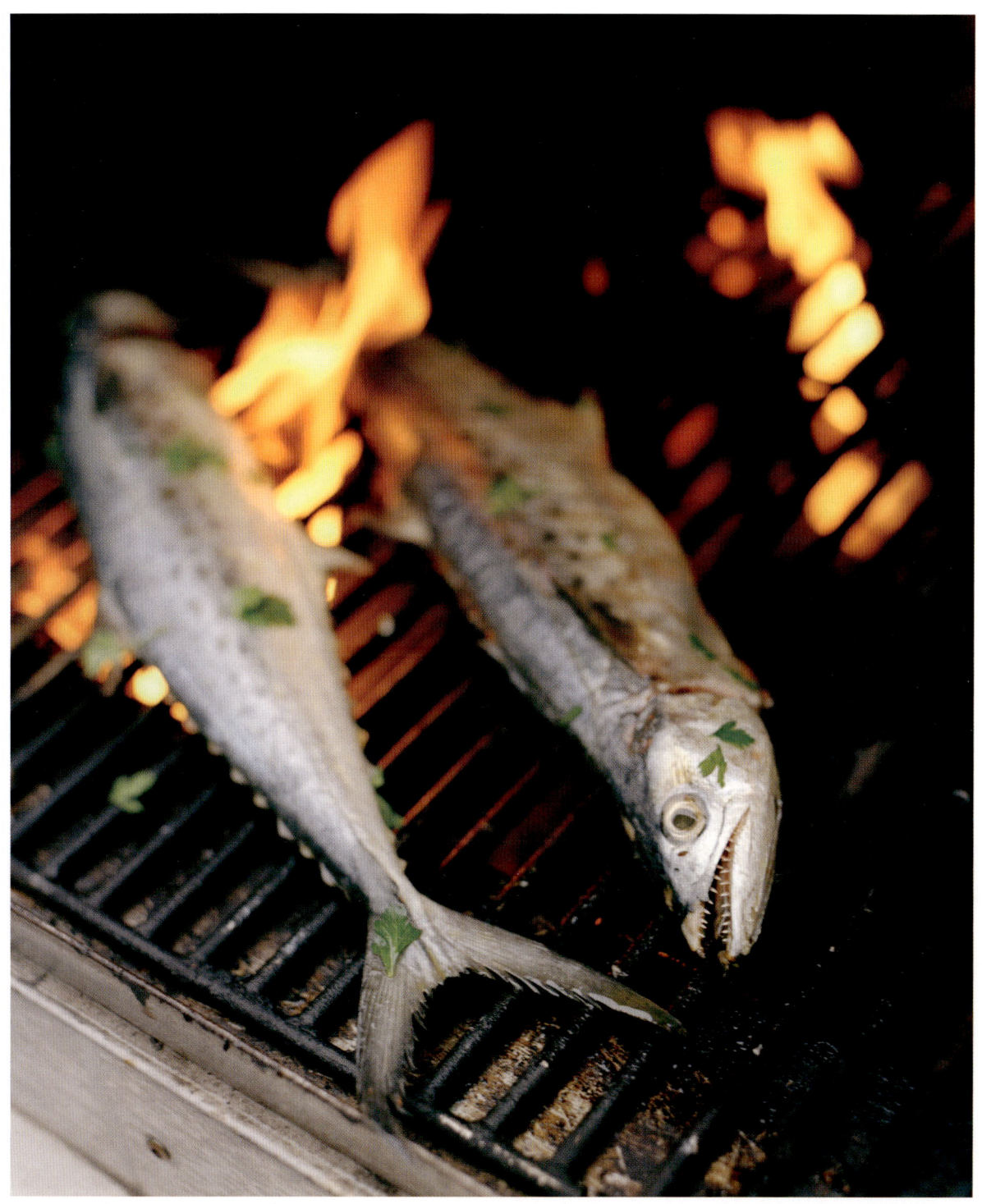

Perfect Grilled Mackerel

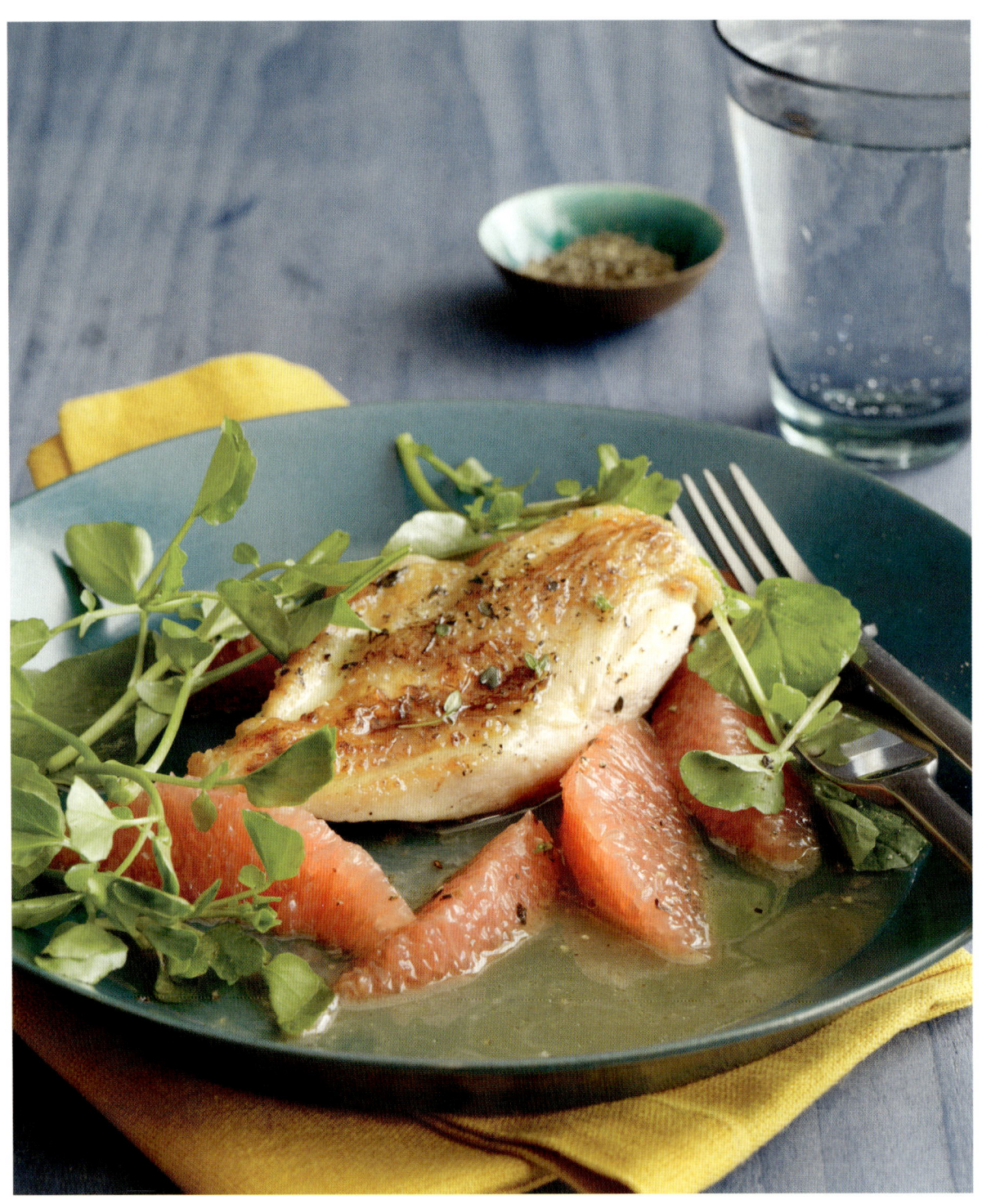

Chicken with Grapefruit

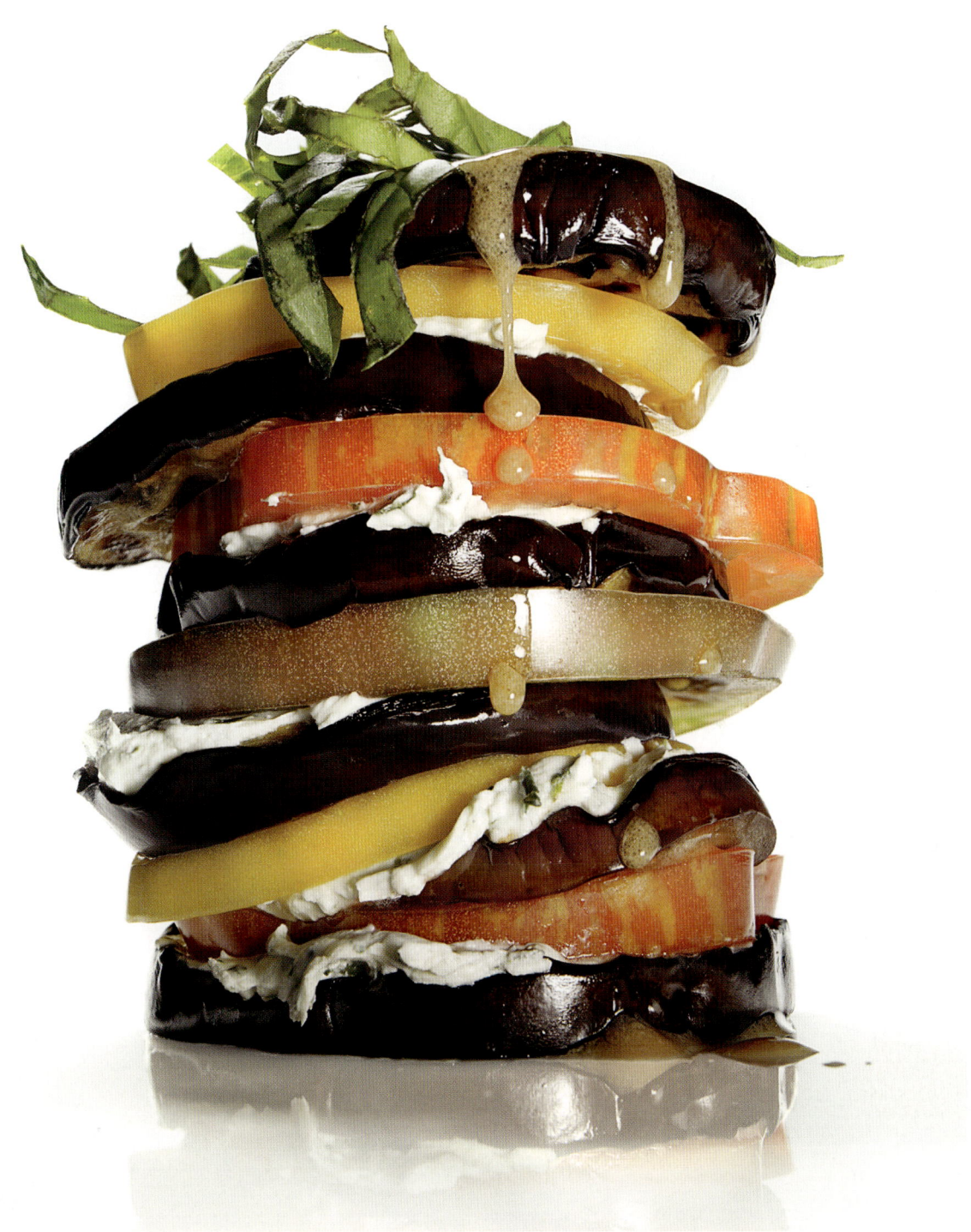

Heirloom Tomato and Eggplant Stacks

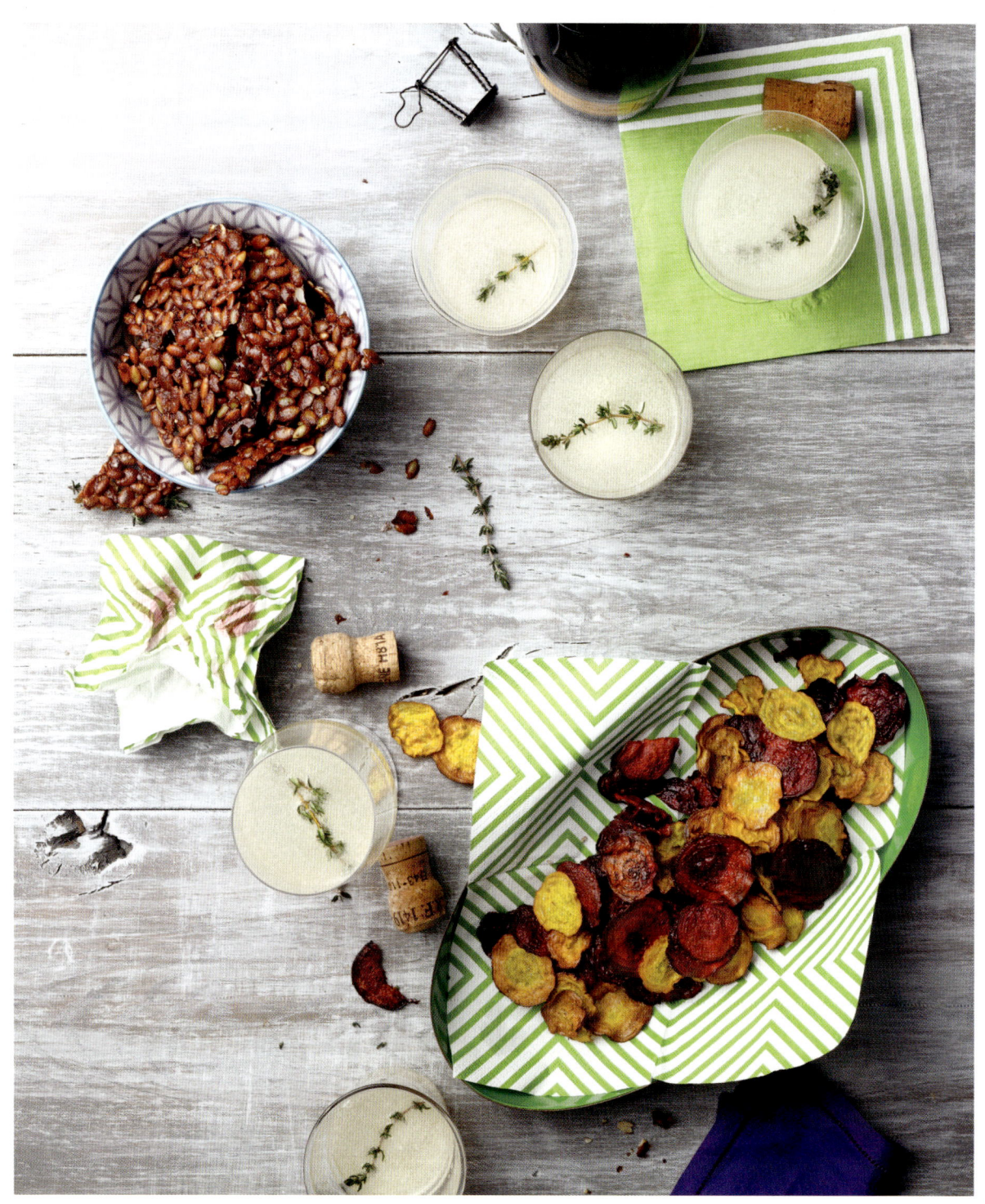

Pear-Thyme Bellini

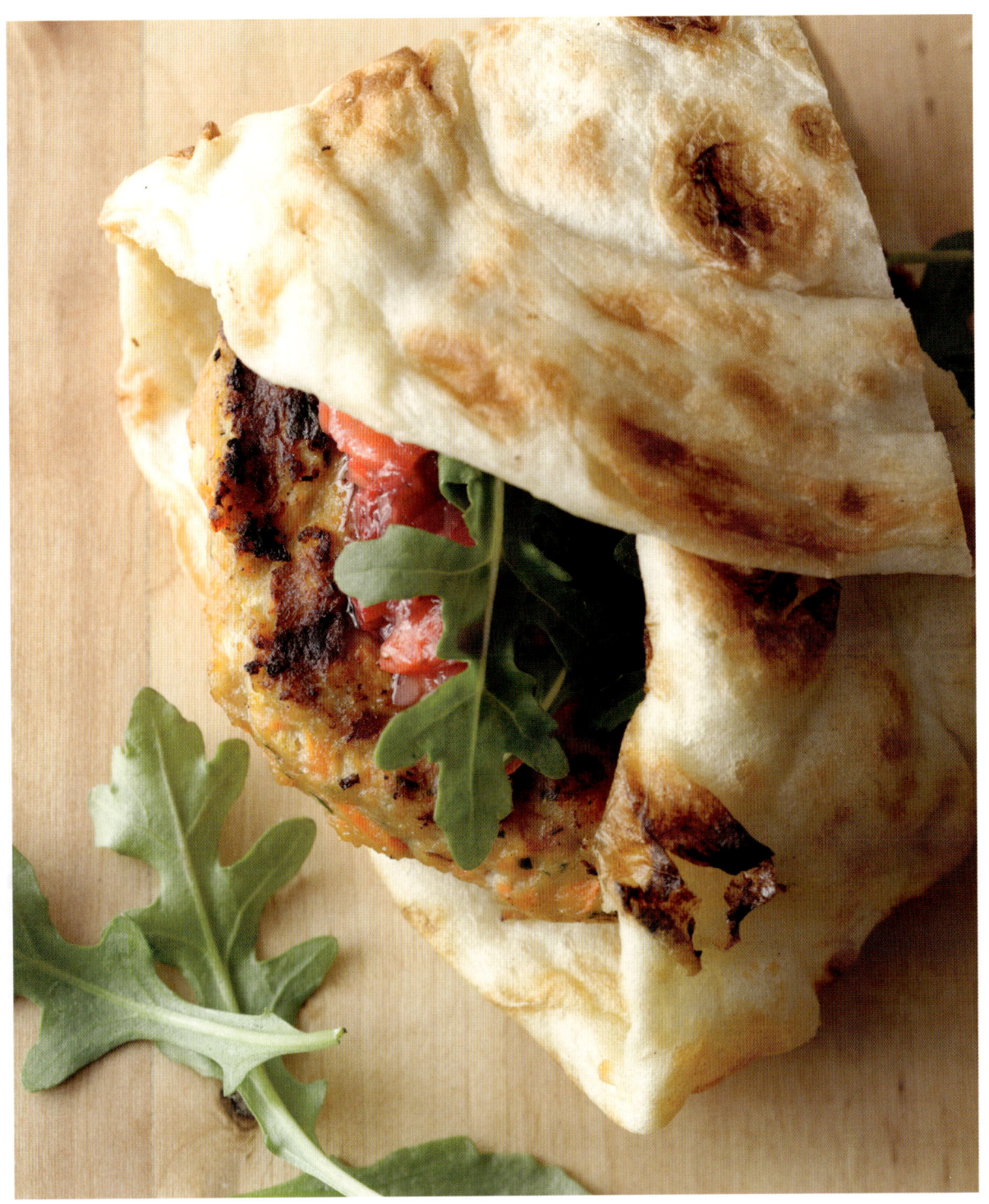

Garden Chicken Burger with Strawberry Sauce

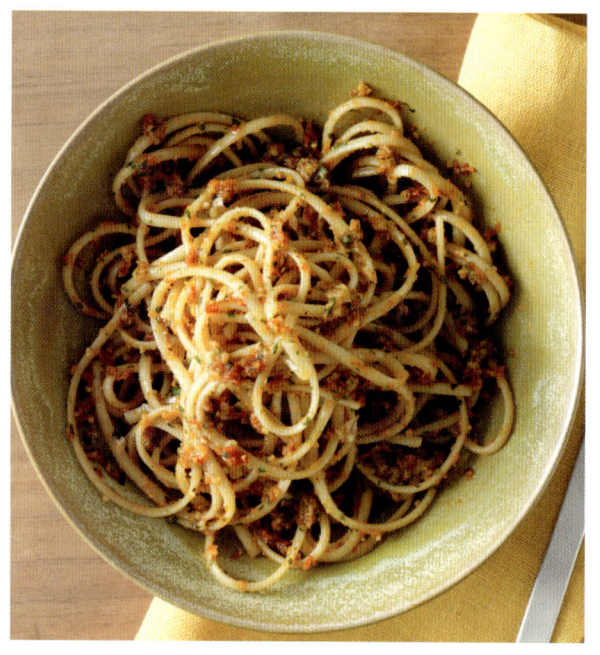

Linguine with Walnut-Tomato Pesto

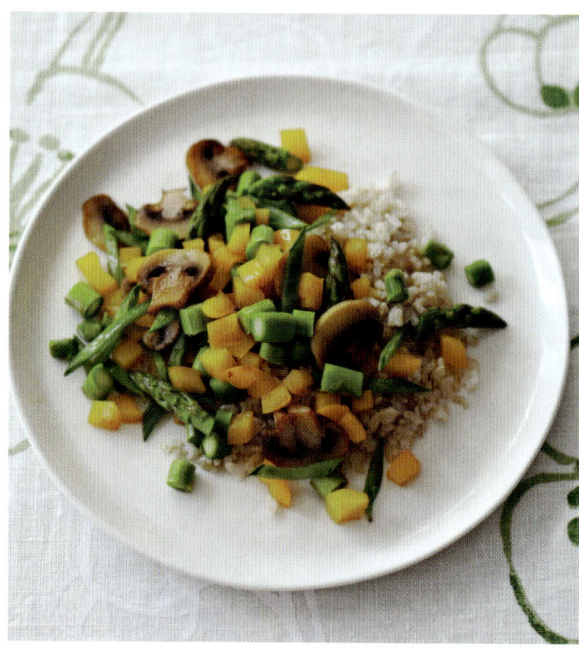

Asparagus Stir-Fry

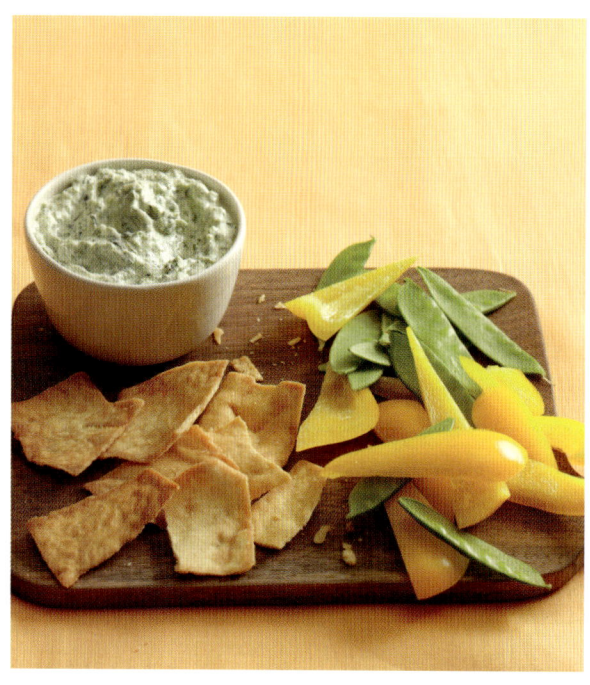

Spinach Dip

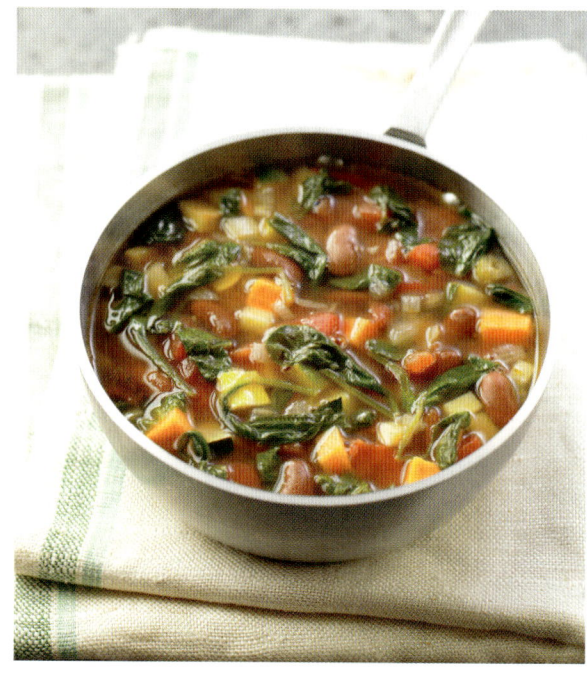

Hearty Minestrone

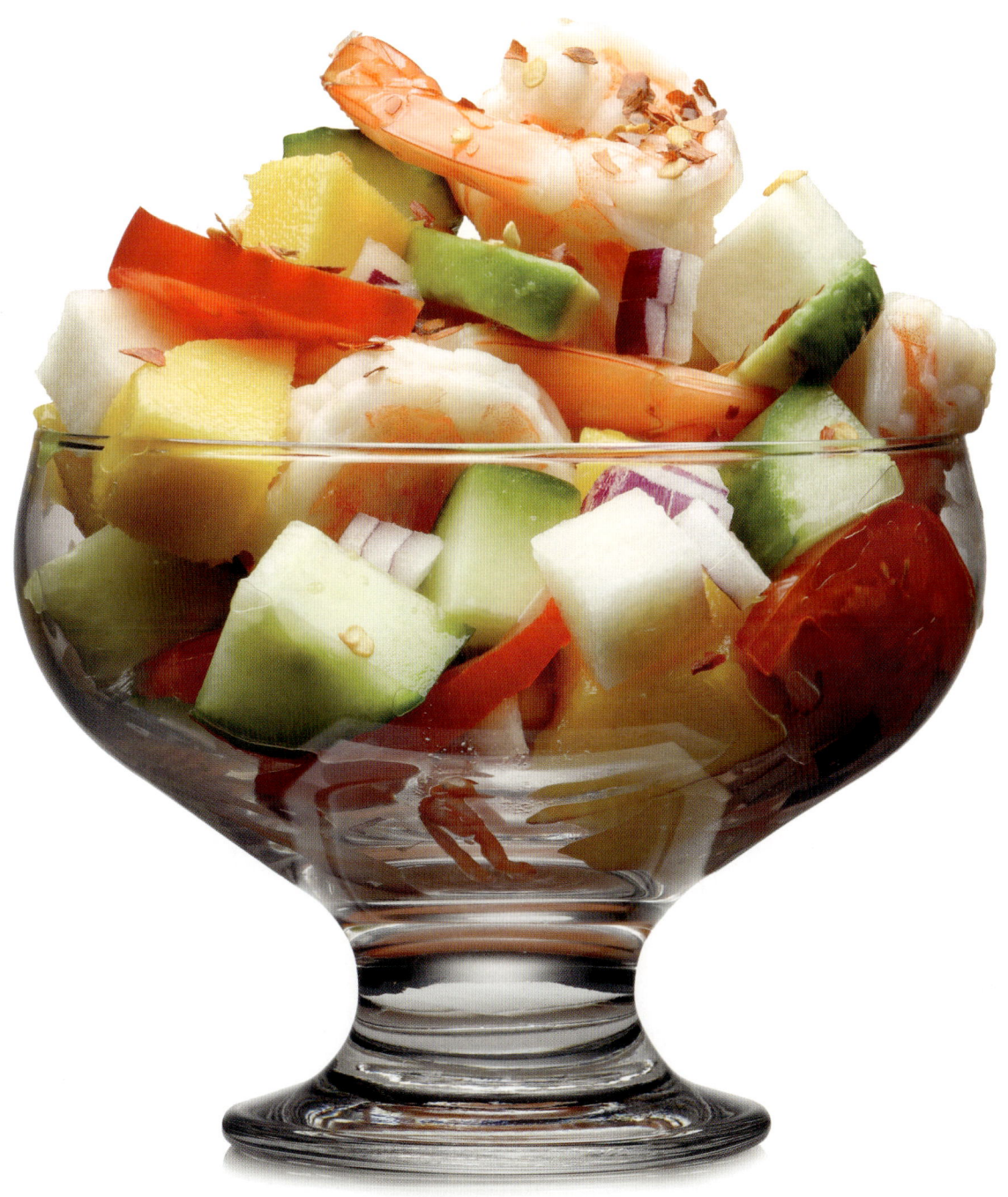

Shrimp Ceviche

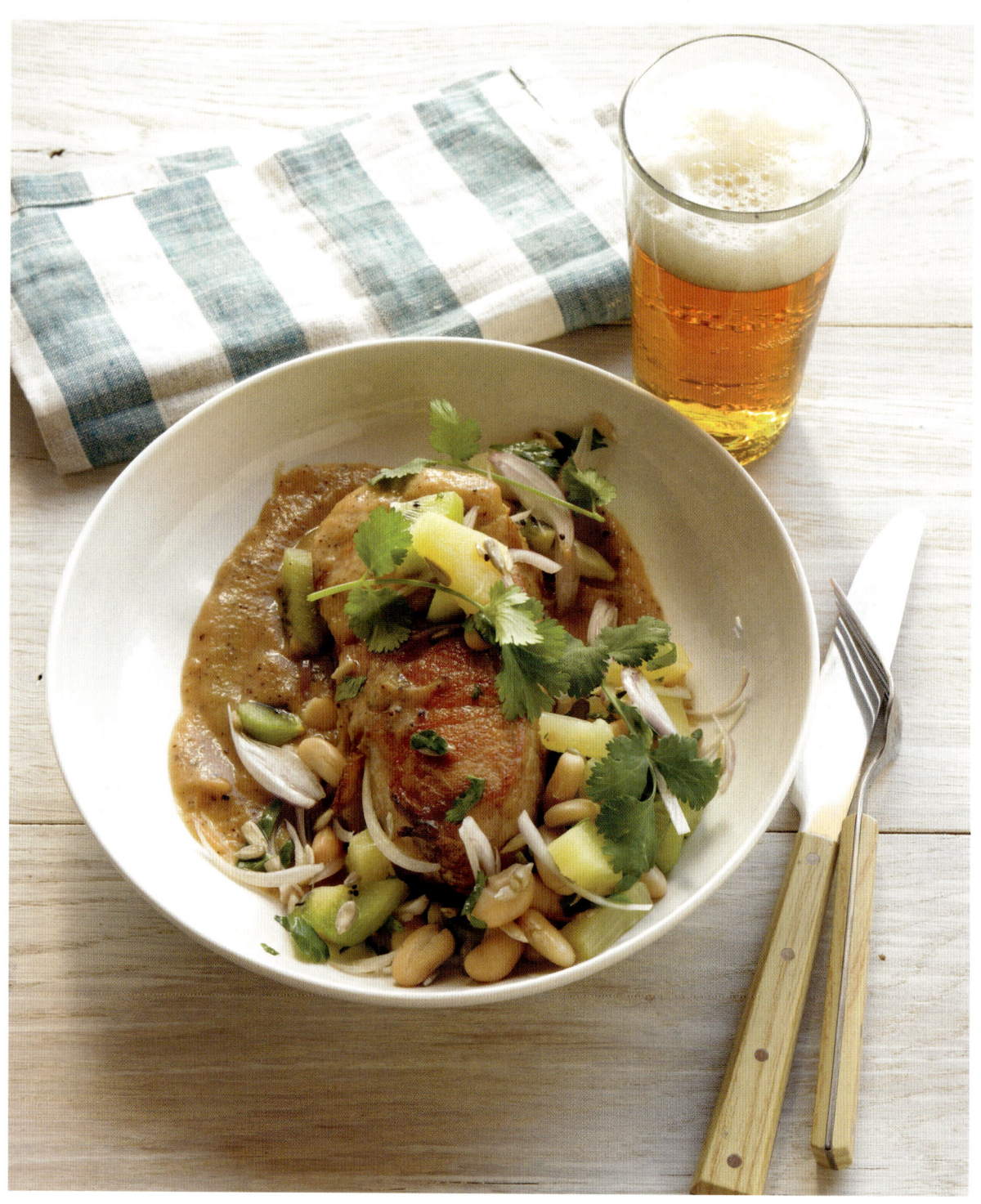

Pork Braised in Kiwi-Coconut Sauce with White Beans

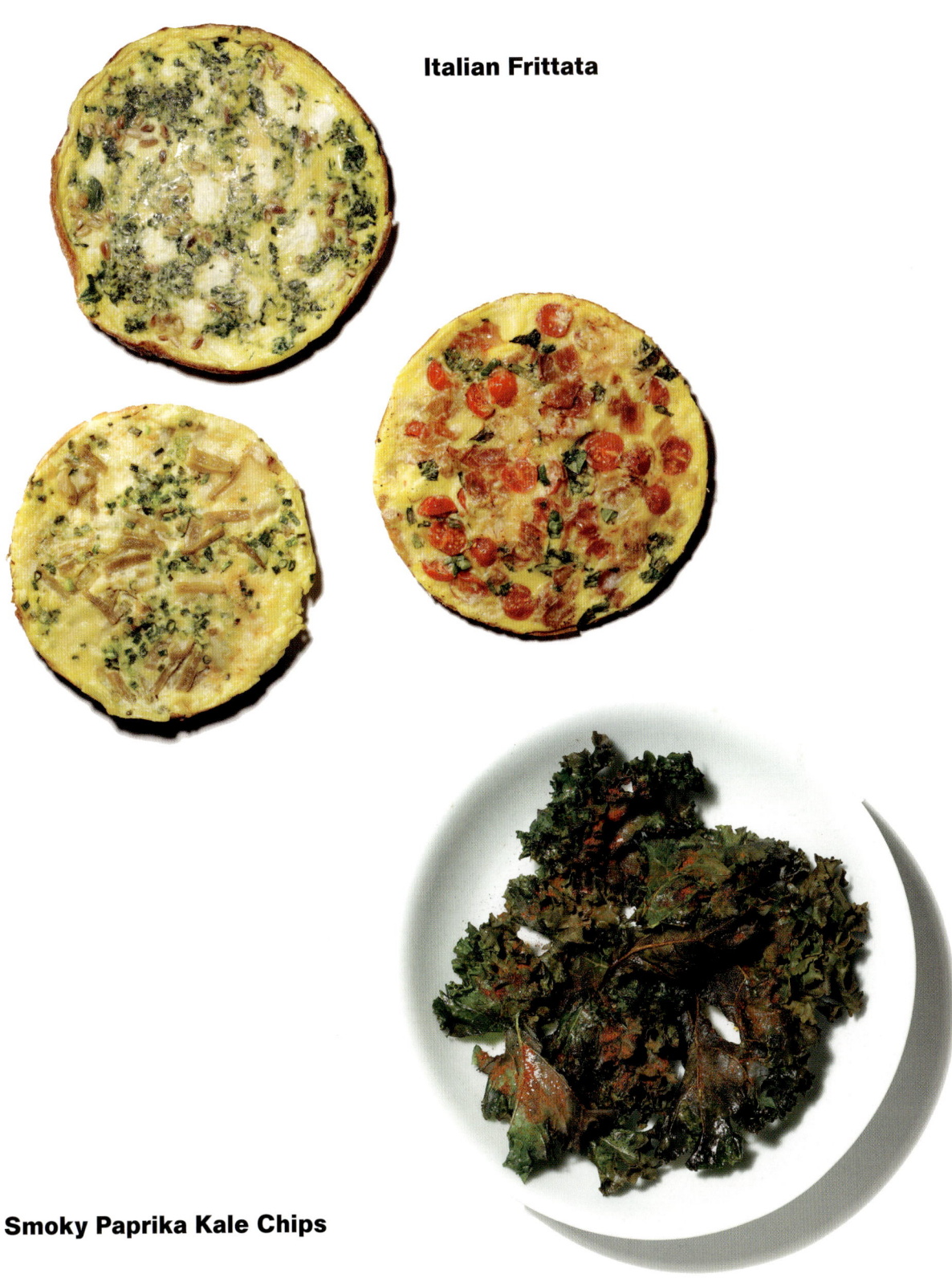

Italian Frittata

Smoky Paprika Kale Chips

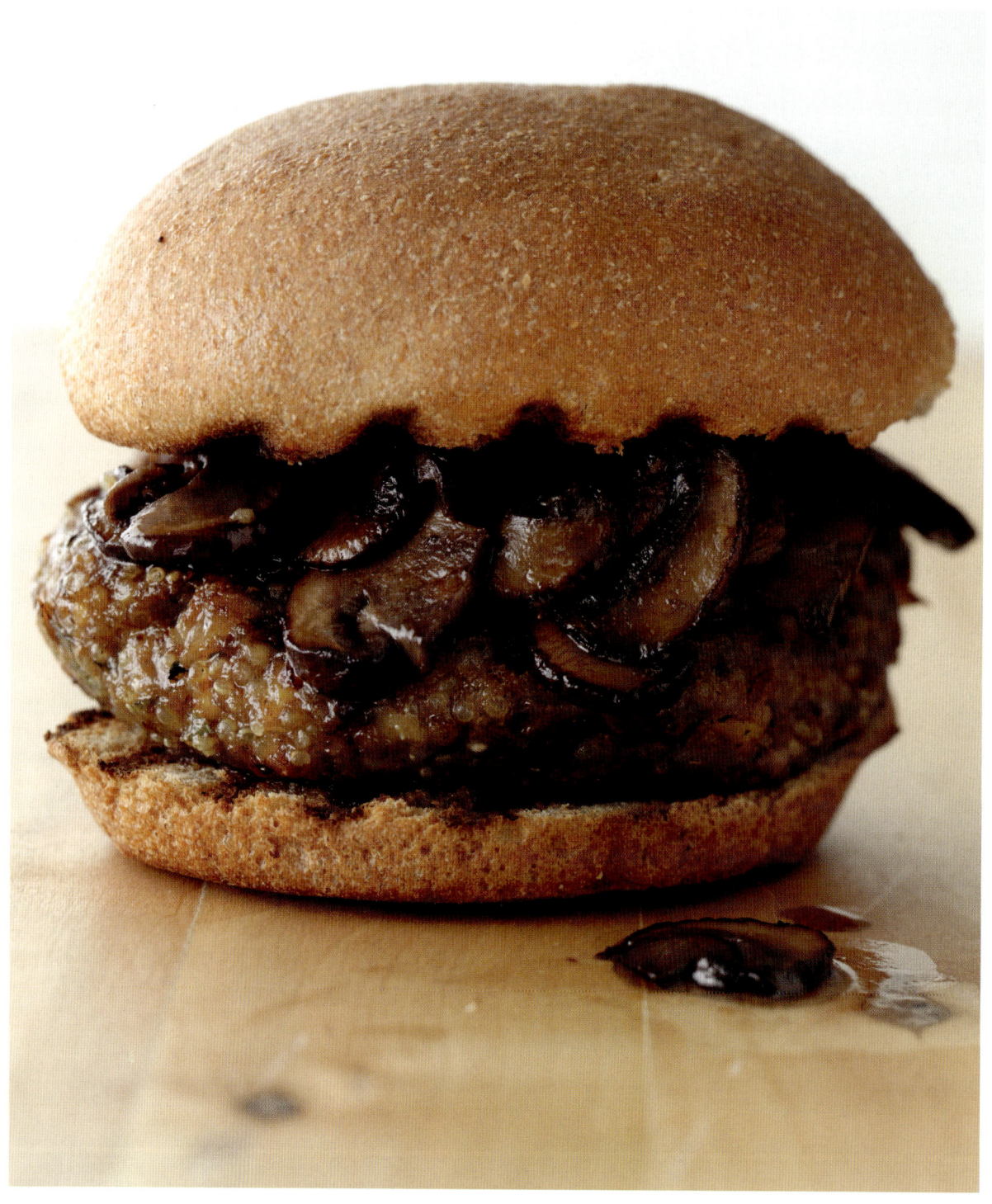

Lentil Quinoa Burgers

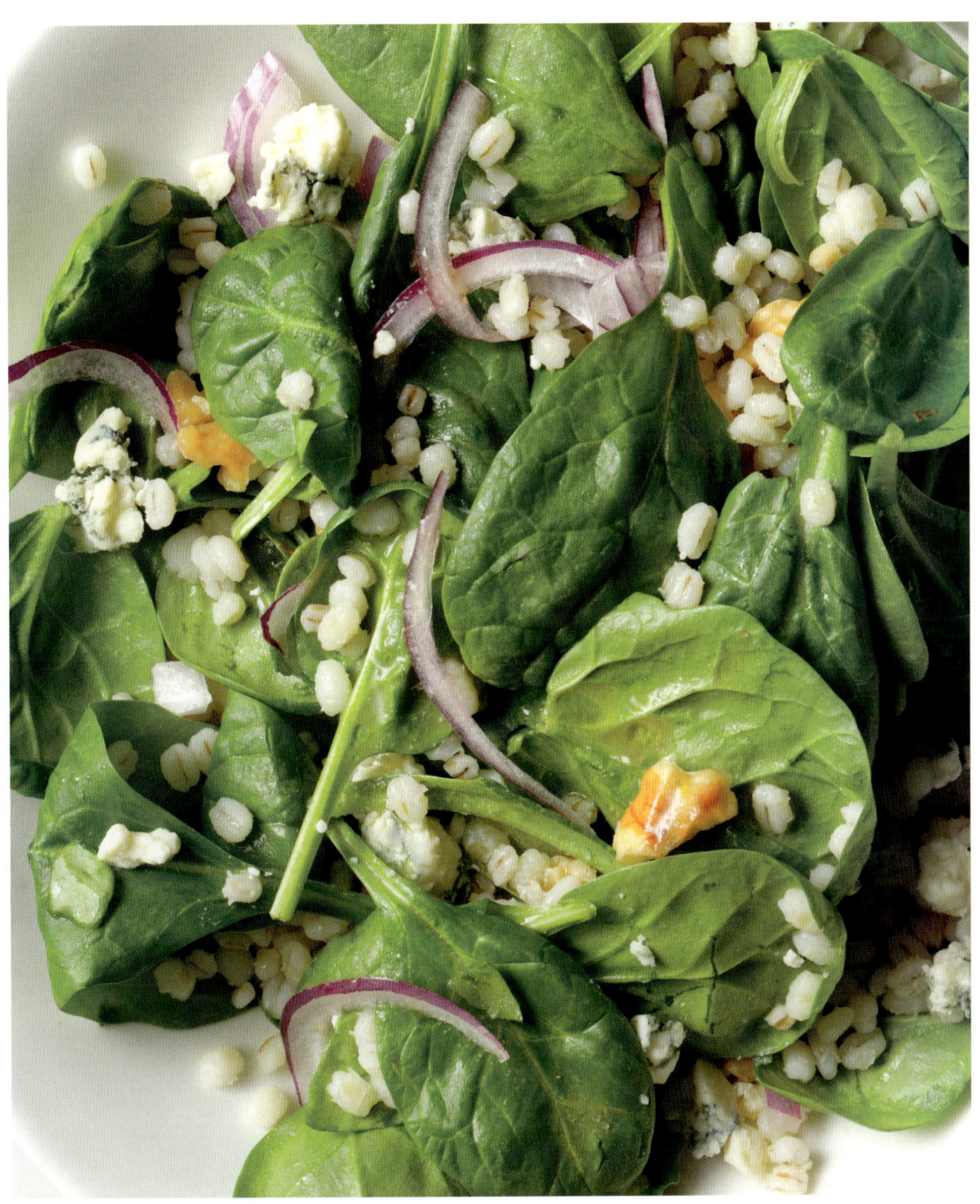

Spinach Barley Salad

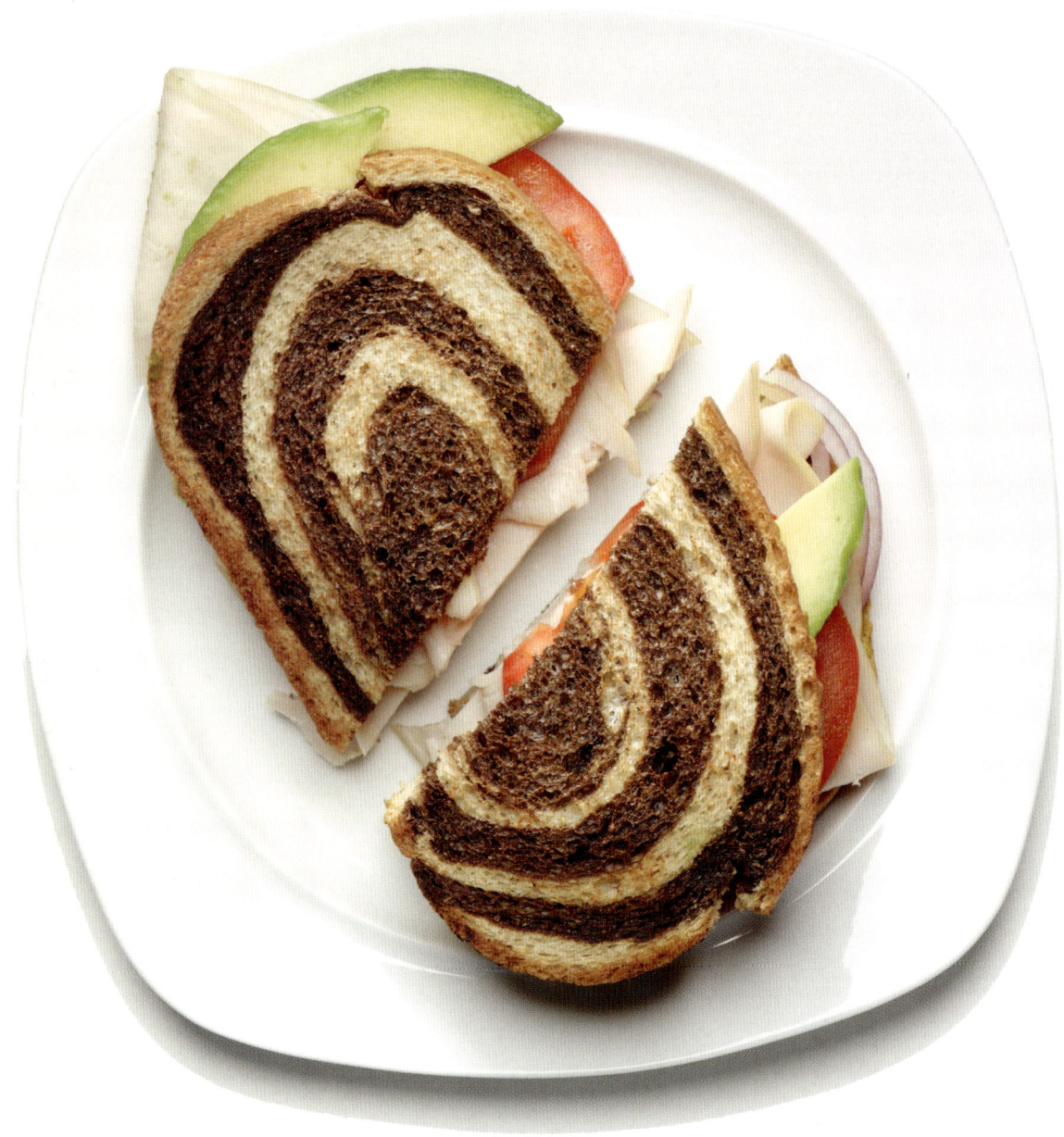

Turkey and Avocado Sandwich

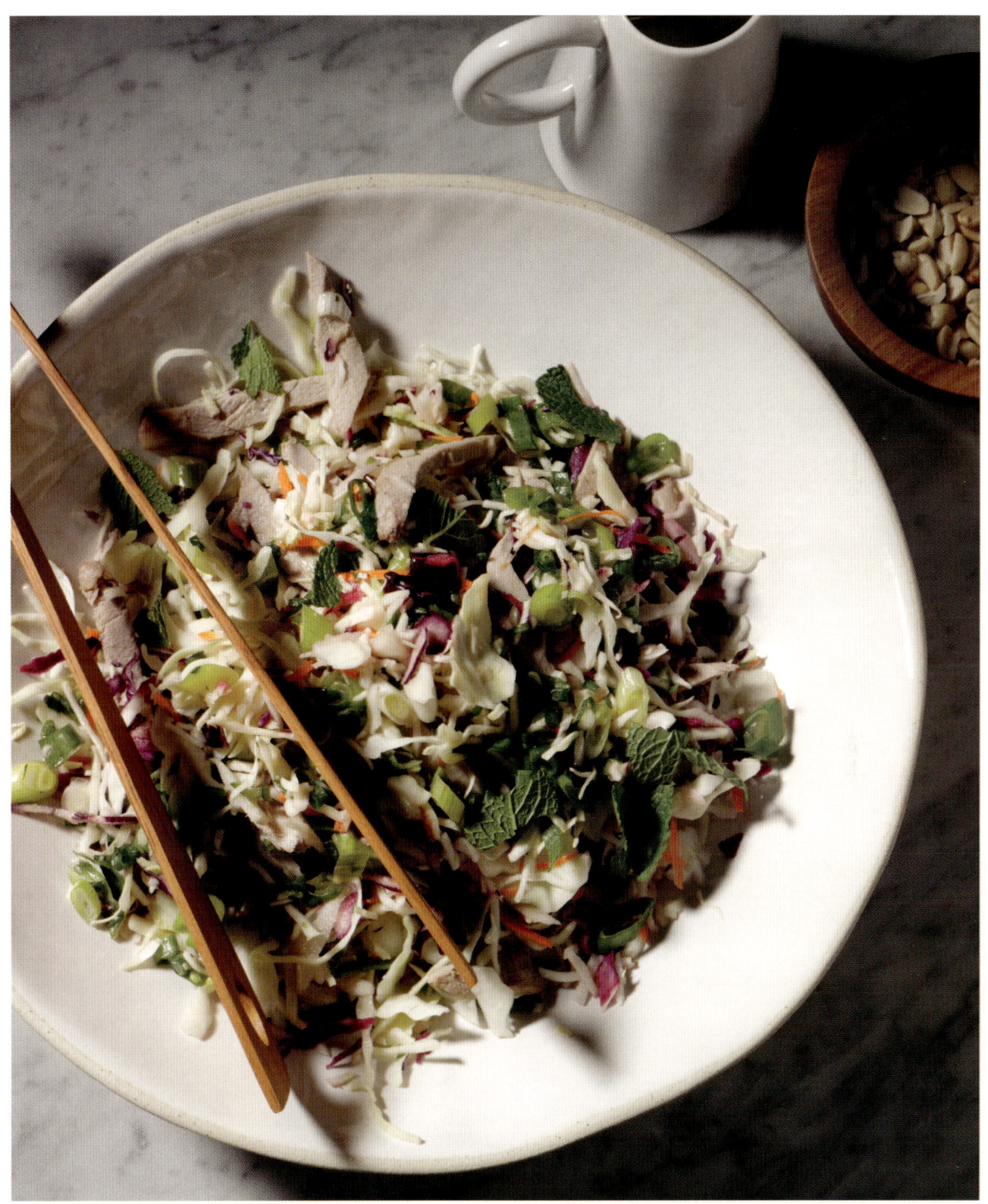

Vietnamese Pork Salad

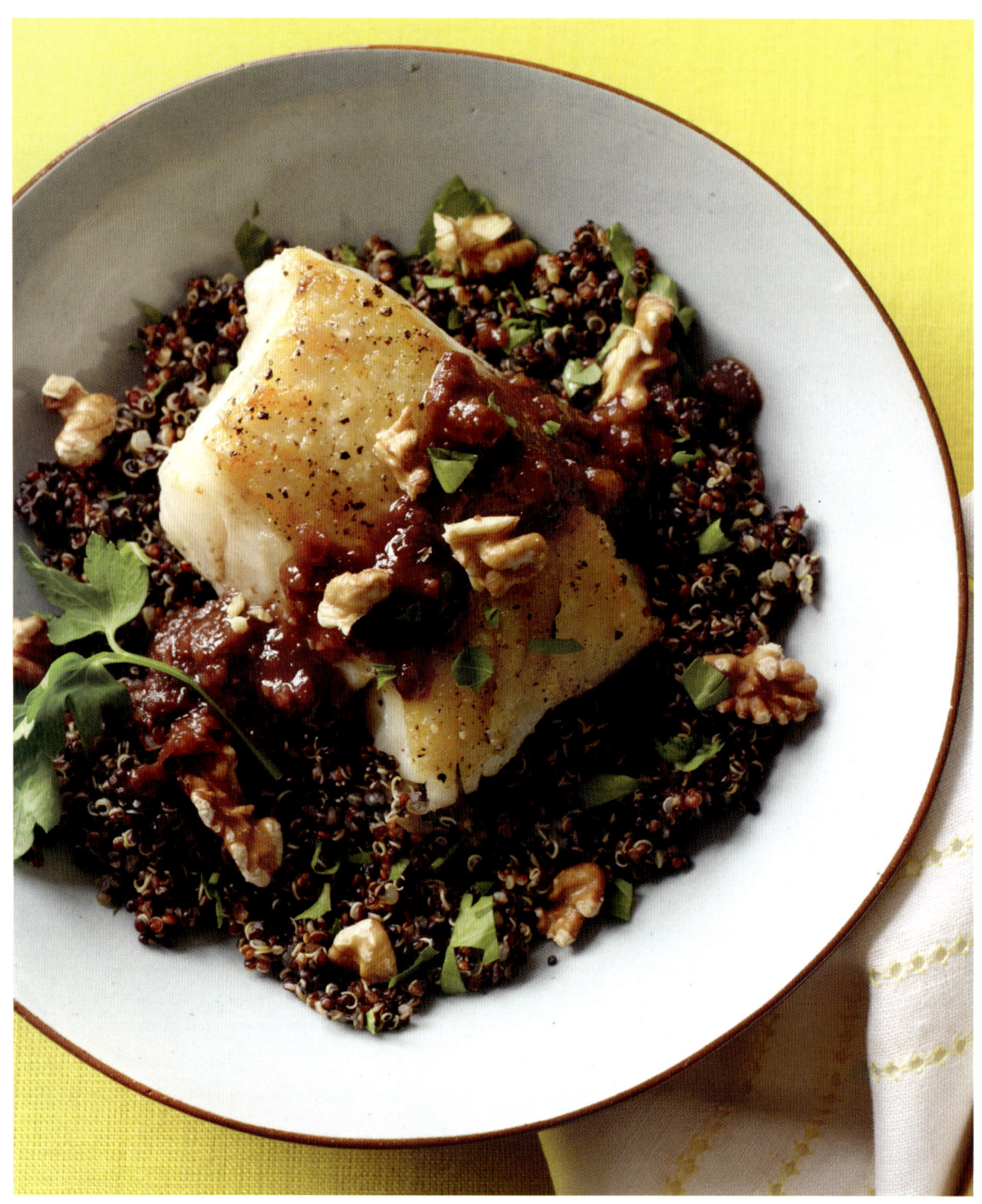

Roast Cod with Pomegranate-Walnut Sauce

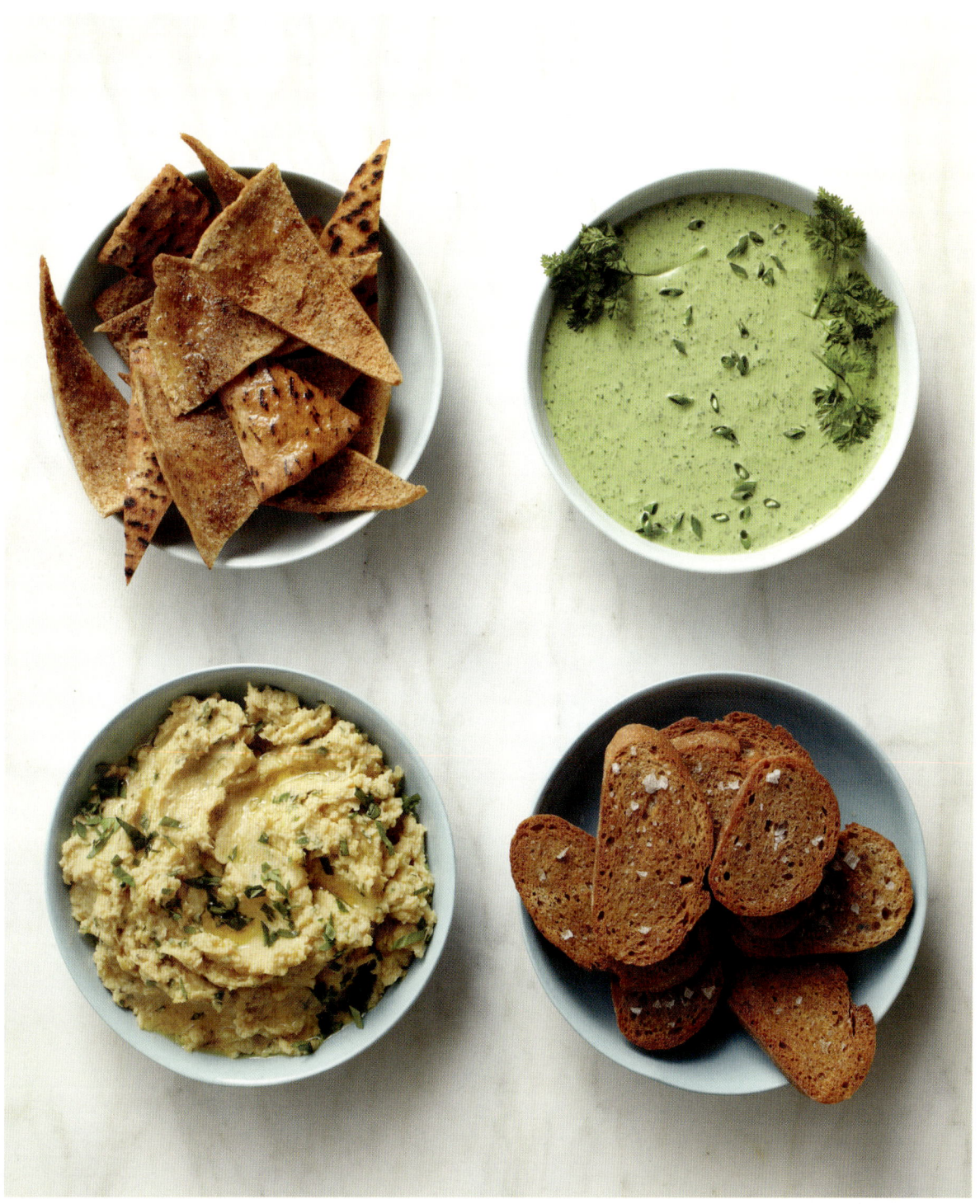

Artichoke Hummus

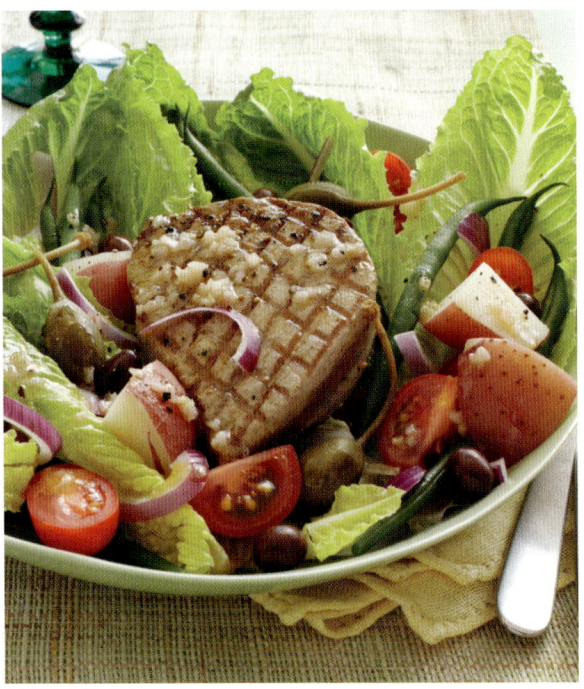

Tuna Niçoise Salad

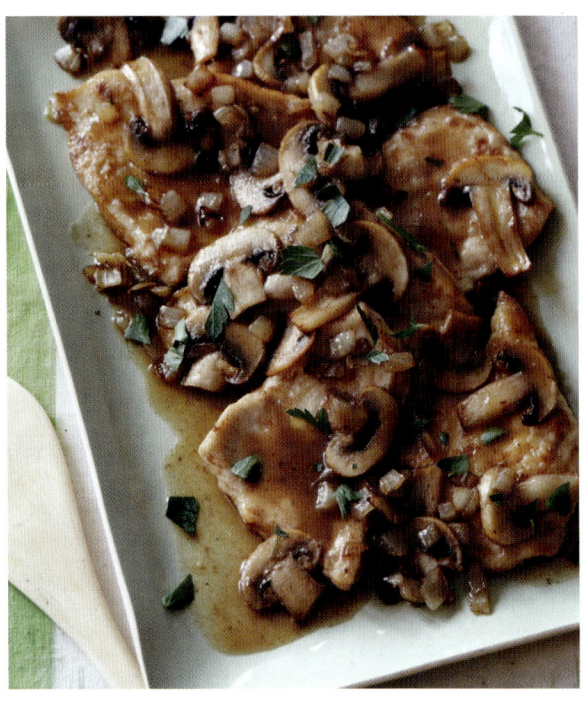

Italian Style Chicken and Mushrooms

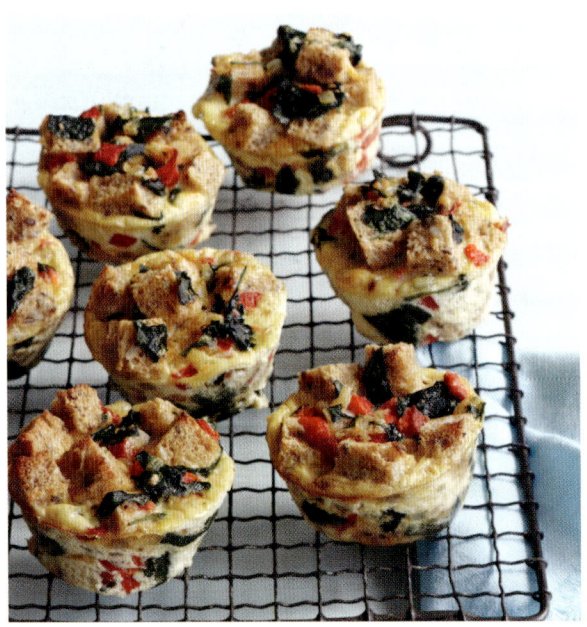

Breakfast Stuffins

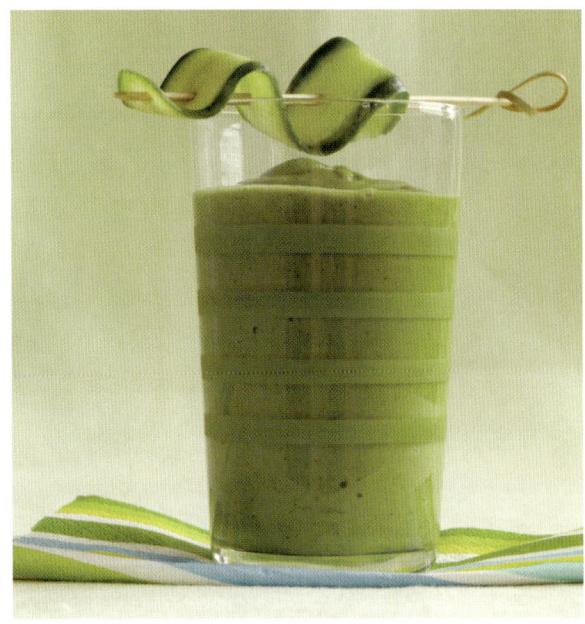

Green Goodness Smoothie

Chicken with Grapefruit

BODY BENEFIT: Grapefruit is a terrific source of vitamins A and B_5, potassium, folate, and fiber. And it's loaded with cancer-fighting lycopene. A half grapefruit has just 53 waistline-friendly calories.

- 4 boneless chicken breasts
- ½ tsp dried thyme
- ½ tsp salt
- ¼ tsp freshly ground black pepper
- 2 Tbsp olive oil
- ¼ cup dry white wine
- ¼ cup chicken broth
- 3 Tbsp grapefruit juice
- 2 tsp honey
- 3 cups trimmed watercress
- 2 grapefruit, cut into segments

1. Season chicken with thyme and half of the salt and pepper.

2. Heat oil in large skillet over medium-high heat. Brown chicken, 6 minutes per side. Add wine, broth, juice, and honey. Simmer until reduced to ⅓ cup. Season with remaining salt and pepper.

3. Put watercress and grapefruit on 4 plates. Top with chicken and sauce.

MAKES 4 SERVINGS.

Per serving:
266 calories, 27 g protein,
15 g carbohydrates (2 g fiber),
10 g fat (2 g sat), 438 mg sodium

Green Goodness Smoothie

BODY BENEFIT: Kefir has more protein and less sugar than yogurt, but with the same creamy texture, tangy taste, and probiotics. These healthy bacteria are a known immune enhancer and may protect against colon cancer, says Tamara Freuman, MS, RD.

- 1 cup baby spinach
- 1 cup cucumber chunks
- ½ avocado, halved, pitted, and peeled
- 1 large kiwi, peeled and chopped
- ½ cup frozen kefir or low-fat vanilla frozen yogurt
- ½ cup fresh orange or tangerine juice
- ¼ cup mint leaves

In blender, combine spinach, cucumber, avocado, kiwi, kefir, juice, and mint. Blend until smooth.

MAKES 1 SERVING.

Per serving:
188 calories, 5 g protein,
29 g carbohydrates (6 g fiber),
8 g fat (1 g sat), 57 mg sodium

Shrimp Ceviche

BODY BENEFIT: Jicama, a slightly sweet and crunchy root veggie, stars inulin, a belly-flattening fiber that acts as a prebiotic to promote helpful bacteria in the gut. It's also an excellent source of vitamin C.

- ½ cup chopped cucumber
- ⅓ cup chopped jicama
- ⅓ cup chopped mango
- 1 Tbsp chopped onion
- ¼ cup sliced avocado
- 1 tomato, sliced
- 1 cup cooked shrimp
- ¼ cup lemon juice
- 1 tsp red-pepper flakes

In large bowl, combine cucumber, jicama, mango, onion, avocado, tomato, shrimp, lemon juice, and pepper.

MAKES 1 SERVING.

Per serving:
295 calories, 29.5 g protein,
30 g carbohydrates (8.5 g fiber),
11 g fat (8 g sat), 1,009 mg sodium

Mango-Coconut Chia Pudding

BODY BENEFIT: One tablespoon of nutty-tasting edible chia seeds has as much fiber as a bowl of oatmeal, plus bone-building calcium and heart-healthy omega-3s. Chia is also a good source of iron and holds up to five times its volume in water, so it helps keep you hydrated.

- 1 can (13.5 oz) light coconut milk
- ⅓ cup white chia seeds
- 2 Tbsp honey
- 1 tsp vanilla extract
- 1 mango, peeled, pitted, and diced
- 1 cup strawberries, diced
- ¼ cup sliced almonds
- 4 tsp coconut flakes

1. In pint-size measuring cup, combine coconut milk, chia seeds, honey, and vanilla. Stir until combined, then refrigerate 1 hour.

2. In each of 4 small serving glasses, layer 2 Tbsp chia pudding mixture and 2 Tbsp mango, and repeat three times. Top with a spoonful of strawberries, sliced almonds, and a sprinkle of coconut.

MAKES 4 SERVINGS.

Per serving:
308 calories, 6 g protein,
32 g carbohydrates (10 g fiber),
20 g fat (10 g sat), 17 mg sodium

Spinach Barley Salad

BODY BENEFIT: Barley is rich in niacin (for healthy hair and skin) and cancer-fighting lignans. Plus "the soluble fiber keeps your cholesterol levels healthy, cutting your risk for heart disease," says Kate Geagan, MS, RD, author of *Go Green, Get Lean*.

- 4 cups quick-cooking pearl barley
- 3 Tbsp sherry vinegar or red wine vinegar
- ½ tsp Dijon mustard
- 2 Tbsp extra-virgin olive oil
- 1 oz Gorgonzola cheese, finely crumbled (about ¼ cup)
- 6 cups baby spinach leaves, shredded
- ¼ cup sliced red onion
- 2 Tbsp toasted chopped walnuts
- Salt and freshly ground black pepper

1. Cook barley according to package instructions.

2. Meanwhile, in medium bowl, whisk together vinegar and mustard. Whisk in oil until well blended, then whisk cheese into the mixture.

3. Put cooked barley in serving bowl. Add spinach, onion, walnuts, and salt and pepper to taste. Toss gently.

4. Stir in vinaigrette. Cover and refrigerate for at least 30 minutes to allow flavors to mix.

MAKES 4 SERVINGS.

Per serving:
325 calories, 7 g protein,
50 g carbohydrates (8 g fiber),
12 g fat (3 g sat), 174 mg sodium

Everything You Need to Know About Energy Foods

Step into any sports store and you're often confronted with a dizzying array of drinks, bars, chews, and gels that promise instant pep in convenient packages. While some are healthy, some are pure hype—or worse. "There's nothing magic about energy foods," says Nancy Clark, MS, RD, author of *Nancy Clark's Sports Nutrition Guidebook*. Lots of foods without energy on their labels boost pep just as well as—or better than—products marketed as such. Here's how to wade through the hype and get the energy you need, while avoiding the junk you don't.

Energy drinks. Energy drinks are caffeine-and-sugar cocktails that come in 8-ounce cans. Caffeine boosts cognitive performance, and glucose (the brain's main source of fuel) gives an added jolt. Many of these drinks also include a rain forest fruit called guarana, which contains still more caffeine. Down a can and it's hard not to feel rocket fueled—but some people also experience anxiety, insomnia, headaches, and increased heart rate and blood pressure from all that caffeine. And the sugar can total 31 grams, as much as a can of soda packs. By comparison, a standard cup of coffee with 2 teaspoons of sugar has about 8 grams and will fortify your body with disease-fighting antioxidants in addition to caffeine.

Energy gels. Think of energy gels as concentrated, Jell-O-like versions of sports drinks. Designed for endurance athletes, they come in plastic pouches that can easily be ripped open and squeezed down the hatch for a superquick fix of carbs, along with electrolytes to replace those lost through sweat. The sugars deliver instant energy because the body can process them so quickly. "They're almost predigested," says Julie Upton, MS, RD, coauthor of *Energy to Burn*. "There's no chewing required because endurance athletes can't eat when they're exercising at such high intensities." If you're running a marathon, an energy gel might help you finish. But if you just want an afternoon lift, there are more satisfying options.

Energy bars. Energy bars are easy to buy and stash in your bag for a pick-me-up on the go. They purport to provide lasting energy, give you the nutrients you need, and power you through a tough workout. Some of them actually are good for you—especially those that contain whole grains, nuts, or fruit. The problem is, many are little better than candy bars, with nearly half their calories coming from various forms of sugar. While these may give you a 15-minute mood boost, you'll get a sugar crash soon after and will have consumed 200 or more calories. So choose carefully or make one yourself.

Energy shots. Your friends the food marketers thought it would be fun to compress a full-size energy drink into a 2-ounce can. Some people gravitate to energy shots because they have fewer calories and are convenient and portable. Manufacturers claim the energy boost acts faster and lasts longer, but there's no proof, says Liz Applegate, PhD, director of sports nutrition at the University of California, Davis, and author of *Eat Smart, Play Hard*. In fact, because the cans are petite (and contain artificial sweeteners instead of sugar, which companies say prevents a crash), you might be tempted to drink more of them, making it easier to OD on caffeine. And the taste . . . well, the label may say lime, but your mouth will know better—metallic and bitter is more like it.

Energy chews. Energy chews or jelly beans are similar to gels but, well, chewable. They're great for endurance athletes who have "bonked" or "hit a wall" and need immediate fuel to complete a race, especially if they can't stomach the taste of gels. But some of these, experts say, are basically gumdrops with added vitamins and minerals. Assuming you get your nutrients from real food, you don't need these, so the only "benefit" is sugar. In the middle of an Ironman? Go ahead and pop a few. Otherwise, think of energy jelly beans and chews as candy. You wouldn't expect sustained energy from a bag of Skittles, so why think these will be any different?

Organic energy drinks. Yep, even energy drinks have gone green. Some companies offer organic beverages that promise to make you alert and focused—naturally. In addition to sugar and various fruit extracts, they usually include yerba maté. The leaves of this tropical tree contain caffeine and two similar stimulants, theophylline and theobromine, and have been used by South Americans to combat fatigue. Lab studies also rate yerba maté high in antioxidants. The downside: The sugar contents are similar to those of other energy drinks—and organic ones cost more and are harder to find. Still, for liquid lightning, they're your best bet among the canned beverages.

Chapter 17

Recipes for Recovery

AFTER A TOUGH WORKOUT, CHOOSE FOODS THAT WILL NOT ONLY REPLENISH YOUR ENERGY STORES, BUT HELP YOUR MUSCLES REBUILD FOR QUICKER GAINS.

When you're working hard to achieve a fitness goal—whether you're focused on shedding excess pounds, building endurance and speed, or packing on muscle—it's easy to forget how important rest is. "It's when you're not exercising that the muscle rebuilds itself and becomes stronger," says Bryan Heiderscheit, PhD, PT, who heads the University of Wisconsin Medical School's Runner's Clinic. "If recovery is insufficient, you'll break down more than you build up." Here's how to make the most of your downtime.

To help you maximize your recovery, check out the menu plan at right, which was designed by Bonci and Therese Franzese (who creates food plans for Olympic cyclists as director of nutrition at the high-end sports club Chelsea Piers in New York City). It provides all the right kinds of energy, vitamins, and nutrients you need to build muscle, recover fast, and incinerate fat: a mix of 65 to 70 percent carbs, 15 percent protein, and 15 to 20 percent fat, plus 7 servings of fruits and vegetables to provide antioxidants, which fight the harmful free radicals that your body produces as it processes oxygen (as it does when you exercise).

The plan's strategy is to divide your plate this way: one-half fruits and veggies, one-quarter protein, and one-quarter carbs. This five-day menu will get you started. Its 2,500 calories per day are for an active 150-pound guy. If you're bigger or smaller, adjust the calories proportionately (so if you're 180 pounds, which is 20 percent heavier than 150 pounds, you need 20 percent more calories). Following the menu are suggestions for customizing the menu five ways: lose weight, follow a vegetarian diet, help heal injuries, gain muscle, or recover fast.

Day 1

BREAKFAST
1 cup oats cooked with 8 oz 1% milk, sprinkled with 1 Tbsp walnuts; banana

MIDMORNING SNACK
1 cup low-sugar cereal with a mini box of raisins and half dozen almonds (eaten dry)

LUNCH
3 oz can or pouch tuna mixed with thumb-size amount of salad dressing on kaiser roll with lettuce and tomato; orange

MIDAFTERNOON SNACK
2 oatmeal-raisin cookies (2 to 3" diameter); banana

DINNER
½ package all-natural, preservative-free frozen dinner, with a palm-size piece of chicken cooked in 2 tsp oil, cut up, and added to the meal

EVENING SNACK
1 cup frozen yogurt in dish or flat-bottomed wafer cone

Day 2

BREAKFAST
8 oz yogurt with ¼ cup granola; 1 slice whole-grain toast with 2 tsp peanut butter; apple

MIDMORNING SNACK
Protein bar

LUNCH
½ can vegetable soup (about 1 cup); 2 slices cheese on toasted English muffin; pear

MIDAFTERNOON SNACK
2 slices whole-grain bread with 2 tsp peanut butter and 1 tsp jelly; nectarine

DINNER
2 cups pasta with pesto and palm-size piece of grilled or broiled salmon; 1 cup steamed veggies

EVENING SNACK
1 cup instant pudding

Day 3

BREAKFAST

English muffin with ¼ cup shredded Cheddar cheese melted on top; pear

MIDMORNING SNACK

Package of peanut butter crackers; apple

LUNCH

6" turkey sub; handful of baby carrots; small bag of baked potato chips; nectarine

MIDAFTERNOON SNACK

Sandwich baggie of microwave popcorn; 8 oz cranberry juice spritzer (½ cranberry juice, ½ seltzer)

DINNER

2 thin ground-turkey burgers on 2 buns; 2 cups salad with 2 Tbsp light dressing

EVENING SNACK

Smoothie: 4 oz 1% skim milk, 4 oz yogurt, and ½ cup fruit

Day 4

BREAKFAST

Quick blintz: spread ½ cup cottage cheese on 2 flour tortillas, cover with 2 Tbsp strawberry jelly, and roll up; 8 oz orange juice (¾ juice, ¼ water)

MIDMORNING SNACK

Granola bar or fruit

LUNCH

3 scrambled eggs; small bagel (Lender's size) with light margarine; 8 oz tomato juice; ½ cup juice-packed canned fruit

MIDAFTERNOON SNACK

¼ cup dried cranberries mixed with 1 Tbsp nuts and handful of mini pretzels

DINNER

Baked potato (about 5" long) with butter or sour cream (you should be able to see the potato after you spread it); 6 oz steak fillet, broiled; 1 cup steamed broccoli

EVENING SNACK

1 cup hot cocoa; 2 thin biscotti

Day 5

BREAKFAST

8 oz milk; small muffin (about 3" diameter); banana

MIDMORNING SNACK

Handful of cheese crackers; handful of grapes

LUNCH

2 handfuls of bagged salad with cold ½ chicken breast (about the size of a computer mouse) and 2 Tbsp light dressing; medium whole-grain roll; tangerine

MIDAFTERNOON SNACK

Protein bar; piece of fruit

DINNER

Chicken fajitas: palm-size piece of chicken sliced and stir-fried in 2 tsp oil with a handful of sliced peppers and a handful of sliced onions; divide into 2 flour tortillas and add salsa

EVENING SNACK

Handful of baked tortilla chips with ¼ cup shredded cheese melted on top

Customize Your Diet

The following suggestions from Liz Applegate show ways you can alter the sample menu to suit your individual needs.

If You Want To . . . Lose Weight

Forget fad and crash diets—you might lose weight, but you won't have adequate energy to train hard. The best and simplest way to lose weight is to pare portions and increase exercise, says Applegate. To lose a pound a week, you need to create a deficit of 500 calories a day.

How easy is that? Eat 250 fewer calories—the amount in one energy bar—a day and burn an additional 250 calories during exercise (run 1 mile or do 25 minutes of strength training, or add 25 more minutes of rigorous mountain biking or road riding at 15 mph). You can slash the entire 500 from food, but we'd rather play harder and eat more.

If You Want To . . . Eat Vegetarian

Often, a big challenge for vegetarians is getting adequate protein, says Applegate. The easiest solution: Add beans to every dish and eat soy products. Other nutrition concerns: vitamin B_{12} (milk, eggs, fortified soy milk, cereal), iron (dried fruit, leafy greens, fortified cereal), and zinc (wheat germ, whole grains, fortified cereal). Here's what a vegetarian day looks like:

BREAKFAST
1½ cups nine-grain cooked cereal topped with 1 oz chopped almonds, ¾ cup blueberries, 2 Tbsp honey, and 8 oz soy milk

MIDMORNING SNACK
2 oz trail mix: raisins, dried papaya, and pumpkin seeds

LUNCH
1 bean burrito: 1 cup black beans, ½ cup rice, 1 oz soy cheese, and ¼ cup salsa; 1 cup fruit salad

MIDAFTERNOON SNACK
1 banana spread with 2 Tbsp peanut butter; 8 oz cranberry juice

DINNER
1 cup spinach pasta with "meat" sauce: ¾ cup red sauce and 2 crumbled soy burgers; 1 cup steamed broccoli; 1½ cups dark greens tossed with 1 Tbsp olive oil vinaigrette; 1 oz dark chocolate

If You Want To . . . Heal Injuries

Whether you're ripped, torn, or broken, your body needs extra nutrients to put you back together, says Applegate. In particular, you want to emphasize bone-, skin- and muscle-healing nutrients such as protein, zinc, calcium, and antioxidants (vitamins C, E, beta-carotene, and other carotenes and flavonoids).

This menu reflects a lower-calorie diet (1,530 calories). To increase calories to 2,500, add a sandwich to lunch, add a snack, and slightly increase portions.

BREAKFAST
½ cup high-fiber cereal mixed with ¼ cup whole-grain cereal, topped with 2 tsp chopped nuts and 6 oz 1% milk; orange; latte made 4 oz 1% milk and sprinkled with 1 tsp chocolate shavings

MIDMORNING SNACK
Energy bar containing 12 grams of protein

LUNCH
1 cup reduced-fat cottage cheese; 1 chopped tomato; 3 Tbsp mixed nuts; 2 medium kiwi

MIDAFTERNOON SNACK
¼ cup dried cherries; 2 chocolate candies

DINNER
1 cup spinach pasta tossed with ⅓ cup tomato sauce and 3 oz clams; 2 cups greens with ¼ cup whole soybeans

If You Want To . . . Gain Muscle

Pumping up your muscles means more time on the leg press and about 50 percent more protein on your plate, as well as more carbs for fuel, says Applegate. Here's what a muscle-building diet looks like.

BREAKFAST

Fruit smoothie: 6 oz pasteurized liquid egg substitute, 4 oz vanilla soy milk, 1 cup frozen blueberries, 4 oz cranberry juice, and crushed ice, blended; 1 whole-wheat English muffin with 1 tsp margarine and 1 Tbsp jam

MIDMORNING SNACK

Energy bar with 1 tsp peanut butter; 8 oz milk

LUNCH

Tuna sandwich: 2 slices whole-wheat bread, 3 oz tuna, 2 tsp reduced-fat mayonnaise, lettuce, and tomato slices; ½ cup baked corn chips; 1 cup fruit salad (pineapple, peaches, kiwi)

MIDAFTERNOON SNACK

Half an energy bar; 16 oz sports drink

DINNER

1½ cups bean and turkey chili; 1 cup brown rice; 1 cup red and green bell pepper slices dipped in 2 Tbsp reduced-fat dressing; 2 oatmeal cookies

If You Want To... Speed Recovery

Most of us exercise (and feel) our best with a diet at the recommended standard of 65 to 70 percent carbs, 15 percent protein, and 15 to 20 percent fat. But some people perform better and feel more satisfied with a little more protein, says Franzese. Protein makes you feel fuller sooner and longer, so you don't have the energy spikes that sometimes accompany high-carb meals. When you're training hard, you also break down muscle tissue, which protein helps repair. And when you exercise, you lose protein, which you need to replenish.

Here are two sample menus with about 20 percent protein (but still about 2,500 calories per day).

Day 1

BREAKFAST

2 cups bran cereal with raisins and 8 oz 1% milk or fortified soy milk

MIDMORNING SNACK

2 slices whole-wheat toast with 2 Tbsp peanut butter

LUNCH

2½ cups pasta; 2 oz grilled chicken (size of about 2 fingers); 1 cup broccoli; apple

MIDAFTERNOON SNACK

Yogurt smoothie: 8 oz low-fat yogurt, 4 oz fruit juice, ½ banana, and 2 Tbsp wheat germ, blended

DINNER

4 oz meat, fish, or low-fat cheese (portion should fit in the palm of your hand) or 2 to 3 eggs; large potato or sweet potato; 1 cup cooked spinach; ½ cup cooked carrots; 1 cup grapes

EVENING SNACK

4 to 5 whole-grain crackers with 3 Tbsp olive spread or hummus

Day 2

BREAKFAST

2-egg omelet with 1 oz feta cheese, a handful of spinach, and tomato; 2 slices toast with 1 tsp butter; 4 oz grapefruit juice

MIDMORNING SNACK

1 oz reduced-fat cheese (about the size of a finger) on 2 slices whole-wheat bread

LUNCH

1⅓ cups brown rice with 1 cup string beans sautéed in 1 tsp olive oil, sprinkled with a small handful of sliced almonds; 1 cup strawberries

MIDAFTERNOON SNACK

Yogurt smoothie (see recipe Day 1)

DINNER

4 oz steak (about palm size); 2 cups pasta with 1 cup chopped tomato sautéed in 1 tsp olive oil with chile pepper and sliced basil leaves; ½ cup Brussels sprouts, cooked; 1 cup melon

EVENING SNACK

Low-fat fruit granola bar; 8 oz reduced-fat yogurt or soy milk

Whip Up the Perfect Postworkout Smoothie

Depending on what you toss in them, smoothies are more than just a refreshing postworkout snack. With the right ingredients, they offer a wide range of immediate heart-saving, muscle-building, brain-juicing, mood-boosting benefits. Here are the building blocks and the blueprints—all you need to do is liquefy.

INGREDIENTS

Peanut butter: Packed with protein, manganese, and niacin, peanuts can help stave off heart disease and, when eaten in moderation, promote weight loss.

1% milk: Contains all the calcium and protein, with less fat.

Blueberries: The huge amounts of antioxidants, such as anthocyanins, in blueberries have been shown to slow brain decline and reverse memory loss.

Reduced-fat vanilla yogurt: Contains a cache of calcium and digestion-aiding probiotics in every scoop.

Raspberries: An antioxidant powerhouse bursting with fiber, manganese, and vitamin C, these berries will keep your heart and brain in top shape.

Fat-free chocolate frozen yogurt: Calcium, phosphorus, and none of the guilt.

Pineapple-orange juice: OJ has vitamin C, and pineapples contain bromelain, a cancer-inhibiting, inflammation-reducing enzyme.

Cherries: In addition to their vitamin C and fiber content, cherries have been linked to reducing arthritis pain.

Bananas: Heavy on potassium, fiber, and vitamin B_6, bananas do wonders for your heart and provide good carbs to keep you full and energized.

Whey protein: Its essential amino acids help pack on the muscle—making whey the best friend of athletes and gym rats.

Frozen mangoes: To their stock of vitamins A and C, mangoes add a healthy dose of beta-carotene, which helps prevent cancer and promotes healthy skin.

Ice: A little H_2O never hurt anyone.

RECIPES

BRAIN BOOSTER
The berries here aren't just superfood for your brain; they offer an important cancer-fighting bonus.

- ½ cup fresh or frozen blueberries
- ½ cup fresh or frozen raspberries
- 1 cup pineapple-orange juice
- ½ cup reduced-fat vanilla yogurt
- 1 cup ice

MUSCLE BUILDER
This mix features the brawn-building power of protein from both peanut butter and whey.

- 2 Tbsp peanut butter
- 1 banana
- ⅓ cup whey protein
- ½ cup reduced-fat chocolate frozen yogurt
- 1 cup 1% milk

HEART HELPER
The fiber from the fruit teams with the artery-protecting antioxidants and healthy monounsaturated fats of the peanut butter to keep your ticker tickin'.

- 1 banana
- ½ cup raspberries
- 1 Tbsp peanut butter
- ½ cup reduced-fat chocolate frozen yogurt
- 1 cup 1% milk

SMOOTH OPERATOR
The yogurt aids digestion, while the mango and juice boost immune response.

- ½ cup pitted cherries
- ½ cup mango
- ½ cup reduced-fat vanilla yogurt
- 1 cup pineapple-orange juice
- 1 cup ice

MOOD MAKER
This all-fruit smoothie is packed with carbs to boost your serotonin levels. Add a handful of flaxseeds for an extra dose of mood-boosting omega-3 fatty acids.

- ½ cup fresh or frozen blueberries
- ½ cup fresh or frozen mango
- 1 cup pineapple-orange juice
- 1 cup ice

The All-Star Diets

Chapter 18

JUST AS YOU WOULDN'T FOLLOW THE SAME REGIMEN AS A BODY BUILDER IF YOU WERE TRAINING FOR A TRIATHLON, YOU DON'T WANT TO BE EATING LIKE HIM, EITHER. HERE'S HOW TO TAILOR THE BEST SPORTS NUTRITION NO MATTER WHAT YOUR FITNESS GOAL.

Sports nutrition is easy, if you're a cartoon character. Take Popeye: The gravel-voiced sailorman would down a can of spinach, and next thing he knew he was shot-putting Bluto. Try that at home and the only thing you'll be heaving is the spinach. "No specific food will make you faster or stronger tomorrow," says Lonnie Lowery, RD, PhD, an exercise and nutrition scientist. Instead, whatever your goal—packing on muscle, going the distance, or losing that gut—you have to think long-term. "Sports nutrition is all about many factors adding up over time," he says. In other words, think marathon, not sprint.

Even though there's nothing that will make you an instant athlete (or substitute for that last set of reps), the right foods and drinks can help you work harder, train longer, and look better. Good nutrition supports good workouts, and good workouts make the most of good nutrition. We've rounded up the latest research to help you fuel the body you have and create the body you want. All you need is enough strength to twist a lid, tear a pouch, and, yes, open a can.

TO INCREASE YOUR ENDURANCE

The right carbs (and occasionally even a dose of salt) can help you go farther, longer. In some ways, your body is one big bundle of fuel wrapped in skin. A man of average size stores enough fat to sustain him for days, weeks, maybe months. So why is it so hard to exercise for much longer than a couple of hours at a time? One word: glycogen. It's glucose in storage form, and your body's most easily accessible source of energy. You can work, sleep, or wander the mall all day without ever making a dent in the glycogen stored in your muscles and liver. But the minute you ramp it up, your energy supply is on the clock.

"Most adults have enough glycogen to exercise 1 to 3 hours at most. If you're exercising at moderate to high intensity, your glycogen levels will sink more rapidly," says Marie Spano, MS, RD, a sports nutritionist in Atlanta who works with pro and college athletes. Your body will never let you use all your glycogen—there's always some in reserve—but you'll start slowing down when the needle nears the E. To train seriously, you need to delay that moment as long as possible.

Load up to go long. Research shows that eating the right amount of carbs several hours before a race or a multihour training session can maximize your glycogen supply, which boosts your endurance. To top off your tank, your preworkout meal should include $\frac{1}{2}$ to 1 gram of carbohydrates per pound of body weight, Spano says. For a 180-pound guy, that's between 350 and 700 calories from carbs (or 2 to 4 cups of cooked spaghetti). Which end of the range is right for you? Depends on how much time you have to digest. The longer the lag before game time, the more you can eat.

Eat right for short workouts. If you're exercising for an hour or less, you don't need to make special dietary accommodations. But you do need fuel to sustain yourself. Lowery recommends eating a simple meal with at least 200 calories, 20 grams of protein, and 30 grams of carbs an hour or two before your workout. A simple grilled-chicken sandwich will set you up.

Drink for endurance. Exercise-induced dehydration slows your motor neurons; it's as if you were making Michael Phelps swim through Jell-O. Not only do you feel fatigue sooner than you otherwise would, but your performance slips as well. Skipping liquids also means missing out on an easy-to-absorb delivery system for the nutrients your body needs during or after exercise.

Knowing how much fluid you need to replace isn't easy. Sweat rates range from a pint an hour to four times that, and of course rates fluctuate with the weather. Whatever you do, don't rely on thirst as a gauge. By the time you're hankering for a drink, you're probably well on your way to dehydration.

There's one way to know for sure if you're drinking enough: Weigh yourself before and after a long race or training session. Almost all the weight you lose is water. Replace each lost pound with 24 ounces (3 cups) of fluid. Another indicator of hydration status is your urine. If your bladder goes longer than 3 hours without a cry for help, you're probably not drinking enough, Spano says. Color matters, too; urine shouldn't be darker than a pale lager.

Go for the fast burn. If you have to be on the starting line first thing in the morning and your window for digesting food is less than an hour, go for easily digestible carbs with high water content, such as bread (which surprisingly contains 35 percent water) and lower-fiber fruits, like melons and bananas. Stay away from foods that are high in protein and fat (nuts, for example), which take longer to digest than quick carbs do. Also, avoid high-fiber fruits and vegetables (beans, broccoli, raisins, berries), which can cause gastrointestinal distress if you eat them just prior to strenuous exercise.

Caffeinate a workout. Caffeine does more than keep you awake. If you're a long-haul athlete, it can boost your performance, help you use more fat for energy (thus sparing your precious glycogen), and reduce post-training pain. Curiously, though, you can't reap these benefits from the world's most popular caffeine-delivery system. "There seems to be a compound in coffee that limits caffeine's benefits," says Jay Hoffman, PhD, a professor of sports and fitness at the University of Central Florida. That's why caffeine studies that demonstrate its benefits have involved people drinking powdered caffeine dissolved in water instead of consuming coffee.

Energy drinks are another source of caffeine. But they also pack a boatload of calories, and you'd need a PhD in chemistry to decipher their ingredient lists. Consider taking a caffeine tablet instead, so you know what you're consuming. Studies show benefits with 1.4 to 2.7 milligrams of caffeine per pound of body weight, which works out to about 252 milligrams for a 180-pound guy (maximum-strength NoDoz contains 200 milligrams). If you aren't a heavy coffee or soda drinker, you'll probably get wired with less.

Add salt for stamina. There's plenty of hype about the evils of salt, but avoiding it is bad advice for any man who does high-volume, high-intensity training, especially in heat and humidity. If you regularly sweat out 2 to 3 percent of your body's weight—3 to 6 pounds, for most of us—you probably need more sodium. Spano recommends SaltStick Caps (saltstick.com), an electrolyte-replacement product developed by a former pro triathlete. Each capsule has double the sodium of a typical sport drink.

Juice up your body. To protect your muscles during intense training, think dark-red fruit. A study at Oregon Health & Science University showed that runners who drank tart cherry juice for a week before an ultra-endurance challenge had less pain after the race. Tart cherries, red grapes, and pomegranates are all available in juice form and are loaded with anthocyanins, a type of antioxidant that helps reduce the muscle inflammation and damage caused by serious exercise. The high level of antioxidants in the fruit might also be good for your heart. In a study in the *Journal of Nutrition*, participants drank about 8 ounces of tart cherry juice or a placebo twice a day for 2 weeks. Researchers found the juice reduced oxidative damage, which can contribute to heart disease.

Refuel on the fly. Along with providing water and carbohydrates, sport drinks replace some of the minerals you lose through heavy sweating. Three of those minerals—potassium, magnesium, and chloride—are called electrolytes for a simple reason: Your body needs them to transmit electrical signals from your brain to your muscles. Those signals travel through your body's fluids, which are regulated by another electrolyte, sodium. If you'll be running or riding continuously for longer than an hour, start replenishing your carbohydrate and electrolyte stores around the 30-minute mark, and every 15 minutes after that, Spano says. You want 30 to 60 grams of carbs for every hour of exertion. So if you tank up with 4 ounces of a sport drink (which usually has about 7 grams of carbs) at 15-minute intervals, you'll reach the low end of that range. Eight ounces every 15 minutes and you'll be at the high end.

TO FEED YOUR MUSCLES

Lifting alone won't build muscle. You need plenty of good-quality protein. Imagine living in a house that's constantly under construction. That's what it's like inside your body, where three shifts of molecular laborers tear down and build up muscle tissue all day, every day. After strength training, your body's construction crew wants to work overtime, but it needs the right building materials. "Consume protein as soon as possible after strength exercise," says Stuart Phillips, PhD, a professor of kinesiology at McMaster University in Ontario. If you eat nothing, your muscle growth will be seriously hampered—you could even lose muscle, in fact. Be strategic with foods and supplements instead, and you'll reap big results from your workout.

Whey to grow. When it comes to muscle growth, one protein source stands out. "Whey protein offers the biggest benefit," Phillips says. You digest it more quickly than other types of protein, so it hits your muscles faster. Whey protein also has the highest concentration of the amino acid leucine, giving it more muscle-building power than anything in the supermarket. Phillips recommends 25 grams of whey protein postworkout. There's no harm in having more, but there's no proven benefit, either.

Combine protein with carbs. Together, they achieve more than either does on its own. Carbs may help protein reach your muscles faster, speeding growth. Meanwhile, some research suggests protein accelerates the buildup of glycogen. Even if you're on a low-carb diet, you should take in some carbs with your postworkout protein. Use a protein supplement that contains carbs or add your own with whole fruit. Mix some in a blender with water and ice for the perfect postworkout treat. You can also use skim milk instead of a protein supplement—24 ounces (3 cups) provides 25 grams of protein, 35 grams of carbs, and a generous dose of muscle-building leucine.

Hit the right ratio. For men who run, lift, or play sports a few hours a week, no postworkout combination of carbs and protein has been shown to work better than any other. But if you're a serious athlete who trains hard for over an hour every day, some research has shown that your best results will come with a ratio of carbs to protein that's at least 2:1. Two supplements that are specially formulated to hit this ratio are Gatorade's G Series Pro 03 Recover (for runners, elite athletes, and aspiring professional athletes) and Biotest's Surge Recovery (for serious lifters).

Pop the muscle vitamin. Back in the day, fitness buffs were really into the benefits of sunlight. Charles Atlas, for example, included daily sunbaths in his famous Dynamic-Tension program. Today, science is starting to figure out what old-school bodybuilders understood intuitively: Vitamin D, created by your body through direct sun exposure without sunscreen protection, has an important role in muscle health and function.

Giving your body more D (through supplements and/or sun exposure) could very well help you grow stronger and avoid injury. Researchers at the University of Wyoming say most people would benefit from taking a supplement with 1,000 to 2,000 international units (IU) of vitamin D each day. You can also learn more about the benefits of vitamin D in Chapter 32.

Don't lift dehydrated. Weight training doesn't cause dehydration; after all, lifters tend to work out in air-conditioned gyms. But if you're dehydrated before a lifting session, you could do more harm than good. A 2008 study in the *Journal of Applied Physiology* found that dehydrated lifters produced more stress hormones, including cortisol, while reducing the release of testosterone, the body's best muscle builder. If you lift first thing in the morning, have a glass of water first. This is especially important if you're dehydrated from the night before.

Boost your results. If you're looking to increase your strength and workout capacity by as much as 10 percent and add muscle size over time, you can't go wrong with the one supplement shown to do both in numerous studies: creatine monohydrate. For the fastest results, the International Society of Sports Nutrition recommends loading with 0.14 gram per pound of body weight a day (about 25 grams for a 180-pound man) for at least 3 days, and then maintaining with 3 to 5 grams a day. If you're not in a hurry, taking 2 to 3 grams a day for a month will achieve the same result. Skip the nitric oxide supplements, though. "They're a waste of money," Phillips says. "I'm stunned that they've stuck around as long as they have."

Fight off fatigue. Beta-alanine is another supplement with solid science behind it. It's an amino acid your body uses to form a compound called carnosine. "Carnosine is found in skeletal muscle and helps you delay fatigue," Hoffman says. Early research suggests it could help improve strength and endurance. There's no firm dosage recommendation yet, but University of Oklahoma researchers suggest taking 6.4 grams a day, spread over four doses.

To see results, however, you need to be patient. It takes 2 to 4 weeks to build up enough carnosine in your muscles to have an effect. The good news: Levels stay elevated for weeks after you stop supplementing.

Mix and match. Combining creatine with beta-alanine can also be a smart move. One of Hoffman's College of New Jersey studies found that college football players who took both supplements (10.5 grams a day of creatine, 3.2 grams a day of beta-alanine) had more productive workouts and less fatigue, and built more muscle than those who took only creatine.

Eat for more energy. If you're following a daily training regimen, don't eat like a guy who's trying to drop pounds. A study in the *Journal of Applied Physiology* showed that athletes who trained to exhaustion after 2 days of low-carb eating slowed down the process of building muscle. "The lower you drive carbohydrates down, the more you need other fuel for energy," Phillips says. "Drop carbs below 40 percent of total calories at that activity level, and you're going to sacrifice performance."

And keep eating. To grow a pound of muscle, your body needs about 2,800 calories. If you want to build it in a week, that means you'll need about 400 extra calories a day, says Lowery. "In our studies, the only times we've seen big gains in muscle are with the men who were the biggest eaters," adds Phillips. Now, if you find yourself struggling to swallow those additional calories (some guys do), the problem could be your go-to protein. While whey is terrific in a postworkout drink, it's also the most satiating type of protein, blunting appetite more than tuna, eggs, or turkey, according to a recent study published in the *British Journal of Nutrition*.

TO BURN FAT

Some men don't work out to lose body fat. They eat and train with the goal of becoming stronger or faster or better at their sport, and a great physique is just part of the deal. In fact, athletes can screw up their chance for glory by focusing too much on appearance—that is, cutting the calories they need to fuel their workouts. But for most of us, better performance is just a nice perk. What we really want is to drop fat without losing muscle.

Calculate your carbs. The key to shedding flab is to adjust your carb intake to your activity level. *Men's Health* nutrition advisor Alan Aragon, MS, has a simple way to calculate how many carbs you need.

Multiply your target body weight by 1 if you have a desk job, work out in a gym several times a week for an hour or less, and your main goal is fat loss. Multiply by 2 if you're a recreational athlete who trains for more than an hour a day. And multiply by 3 if you're a competitive athlete who trains multiple hours a day, or if you're a guy with a Mini Cooper body and a Corvette metabolism who is struggling to gain weight.

The number you end up with indicates how many grams of carbs you should eat every day. If you're in category 1 and weigh 180 pounds, that's the equivalent of about two Chipotle burritos.

Eat to lose weight. Don't forget the protein. About 25 percent of the protein calories in your food are burned off in digestion, absorption, and chemical changes in your body, so protein has less of a caloric impact. And perhaps best of all, it defends your hard-earned muscle tissue when you're trying to lose fat. A study in *Medicine & Science in Sports & Exercise* found that a weight loss diet with 35 percent of its calories from protein preserved muscle mass in athletes, while a diet with just 15 percent protein led to an average loss of $3\frac{1}{2}$ pounds of muscle in just 2 weeks. Aim for a daily intake of about 1 gram of protein per pound of target body weight when you're working to lose fat.

Blend the best shake. You can boost the appetite-suppressing effect of a whey shake by whipping it to a froth. When Penn State researchers had men drink blended shakes of various volumes, they found that the men who drank the more-aerated shakes ate 12 percent less food at their next meal. The scientists speculate that the larger appearance of the shakes made men think they were drinking more.

Fight fat with fat. A lean body is a well-oiled machine. A 2007 study in *The American Journal of Clinical Nutrition* showed that people who swallowed 1.9 grams of omega-3s daily and did cardio a little more than 2 hours a week reduced their body fat, lowered their triglycerides, and raised their HDL cholesterol. Here's the kicker: When another group with the same exercise regimen was given sunflower oil (which has mostly omega-6 fats) instead, they lost hardly any fat. Omega-3s are powerful body sculptors in their own right.

Fixing the omega imbalance is a two-step process. First, says Aragon, take three to six fish oil capsules a day, for a total of 1 to 2 grams of DHA and EPA. Second, cut back on omega-6s. Many salad dressings and mayonnaises are packed with soybean oil, the source of more omega-6 fats than any other food. Choose salad dressings made with extra-virgin olive oil (rich in heart-healthy monounsaturated fats), and use mustard instead of mayo.

20 Instant Pre- or Postworkout Bites

Sliced tomato with a sprinkle of feta and olive oil
Lunch left something to be desired? This savory dish will make your tastebuds happy.

Banana
This is naturally pre-packaged goodness you can take anywhere, with the added benefit of cramp-preventing potassium.

½ cup edamame (shelled)
Eating this protein-packed pick-me-up out of the shell will help make the snack last longer.

Light yogurt (fruit flavors)
This bone-building goodie provides 20 percent of your RDA for calcium and vitamin D.

4 shrimp with cocktail sauce
The perfect appetizer—and no one at the table will know you're counting calories.

2 light string cheese snacks
Any food you can play with is a great distraction—plus, the protein battles midafternoon hunger pangs.

Granola bar
Stash chocolate-peanut or strawberries-and-cream bars in your glove box to help you resist the lure of the drive-thru when you're on the road.

1 cup baby carrots with 2 Tbsp hummus
The crunchy texture keeps choppers busy, and tangy hummus feeds your need for comfort food.

1¼ oz turkey jerky
When you must have meat, chew on this low-cal, low-fat power snack.

½ cantaloupe
Like most fruit, melon contains a lot of water. So you get a lot of food—and beta-carotene—for not a lot of calories.

1 cup vegetable juice and 2 oz oven-roasted turkey breast
Here's an antioxidant- and protein-rich hunger buster.

1 Tbsp peanuts and 2 Tbsp dried cranberries
Toss together this pared-down trail mix and premeasure into plastic baggies.

1 cup strawberries and 3 Tbsp fat-free whipped topping
For a totally guiltless dessert, dish up a bowl of this sweet, fiber-rich combo.

1 cup raspberries with 2 Tbsp plain yogurt and 1 tsp honey
This sweet mix does the job until you can break away from your desk for a full meal.

2 egg whites with 1 slice whole-wheat toast
This protein-and-carb duo gives you a light but energizing start when you have a belly-busting lunch on your calendar.

1 oz yellowtail and 1 oz tuna sashimi
The protein will keep you from getting ravenous later.

18 mini pretzel twists
This kill a carbs-and-salt craving in a single snack session. Plus, this smart munchie will keep you fuller longer, so you won't reach for a higher-calorie food.

Chocolate milk (1 cup fat-free milk plus 1 Tbsp chocolate syrup)
Quell your inner cocoa monster and get a hit of calcium.

¼ cup sunflower seeds
They're packed with nutrients, and snacking on a handful may regulate your nerves and muscles.

1½ cups plain frozen yogurt with fresh fruit
It has less fat than ice cream but 5 grams of filling protein per serving. Fruit gives it more flavor, texture, and vitamins.

30 in-shell pistachios
Just one helping will satisfy a salt craving while delivering more natural antioxidants than most other nuts. Plus, the shells will slow you down.

Stock Up, Shape Up

Part Five

It's easy to tell someone how to eat. And for you, the reader, it's even easier to scan through the previous pages and be psyched about the new possibilities in how you approach eating. But then you walk into your kitchen and the questions hit hard and fast: Whoa, what foods should I buy? How do I stock up? Where do I start? Start here. This section is all about showing you how to navigate the supermarket, how to choose the best foods, and how to make your shopping trips quick, easy, and stress free. It's pretty simple: If the right foods aren't in your home, you can't eat them. Use this guide to keep your cupboards filled with the very best.

Chapter 19

Master the Market

LEARN TO NAVIGATE YOUR WAY THROUGH EACH AISLE OF THE GROCERY STORE SO YOU DON'T WASTE TIME, MONEY, OR CALORIES ON SUBPAR INGREDIENTS.

A hundred years ago, people didn't worry about trans fats in their cheese crackers or artificial colors in their fruit snacks. They didn't have to—they were eating real cheese and real fruit. And food companies used to focus more on making food than on enticing people to buy it. That's why supermarkets are so daunting today: It's easy to make a false move, even when you're trying to eat healthfully.

"The influence of marketing on what Americans eat has been gigantic," says Frederick J. Zimmerman, PhD, chairman of the health services department at UCLA's School of Public Health. "We tend to eat 'typical' meals, but marketers are the ones who define what that is." It's time to regain control over what you're eating. The first step? Learning how to navigate the aisles of the grocery store. Here's how.

MARKET STRATEGY #1: IGNORE THE PACKAGING BILLBOARDS

Time for a turnaround. "The front of a food package is real estate owned by the manufacturer, whose goal is to sell you something," says *Men's Health* weight loss advisor David Katz, MD, MPH. Flip the package over to find the information you need on the part that's well regulated by the FDA: the Nutrition Facts label.

Calories
A University of Minnesota study showed that 91 percent of shoppers often bypass the calorie count before buying an item. That's bad: If each meal exceeds your energy needs by just 170 calories, you can gain a pound a week.

Fat
Plenty of men still assume that if a food is low in fat, it's good for them and vice versa. Far from it, says Katz. A better approach: Seek out healthier omega-3 and monounsaturated fats to reap heart-health benefits.

Sodium
Some studies suggest that healthy men don't need to watch their sodium, but the more sodium a food has, the more processed it's likely to be. Rule of thumb: Don't buy foods with higher sodium counts than calories.

Protein
An average active guy should take in at least 115 grams of protein a day, says *Men's Health* nutrition advisor Alan Aragon, MS. Plus, protein-rich foods keep you full longer, so they may help prevent overeating.

Serving Size
"Don't assume the amount listed is an accurate serving size for you," says Chris D'Adamo, PhD, a nutritional epidemiologist at the University of Maryland School of Medicine. Assess how much you'll actually eat and judge the impact accordingly, D'Adamo says.

Fiber
The USDA recommends 38 grams a day for men. To reach that, be sure to eat grain products that contain at least 2 grams of fiber per 100 calories.

Sugar
We consume about 10 percent more caloric sweeteners today than we did 30 years ago, the USDA reports. In that same period, adult obesity has doubled. Coincidence? Keep the sugars below 10 percent of total calories—that's $2^1/_2$ grams of sugar per 100 calories, says Katz.

MARKET STRATEGY #2: CHALLENGE THE CASHIER

Every industry employs tools that make routine tasks easier. For register jockeys, it's the UPC bar code. UPCs let the cashier become a brainless automaton that dutifully drags cans and boxes over a static scanner. Fruits and vegetables are the cashier's enemy—no bar codes. "I tell clients all the time to move from bar codes to bags," says nutrition consultant Mike Roussell, PhD. In other words, the harder your cashier works, the healthier your purchase tends to be. You'll reap the rewards when you step on the scale: A 2009 *Journal of Nutrition* study of nearly half a million people found that men with diets high in vegetables, seafood, legumes, fruits, nuts, and cereal grains—all foods typically purchased in bulk and without bar codes—had smaller waist circumferences.

MARKET STRATEGY #3: CONSIDER THE RECIPE

Twinkies, Pop-Tarts, French's Classic Yellow Mustard—they all have their recipes printed right on the package. It's near the Nutrition Facts label under the word "Ingredients." "If the contents cannot be placed in any part of the universe you're familiar with—animal, vegetable, or mineral—then step away from the box and nobody will get hurt," says Katz. Here are three companies that have come clean and eliminated certain mystery additives.

Eden Foods
What it eliminated: Bisphenol A
Why: UK scientists have linked BPA, a chemical used to line metal cans, with heart disease and diabetes. Worse, a CDC study detected it in the urine of 95 percent of Americans tested. Recently, Eden Foods became the first US producer of BPA-free canned goods.

Hormel Natural Choice
What it eliminated: Added nitrates and nitrites
Why: A Harvard meta-analysis from 2010 linked processed meats (not red meat itself) to coronary heart disease and listed nitrates and their by-products as some of the likely culprits. Hormel's Natural Choice line uses a high-pressure processing method instead.

Oh Boy! Oberto
What it eliminated: Hydrolyzed protein
Why: Oberto's new all-natural jerky line skips this additive, which is chemically similar to MSG. That's good news: A study in Obesity found that people who consumed the most MSG were almost three times as likely to be overweight as MSG avoiders were.

MARKET STRATEGY #4: CALL YOUR REP IN CONGRESS

The average US household kicks in about $1,500 in annual subsidies, and the foods we subsidize most are among the least healthy, says Thomas Kostigen, author of *The Big Handout*. Check out the foods (and nonfoods) your tax dollars support.

CORN
$77.1 billion

WHEAT
$32.4 billion

SOYBEANS
$24.3 billion

SORGHUM
$6.1 billion

DAIRY
$4.9 billion

TOBACCO
$1.1 billion

OATS
$267 million

APPLES
$262 million

POTATOES
$665,698

BLUEBERRIES
$207,659

AVOCADOS
$6,984

TOMATOES, BROCCOLI, LETTUCE: $0

US subsidies from 1995 to 2010, according to the Environmental Working Group

MARKET STRATEGY #5: MASTER YOUR IMPULSES

Easy-grab items at the market tend to be built from bottom-of-the-barrel ingredients—sugar, starch, and cheap fats. Use these strategies to resist their siren song.

Grab a cart. A study in the *Journal of Marketing Research* shows that shopping with a basket instead of a cart makes you nearly seven times more likely to purchase vice foods like candy and chocolate. The researchers say that curling your arm inward to carry a basket increases your desire to embrace instant rewards—like sweet foods. With a cart, you tend to extend your arm—a motion associated with avoiding negative outcomes. That makes you more likely to shop smart.

Avoid lines. The longer you're exposed to tempting snacks at the checkout, the more likely you are to succumb to them, say University of Arizona researchers. Avoid the wait by shopping during off-peak hours, such as the middle of the week or late at night.

Leave the kids at home. "Children shouldn't have a vote in supermarket decisions," says Greg Critser, author of *Fat Land: How Americans Became the Fattest People in the World*. About 80 percent of parents report they'll probably buy snacks or frozen desserts if their kids ask for them at the grocery store, according to a 2011 Mintel report.

MARKET STRATEGY #6: DISCOVER THE CHEAPEST HEALTHY FOODS

To save cash, we compared prices of foods that scored 90 or higher on the NuVal scale, a sophisticated system used to rank their overall nutritional values. Then we chose the cheapest common items per serving from five spots on the color wheel. Prices shown are per serving.

Purple
Red cabbage, 15¢
- A dose of vitamin A, fiber, and glucosinolates, which may help prevent some types of cancer

Black
Dry black beans, 12¢
- Loaded with fiber and plenty of brain-boosting anthocyanins

Orange
Butternut squash, 19¢
- Lots of beta-carotene and less than half the calories of a sweet potato

Green
Spinach, 38¢
- Packed with folate, a B vitamin shown to bolster cognitive performance

Yellow
Banana, 13¢
- Potassium rich, with prebiotic fiber that promotes good gut bacteria

MARKET STRATEGY #7: SHOP FOR SHORTCUTS

Not all boxed, bagged, and jarred foods are terrible, says J. Lynne Brown, PhD, RD. (Case in point: the 125 best packaged foods in Chapter 23.) Shortcut products with honest ingredient lists can save you time—and make a home-cooked dinner on a weeknight a viable option. Start with these meals. They all take less than 5 minutes, use a healthy shortcut ingredient, and use five ingredients, max.

Pasta Dinner
Cook whole-wheat pasta. Simmer tomato sauce with crumbled tuna for 5 minutes. Toss together and top with chopped parsley.

Shrimp Stir-Fry
Stir-fry shrimp and asparagus in olive oil. Add minced garlic at the last minute if you like. Top with a squeeze of lemon and serve over rice.

Mushroom And Dumpling Soup
Cook dumplings in simmering broth. Add sliced shiitake mushrooms for the last 3 minutes and stir in spinach right before serving.

Eggs and Salsa
In a small pan, heat salsa to simmering. Crack in eggs, cover, and cook until the whites are set. Serve with avocado and Wasa crispbread.

Easy Chicken with Slaw
Skin and shred rotisserie chicken and toss with bagged coleslaw mix. Add sriracha to yogurt and toss with the chicken slaw.

MARKET STRATEGY #8: INVEST IN NUTRIENTS, NOT CALORIES

Conventional wisdom says that healthy food costs more than junk food. "The notion of food value that everyone embraces is calories per dollar," says Katz. The problem is, we live in an age of pandemic obesity, and processed foods have made calories abundant and nutrients scarce. Shop for nutrients, not calories, and see where the real value lies.

EAT $1 OF	INSTEAD OF $1 OF	YOU EARN
Sweet potatoes, 1 lb	Ore-Ida Sweet Potato Fries, 5.3 oz	More than quadruple the fiber, nearly five times the bone-building calcium, and more than 19 times the vitamin A
Broccoli, 0.6 lb	Campbell's Cream of Broccoli Condensed Soup, 7.75 oz, unprepared	Almost four times the fiber, twice the muscle-building protein, and an extra dose of vitamin K
Blueberries, 2.9 oz	Kellogg's Blueberry Pop-Tarts (unfrosted), 3½ tarts	A dose of vitamins C and K, plus plenty of disease-fighting phytonutrients
Tomatoes, 0.4 lb	Heinz Ketchup, half of a 20-oz bottle	Twice the fiber and less of a post-eating blood-sugar spike
Oats, 3 cups (uncooked)	Nature Valley Oats 'n Honey Crunchy Granola Bars, 4 bars	Four times the protein, six times the fiber, and nearly six times as much iron
Strawberries, 4 oz	Smucker's Strawberry Topping, 7½ Tbsp	Your RDA of vitamin C and a dose of plant protein and fiber in the bargain

MARKET STRATEGY #9: FILL YOUR CART WITH DARK

When it comes to whole foods, more pigment often means more nutrient power.

	FROM	TO	THE PAYOFF
UPGRADE	Light beer	Dark beer	More iron and cancer-fighting polyphenols
	Honeydew melon	Cantaloupe	Double the vitamin C, plus nearly 70 times the vitamin A and beta-carotene
	White wine	Red wine	A dose of sleep-regulating hormone melatonin and the heart-healthy antioxidant resveratrol
	Chicken breast	Dark-meat chicken	Nearly triple the iron, 245 percent more zinc, and extra vitamin B_{12}
	Iceberg lettuce	Spinach	Triple the protein, a higher concentration of powerful antioxidants like beta-carotene, and loads of vitamin A
	White rice	Brown rice	Thirty percent more of the antioxidant selenium and 4½ times the fiber
	Table sugar	Maple syrup	One hundred times the heart-healthy potassium
	Apple juice	Pomegranate juice	Vitamin K, cell-building folate, abundant antioxidants
	Potato	Sweet potato	More than a day's worth of vitamin A, 2½ times the calcium, and 50 percent more fiber
	Milk chocolate	Dark chocolate	Three and a half times the iron, plus extra antioxidants
	White mushrooms	Baby bellas	Six times the calcium, 40 percent more potassium, and almost triple the selenium

MARKET STRATEGY #10: BEWARE THE NATURAL FOOD STORE

Fancy food shops can still wreck your waistline.

Don't Assume It's Healthier

In a study in the *Journal of Consumer Research*, people estimated familiar foods to have up to 35 percent fewer calories when they came from a "healthy" place. But be warned: Trader Joe's, Whole Foods Market, and Fresh Market all stock plenty of stuff that can make you fat. One cup of Trader Joe's Pecan Praline Granola has as many calories as two twin-wrapped packages of Reese's Peanut Butter Cups.

Watch Out for the Free Samples

Stanford researchers discovered that a tasty sample can make you more likely to engage in reward-seeking behavior, like buying foods you normally wouldn't go for.

Don't Fall for Fads

Just because that scone is vegan, lactose-free, and made with positively charged ions doesn't mean it isn't still loaded with calories. Whole Foods' Gluten Free Vanilla Cupcake has 480 calories, but you wouldn't know that, because foods prepared in-house don't have to carry nutrition labels.

BONUS MARKET STRATEGY: UNDERSTAND SUPERMARKET RATING SYSTEMS

The theory behind these scorecards is that people are more likely to buy healthy foods if they can identify them at a glance rather than, say, freezing their fingers comparing the Nutrition Facts on three different brands of frozen pizza. About 1,600 supermarkets feature NuVal, a system that ranks a food's nutritional value from 1 (poor) to 100 (excellent), while about the same number of stores use Guiding Stars to rank foods from zero stars (poor) to three stars (excellent). Both use algorithms to crunch nutrition data down to a simple score.

The two systems haven't been compared head-to-head, but research suggests that each has its benefits. A 2011 Harvard study linked the consumption of foods with higher NuVal ratings to a 9 to 12 percent lower risk of developing a chronic disease. As for Guiding Stars, a 2010 study published in *The American Journal of Clinical Nutrition* found that people using these rankings purchased a significantly higher percentage of healthy food. "Summary ratings can help you quickly figure out what's in packaged foods, which are often covered in marketing phrases like 'low in fat' or 'all natural,'" says James C. Hersey, PhD, a nutrition researcher at RTI International, a nonprofit institute.

Pick Your Produce

THE TASTIEST, MOST WHOLESOME FRUITS AND VEGETABLES AREN'T ALWAYS THE BEST-LOOKING ONES. HERE'S HOW TO SEPARATE THE NUTRITIONAL ALL-STARS FROM THE DUDS.

The best-tasting, most nutritious produce is easy to find—if you know how to look. Imperfections can be attractive, hinting at surprising sweetness and depth of character. We're talking about food, by the way. Too many supermarkets sell produce bred not just for taste but to withstand shipping—it's well-shaped but not flavorful. You want your fruit to be naturally voluptuous; the farmer's daughter, not the plasticized porn star. Employ your senses. Look: Prime fruits and vegetables are often irregularly shaped and blemished. Touch: Heavy, sturdy fruits and vegetables with taut skin are freshest. Smell: Many fruits can be sniffed for ripeness. And shop seasonally. The foods are tastier and cheaper. We asked Aliza Green, the author of *Field Guide to Produce,* how to find the best.

Decoding Color

Green
Green vegetables are often good sources of magnesium, which helps to protect your bones. Other greens, like Brussels sprouts, are rich in vitamin K, needed for blood clotting.

Yellow
Yellow fruits and vegetables, including pineapples, lemons, and certain tomatoes, often contain vitamin C, which helps heal wounds and clears out free radicals.

Orange
Orange often means caratenoid-rich foods. Carrots are a source of immunity-boosting vitamin A, while vitamin C in orange citrus fruits promotes oral health.

Red
Red produce usually contains anthocyanins, which may fight cancer. Tomatoes have potassium to control blood pressure, and vitamin A in red peppers keeps eyes healthy.

Blue and Purple
Blue and purple fruits and vegetables, like grapes and purple cabbage, have anthocyanins that may protect cells from oxidative damage.

A Field Guide to Fruits and Vegetables

ARTICHOKES
Look for: Deep-green, heavy artichokes, with tightly closed leaves that squeak when pinched together

Peak: March to May

Storage: In the fridge, in a plastic bag, up to 5 days

Payoff: The highest antioxidant capacity of most common vegetables

ASPARAGUS
Look for: Vibrant green spears with tight, purple-tinged buds; thin spears are sweet and tender

Peak: February to June

Storage: Trim the woody ends; stand the spears in a bit of water in a tall container and cover the tops with a plastic bag; cook within a few days

Payoff: Folate, which may protect the heart

AVOCADOS
Look for: Firm ones with no sunken, mushy spots, and a waxy rather than a shiny appearance; shake it—a rattle means the pit has pulled away from the flesh, which is not good

Peak: Year-round

Storage: To ripen, place in a paper bag and store at room temp for 2 to 4 days; add an apple to the bag to speed things up; ripe ones can go in the fridge for up to a week

Payoff: Cholesterol-lowering monounsaturated fat

BELL PEPPERS
Look for: Lots of heft for their size, and brightly colored, wrinkle-free exteriors; the stems should be a lively green

Peak: Year-round

Storage: Refrigerate in the crisper for up to 2 weeks

Payoff: All are loaded with antioxidants, especially vitamin C, but yellow peppers lead the pack

BLUEBERRIES
Look for: Plump, uniform, indigo berries with taut skin and a dull white frost

Peak: May to October

Storage: Transfer them unwashed to an airtight container and refrigerate for 5 to 7 days

Payoff: More disease-fighting antioxidants (especially in wild berries) than most common fruits

BROCCOLI
Look for: Rigid stems with tight floret clusters that are deep green or tinged purple; pass on any with yellowing heads—they'll be more bitter

Peak: October to April

Storage: Refrigerate in a plastic bag for up to 1 week

Payoff: Cancer-fighting sulforaphane

BUTTON MUSHROOMS

Look for: Tightly closed, firm caps that aren't slimy or riddled with dark, soft spots; eat those with open caps and visible gills soon

Peak: September to March

Storage: Spread them on a flat surface, cover with a damp paper towel, and refrigerate for 3 to 5 days

Payoff: Polysaccharides in white button mushrooms may boost immunity and combat tumors

EGGPLANT

Look for: A heavy weight and tight, shiny skin; when pressed, should be springy, not spongy; stem should be bright green

Peak: August to September

Storage: Keep in a cool location (not the fridge) for up to 3 days; eggplants are sensitive to the cold and don't keep well

Payoff: Chlorogenic acid, which scavenges free radicals

GRAPES

Look for: Plump, wrinkle-free grapes that are firmly attached to stems; a silvery white powder on the fruit ("bloom") means they'll stay fresher longer; green grapes with a yellowish hue are the sweetest

Peak: May to October

Storage: Keep unwashed, in a shallow bowl in the fridge, for up to 1 week

Payoff: Resveratrol, which may protect against cardiovascular disease

GREEN BEANS

Look for: Beans with vibrant, smooth surfaces; the best are thin, young, and velvety, and snap when gently bent

Peak: May to October

Storage: Refrigerate unwashed in an unsealed bag for up to 1 week

Payoff: Fiber (almost 4 grams in 1 cup), which is associated with a lower risk of all-cause mortality

KIWIFRUIT

Look for: A ripe kiwi that is slightly yielding to the touch; avoid mushy or wrinkled ones with an "off" smell

Peak: Year-round

Storage: Leave at room temperature to ripen; to quicken the process, place kiwis in a paper bag with an apple or a ripe banana; once ripe, refrigerate in a plastic bag for up to a week

Payoff: 65 percent more vitamin C than a small orange has

PAPAYAS

Look for: Papayas that are starting to turn yellow and yield a bit when lightly squeezed

Peak: June to September

Storage: Once ripe, eat immediately or refrigerate for up to 3 days; green papayas should be ripened at room temperature in a dark setting until yellow blotches appear

Payoff: Lots of fiber and vitamins C, A, E, and K

PEACHES

Look for: A fruity aroma and a yellow or warm cream background color, without green shoulders; they're ready when they yield to gentle pressure on the seams

Peak: May to October

Storage: Leave unripe ones out at room temperature; ripe ones go in the fridge, but eat within 2 to 3 days

Payoff: Vitamin C, beta-carotene, fiber, potassium

PEARS

Look for: A pleasant fragrance and some softness at the stem end; some brown discoloration is fine

Peak: August to March

Storage: Ripen at room temperature in a loosely closed paper bag

Payoff: Fiber and vitamin C, if eaten with the skin

PINEAPPLE

Look for: Vibrant green leaves, a bit of softness to the fruit, and a sweet fragrance at the stem end; avoid spongy fruit

Peak: March to July

Storage: If it's unripe, keep it at room temp for 3 to 4 days until it softens and gives off a pineapple aroma; refrigerate for up to 5 days

Payoff: Niacin for skin and GI health, and manganese for bones

RASPBERRIES

Look for: Plump and dry berries; seek out good shape and intense, uniform color

Peak: May to September

Storage: Place unwashed berries in a single layer on a paper towel; cover with a damp paper towel and refrigerate 2 to 3 days

Payoff: More fiber (8 grams per cup) than any other commonly eaten berry

ROMAINE LETTUCE

Look for: Crisp leaves free of browning edges and rust spots

Peak: Year-round

Storage: Refrigerate for 5 to 7 days in a plastic bag

Payoff: Vitamin K, which is needed for blood clotting and bone health

STRAWBERRIES

Look for: Unblemished berries with a bright-red color extending to the stem and a strong fruity smell; they should be neither hard nor mushy

Peak: April to September

Storage: Place unwashed berries in a single layer on a paper towel in a covered container

Payoff: The most vitamin C of all commonly eaten berries

TOMATOES

Look for: Heavy ones with rich color and no wrinkles, cracks, bruises, or soft spots; they should have some give

Peak: June to September

Storage: Never in a fridge as cold destroys flavor and texture; keep them out of direct sunlight for up to a week

Payoff: Lycopene for prostate health

WATERMELON

Look for: A dense melon free of cuts and sunken areas; the rind should be dull, with a creamy-yellow underside; a slap produces a hollow thump

Peak: June to August

Storage: Keep whole in the fridge for up to a week to prevent flesh from drying out and turning fibrous

Payoff: Citrulline, an amino acid that can help improve blood flow

GET YOUR FILL
In hot or cold dishes, fruits and vegetables add antioxidants, fiber, and tons of luscious flavor. So go ahead—take your pick from these recipes!

Artichoke Hummus

- 1 can (14 oz) artichoke hearts, rinsed and drained
- 1 can (15 oz) chickpeas, rinsed and drained
- 1 Tbsp tahini
- 2 Tbsp lemon juice
- 1 Tbsp minced garlic
- 1 Tbsp extra-virgin olive oil
- ½ tsp cumin
- ½ tsp hot paprika
- 1 cup chopped fresh basil

1. In food processor, combine artichoke hearts, chickpeas, tahini, lemon juice, garlic, oil, cumin, and paprika. Pulse until smooth.

2. Transfer to serving bowl. Stir in basil. Season to taste with salt and pepper.

MAKES 8 SERVINGS.

Per serving (¼ cup):
88 calories, 3 g protein,
9 g carbohydrates (2 g fiber),
4 g fat (0.5 g sat), 172 mg sodium

Asparagus Stir-Fry

1½ Tbsp grapeseed or canola oil
4 oz sliced mushrooms
¾ lb asparagus, trimmed and roughly chopped
1 yellow bell pepper, chopped
2 oz snow peas, sliced
3 Tbsp seasoned rice vinegar
1½ Tbsp reduced-sodium soy sauce
2 tsp dark sesame oil
2 Tbsp chopped cilantro (optional)
    Cooked brown rice

1. Heat oil in large skillet or wok over medium-high heat. Add mushrooms and cook, stirring, until golden, 4 minutes. Add asparagus, bell pepper, and snow peas and cook, stirring, until tender, about 6 minutes.

2. Drizzle with rice vinegar, soy sauce, and sesame oil. Top with cilantro, if desired. Cook 1 minute.

3. Serve over brown rice.

MAKES 4 SERVINGS.

Per serving:
115 calories, 4 g protein,
10 g carbohydrates (3 g fiber),
8 g fat (1 g sat), 427 mg sodium

Turkey and Avocado Sandwich with Slaw

- 1 Tbsp brown mustard
- 2 slices rye bread
- 3 oz low-sodium skinless turkey breast
- 2 slices tomato
- 1 slice red onion
- ¼ cup sliced avocado
- 2 Tbsp golden raisins
- 1 cup shredded cabbage
- 1 cup shredded red cabbage

1. Spread mustard on bread and top with turkey, tomato, onion, and avocado.

2. In large bowl, toss together raisins and cabbages.

MAKES 1 SERVING.

Per serving:
495 calories, 29 g protein,
69 g carbohydrates (14 g fiber),
14 g fat (2g sat), 1,270 mg sodium

Spaghetti with Roasted Red Pepper Sauce

- 2 Tbsp olive oil
- 1 onion, chopped
- 2 cloves garlic, minced
- 1 can (14.5 oz) crushed tomatoes
- 1 jar (12 oz) roasted red bell peppers, rinsed and drained
- 2 Tbsp sherry vinegar or red wine vinegar
- ½ cup finely grated Parmesan cheese
- 2 pkg (8 oz each) quinoa spaghetti
- ¼ cup sliced almonds, toasted

1. Heat 1 Tbsp of the oil in large saucepan over medium heat. Add onion and cook, stirring, until softened, 4 minutes. Add garlic and cook, stirring, 1 minute.

2. Transfer to food processor along with tomatoes, bell peppers, vinegar, and $1/3$ cup of the cheese. Process until smooth. Return to pan. Bring to a simmer, season with salt and pepper, remove from heat, and cover.

3. Cook pasta according to package directions. Drain and place in large serving bowl. Toss with some sauce to coat. Top with almonds and remaining cheese and oil. Serve with remaining sauce.

MAKES 6 SERVINGS.

Per serving:
403 calories, 10 g protein,
72 g carbohydrates (8 g fiber),
10 g fat (2 g sat), 226 mg sodium

Almond-Blueberry Oatmeal

- ¼ cup steel-cut oats
- ¼ cup 1% milk
- 1 Tbsp slivered almonds
- ⅓ cup fresh or frozen blueberries
- 1 tsp ground flaxseeds

1. Prepare oatmeal per package directions.

2. Add milk, almonds, blueberries, and flaxseeds. Mix and serve.

MAKES 1 SERVING.

Per serving:
178 calories, 7 g protein,
26 g carbohydrates (5 g fiber),
6 g fat (0.5 g sat), 40 mg sodium

Chicken with Cheesy Broccoli Soup

- 1 cup chopped broccoli
- 1 cup chopped parsnips
- ¾ cup fat-free chicken broth
- ¼ cup reduced-fat shredded Cheddar cheese
- 1 Tbsp sliced almonds
- 4 oz chicken breast
- 1 tsp lemon juice
- Salt and freshly ground black pepper

1. Place broccoli and parsnips in steamer and set over saucepan of boiling water. Steam 10 minutes. Transfer to blender and add broth and cheese. Puree until smooth. Transfer to saucepan, sprinkle with nuts, and keep warm.

2. Cook chicken however you prefer (grill, bake, sauté, etc.). Drizzle with lemon juice and season to taste with salt and pepper.

3. Add chicken to soup, and serve.

MAKES 1 SERVING.

Per serving:
361 calories, 40 g protein,
32 g carbohydrates (10 g fiber),
8.5 g fat (2 g sat), 794 mg sodium

Lean Turkey Chili

- 1 tsp olive oil
- ½ onion, chopped
- 2 cloves garlic, minced
- 1 Tbsp mixed fresh herbs
- 4 oz ground turkey
- 2 tomatoes, diced
- 2 cups pinto beans
- 1 cup button mushrooms
- 2 bay leaves
- Dash of freshly ground black pepper
- 1 Tbsp paprika
- 2 chile peppers, chopped (wear plastic gloves when handling)

1. Heat oil in large skillet over medium-high heat. Add onion, garlic, and herbs and sauté 5 minutes. Add turkey and sauté 10 minutes.

2. Add tomatoes, beans, and mushrooms to skillet and simmer 5 minutes. Add bay leaves, black pepper, paprika, and chile peppers. Simmer 20 minutes.

3. Remove bay leaves. If you can bear the wait, let it sit for a day—it tastes even better the next day.

MAKES 2 SERVINGS.

Per serving:
367 calories, 25 g protein,
49 g carbohydrates (14 g fiber),
10 g fat (2 g sat), 770 mg sodium

Heirloom Tomato and Eggplant Stacks

- 1 log (4 oz) soft goat cheese, softened
- 2 Tbsp finely chopped fresh basil
- 1 Tbsp chopped fresh thyme
- 1 large eggplant (about 1 lb)
- ¾ tsp salt
- 3 tsp extra-virgin olive oil
- 1 Tbsp balsamic vinegar
- ¼ tsp Dijon mustard
- ¼ tsp freshly ground black pepper
- 2 medium heirloom tomatoes in assorted colors, each cored and thinly sliced crosswise into 4 rounds

1. In medium bowl, combine goat cheese, basil, and thyme. Set aside. Preheat grill.

2. Cut eggplant crosswise into twelve ½"-thick slices. Place in colander, sprinkle with ½ tsp of the salt, and toss to mix. Let stand 10 minutes. Rinse and pat dry. Brush slices with 1 tsp of the oil and grill 4 minutes. Turn slices over and grill until tender, 4 to 5 minutes.

3. In small bowl, combine vinegar, mustard, and remaining 2 tsp oil and whisk to blend. Stir in pepper and remaining ¼ tsp salt.

4. To assemble stacks, place 1 eggplant slice on a plate. Top with ⅛ of the cheese mixture and 1 slice of tomato. Drizzle with ½ tsp vinaigrette. Add another slice of eggplant, cheese, tomato, and a final slice of eggplant. Top with 1 tsp vinaigrette. Repeat to make three more stacks. Let stand 5 minutes to allow cheese to melt.

MAKES 4 SERVINGS.

Per serving:
178 calories, 8 g protein,
11 g carbohydrates (5 g fiber),
12 g fat (6 g sat), 596 mg sodium

Pomegranate-Cranberry Soda

1½ cups 100% unsweetened cranberry juice
½ cup pomegranate juice concentrate
½ cup red or green grapes
3 Tbsp maple syrup
   Seltzer or soda water

1. In medium saucepan, combine juice, juice concentrate, grapes, and maple syrup. Cover and bring to a gentle boil over medium-high heat, then reduce heat to low and simmer, uncovered, 10 minutes, muddling grapes with wooden spoon to break them up.

2. Remove from heat and let mixture sit 15 minutes. Pour mixture through strainer lined with double layer of cheesecloth and squeeze to extract as much liquid as possible.

3. Chill in sealed glass jar in fridge. Syrup will stay fresh up to 3 days. To serve, pour ¼ cup syrup into tall glass, top with 6 to 8 ounces chilled seltzer or soda water, and stir.

MAKES 6 SERVINGS.

Per serving:
117 calories, 0.5 g protein,
31 g carbohydrates (<1 g fiber),
<1 g fat (0 g sat), 2 mg sodium

Lemony Green Beans

½ lb green beans
2 tsp olive oil
¼ cup chopped hazelnuts
1¼ tsp lemon juice
1¼ tsp grated lemon zest
   Salt and freshly ground black pepper

1. Bring a medium saucepan of salted water to a boil and add green beans. Cook until tender, 5 minutes, then drain.

2. Heat oil in large skillet over medium heat. Add beans and hazelnuts and cook 2 minutes. Stir in lemon juice and zest. Season to taste with salt and pepper.

MAKES 4 SERVINGS.

Per serving:
86 calories, 2 g protein,
6 g carbohydrates (3 g fiber),
7 g fat (1 g sat), 133 mg sodium

Pork Braised in Kiwi-Coconut Sauce with White Beans

- 1 Tbsp canola oil
- 6 (1¼" thick) boneless pork loin chops
- ¼ tsp salt
- Freshly ground black pepper
- ½ large red onion, chopped
- 1 can (14 oz) light coconut milk
- 1 Tbsp green curry paste
- 11 kiwis, peeled and chopped (about 4 cups)
- 1 can (15.5 oz) cannellini beans, rinsed
- 1 can (8 oz) pineapple chunks, drained and chopped
- 6 Tbsp sunflower seeds
- 3 Tbsp sliced shallots
- 2 Tbsp chopped cilantro

1. Heat oil in large pot over medium-high heat. Sprinkle pork with salt and season with pepper. Cook chops until bottoms are browned, 2 to 3 minutes. Turn and repeat on opposite sides. Transfer to plate.

2. Reduce heat to medium-low. Add onion and cook, stirring, until soft, 6 minutes. Add coconut milk, curry paste, and 1⅓ cups of the kiwi. Bring to a simmer, cover, and cook until fruit is very soft, 5 minutes. Remove from heat. Working in batches, carefully puree in blender.

3. Return coconut mixture to pot and simmer. Add pork and any juices. Cover and simmer, turning halfway through, until pork is cooked through, 12 minutes.

4. In large bowl, mix beans, pineapple, sunflower seeds, shallots, cilantro, and remaining kiwi. Serve with pork and sauce.

MAKES 6 SERVINGS.

Per serving:
501 calories, 37 g protein,
45 g carbohydrates (9 g fiber),
20 g fat (7 g sat), 427 mg sodium

Golden Gazpacho

2½ cups diced mango (½" chunks), about three 7-oz mangoes total
1 cup orange juice
½ cup diced pineapple (½" chunks)
½ cup diced melon, any variety (½" chunks)
½ cup diced cucumber (½" chunks)
½ cup diced papaya (½" chunks)
6 mint leaves, chopped, plus additional mint leaves for garnish
Juice of ½ lime
1 drop hot-pepper sauce

1. In blender, combine mango, orange juice, pineapple, melon, cucumber, papaya, mint, lime juice, and hot-pepper sauce. Blend until smooth.

2. Pour mixture through sieve into large bowl. Discard pulp.

3. Chill in fridge, then serve, garnished with mint leaves.

MAKES 6 SERVINGS.

Per serving:
102 calories, 1 g protein,
26 g carbohydrates (2.5 g fiber),
0.5 g fat (0 g sat), 5 mg sodium

Grilled Salmon with Peach Salsa

- 3 peaches, pitted and cut in half
- 1 large red bell pepper, cut in half and seeded
- 2 Tbsp canola or grapeseed oil
- ½ red onion, finely diced
- 1 jalapeño chile pepper, seeded and minced (wear plastic gloves when handling)
- ⅓ cup chopped fresh cilantro
- ⅓ cup chopped fresh mint
- 2 tsp honey
- Zest and juice of 1 lime
- 4 wild Alaskan salmon fillets (4 oz each)
- ¼ tsp sea salt

1. Preheat grill to medium. Brush peaches and red pepper with 1 Tbsp of the oil. Grill peaches 4 minutes per side. Grill red peppers until slightly charred all over, turning every 2 minutes. Remove from grill and let cool.

2. In medium bowl, toss together red onion, chile pepper, cilantro, mint, honey, and lime zest and juice. Remove skin from cooled peaches (it will slip off). Chop peaches and red pepper and stir into onion mixture.

3. Brush both sides of salmon fillets with remaining 1 Tbsp oil, then sprinkle with salt. Place on grill, skin side down first, and grill until flesh is light pink throughout and flakes easily, 5 minutes per side. Serve with peach salsa.

MAKES 4 SERVINGS.

Per serving:
380 calories, 25 g protein,
20 g carbohydrates (4 g fiber),
23 g fat (4 g sat), 171 mg sodium

Pear-Thyme Bellini

2 pears, peeled, cored, and chopped
Juice of 2 lemons (about 6 Tbsp)
Fresh thyme sprigs
Chilled sparkling dry wine

1. In food processor, combine pears and lemon juice. Puree until smooth.

2. Divide mixture among 6 champagne glasses, add thyme sprig to each, and top with wine.

MAKES 6 SERVINGS.

Per serving:
135 calories, 0.5 g protein,
12 g carbohydrates (2 g fiber),
<1 g fat (0 g sat), 1 mg sodium

Tropical Guac

- ½ avocado, pitted, peeled, and chopped
- ⅛ tsp salt
- 2 Tbsp chopped red onion
- 1½ Tbsp chopped fresh cilantro
- 2 tsp chopped jalapeño chile pepper (wear plastic gloves when handling)
- 2 tsp lime juice
- ¼ cup chopped pineapple
- ¼ cup chopped mango
- ¼ cup chopped cantaloupe

1. In large bowl, mash avocado and salt together with fork.
2. Gently stir in onion, cilantro, chile pepper, and lime juice.
3. Fold in pineapple, mango, and cantaloupe.

MAKES 4 SERVINGS.

Per serving:
59 calories, 1 g protein,
7 g carbohydrates (2 g fiber),
4 g fat (1 g sat), 77 mg sodium

Rum Berry Sherbet

- ¼ cup honey
- ¼ cup 1% milk
- 2 cups raspberries
- 2 tsp rum (100 proof)

1. In small microwaveable bowl, mix honey and milk and microwave until honey melts.

2. In blender, combine honey-milk mixture with berries and rum. Blend until smooth.

3. Divide among 4 dessert bowls, freeze, and serve.

MAKES 4 SERVINGS.

Per serving:
99 calories, 1 g protein,
24 g carbohydrates (1.5 g fiber),
<1 g fat (0 g sat), 8 mg sodium

Tuna Niçoise Salad

- 2 Tbsp champagne vinegar or white wine vinegar
- 2 Tbsp extra-virgin olive oil
- 1 large shallot, minced
- 1 tsp Dijon mustard
- 4 tuna fillets (6 oz each)
- 1 large head romaine lettuce (8 oz), trimmed
- 4 oz cooked green beans
- 1½ cups cherry tomatoes, halved
- 4 cooked new potatoes, quartered
- ¼ cup sliced red onion
- 12 caper berries
- 28 niçoise olives

1. Preheat grill to medium.

2. In small bowl, whisk together vinegar, oil, shallot, and mustard.

3. Season tuna with salt and pepper to taste. Grill tuna, turning, until golden brown and cooked through, 8 to 10 minutes.

4. Arrange romaine, green beans, tomatoes, potatoes, onion, berries, olives, and tuna in 4 bowls. Drizzle with vinaigrette.

MAKES 4 SERVINGS.

Per serving:
436 calories, 43 g protein,
39.5 g carbohydrates (7 g fiber),
12 g fat (2 g sat), 662.5 mg sodium

Garden Chicken Burgers with Strawberry Sauce

- 3 tsp vegetable oil
- ½ medium onion, finely chopped
- 2 Tbsp brown sugar
- 2 cups strawberries, sliced
- 1½ tsp balsamic vinegar
- ¼ tsp freshly ground black pepper
- 1 Tbsp chopped fresh mint
- 1 medium carrot, peeled
- 1 medium zucchini, peeled
- 1 lb lean ground chicken breast
- ½ cup bread crumbs
- 2 tsp Worcestershire sauce
- 1 egg, lightly beaten
- ⅓ cup fresh parsley, chopped
- Salt and freshly ground black pepper
- 6 flatbreads or naan
- 1 cup arugula or baby spinach

1. Warm 1 tsp of the oil in skillet over medium heat. Add onion and sauté until soft, about 4 minutes. Add brown sugar and cook 2 minutes. Add strawberries, vinegar, and pepper and cook 1 minute. Stir in mint and remove from heat.

2. Preheat grill to medium.

3. Using a box grater or mandoline, shred carrot and zucchini, then chop into small pieces. In large bowl, lightly mix shredded vegetables, chicken, bread crumbs, Worcestershire sauce, egg, parsley, and salt and pepper. Form into 6 patties and brush with remaining 2 tsp oil.

4. Place burgers on grill and cook until internal temperature reaches 165°F, 4 to 5 minutes per side.

5. Meanwhile, toast flatbreads 1 to 2 minutes per side. Line flatbreads with arugula, add burgers, top with strawberry sauce, and fold bread over burgers.

MAKES 6 SERVINGS.

Per serving:
401 calories, 28 g protein,
54 g carbohydrates (7 g fiber),
9 g fat (2 g sat), 490 mg sodium

Italian Frittata

- 8 large eggs
- ⅓ cup 1% milk
- ½ cup chopped prosciutto
- ½ cup grated Parmesan cheese
- ½ cup halved cherry tomatoes
- ¼ cup chopped fresh basil
- ½ tsp salt
- ½ tsp freshly ground black pepper

1. Preheat oven to 375°F. Grease 8" or 10" ovenproof skillet or round cake pan.

2. In large bowl, gently whisk eggs and milk until blended. Stir in prosciutto, cheese, tomatoes, basil, salt and pepper.

3. Pour mixture into skillet or pan and bake until frittata is set, about 25 minutes. Let cool 10 minutes before cutting into wedges.

MAKES 4 SERVINGS.

Per serving:
262 calories, 25.5 g protein,
4 g carbohydrates (<1 g fiber),
16 g fat (6 g sat), 1,354 mg sodium

Watermelon, Spinach, and Bacon Salad

- 2 Tbsp sweet Asian chili sauce
- 2 Tbsp lime juice
- 1 Tbsp olive oil
- 1 package (5 oz) baby spinach
- 2 cups cubed watermelon
- 3 slices bacon, cooked and crumbled
- 2 Tbsp sliced red onion

1. In large bowl, whisk together chili sauce, lime juice, and oil.

2. Add spinach, watermelon, bacon, and onion. Toss to combine.

MAKES 4 SERVINGS.

Per serving:
111 calories, 3 g protein,
13.5 g carbohydrates (2 g fiber),
5.5 g fat (1 g sat), 227 mg sodium

Pantry Must-Haves

STOCK YOUR KITCHEN WITH THESE INGREDIENTS AND SLIMMING, GOOD-FOR-YOU MEALS WILL ALWAYS BE JUST MINUTES AWAY.

You probably know by now that eating at home is healthier and cheaper than dining out. To make this mission even easier for you, this chapter contains a cheat sheet of staples and cooking hints. Everything here is crazy good for you, including the most antioxidant-packed spices, the best fruits and vegetables for fighting disease, even the healthiest bread crumbs.

When you're finished shopping, put some thought into how you store your provisions. Haphazardly throwing things into the cupboards, fridge, or freezer is a surefire way to diet destruction. That's because how you position your groceries may shape the way you eat.

SHELVE STRATEGICALLY

Store fruits, vegetables, and other nutritious snacks at eye level. You're 2.7 times more likely to eat healthy food if it's in your line of sight, a Cornell University study says. "That's also why manufacturers pay a premium to have their products at eye level in stores," says Kit Yarrow, PhD, a professor of psychology and marketing at Golden Gate University.

PACK SMART

Combine leftover entrées and sides so that each container has one meal's worth. A variety of small leftover containers tempt you to eat more than you planned, says Brian Wansink, PhD, director of the Cornell University Food and Brand Lab and author of *Mindless Eating*.

HIDE THE JUNK

All stocked up on snacks? Now make sure you eat the good ones. In a 2009 Danish study, one in four participants who chose a healthy snack over an unhealthy one later reached for the junk anyway. So place the healthy stuff front and center, and stash small guilty pleasures out of sight.

Healthy Picks for your Pantry, Fridge, and Freezer

HERBS & SPICES

Chili powder: Can relieve congestion.

Cinnamon: Helps control blood sugar; stir it into tea.

Cumin: Boosts immunity.

Oregano: Contains up to 20 times the antioxidant levels of other herbs.

Paprika: Sprinkle on chicken before cooking, for a zesty dose of vitamin C.

Red-pepper flakes: Spice up a meal with metabolism-boosting capsaicin.

Rosemary: Great for savory chicken, pork, and salmon.

Thyme: Use this antioxidant-filled herb in soups.

OILS & VINEGARS

Balsamic vinegar: Sweeter than basic vinegar, full of flavor, and low cal.

Canola oil: Loaded with heart-healthy monounsaturated fatty acids; has a mild taste that makes it good for both cooking and baking.

Olive oil: Extra-virgin for salad dressings and bread dips; regular for cooking.

Red or white wine vinegar: Salad essentials that also add zing to vegetables.

GRAINS

Brown rice: Has about six times as much fiber as white.

Panko bread crumbs: These crispy morsels give a faux fried crunch to oven-baked chicken.

Whole-wheat couscous: With 7 grams of fiber per serving, it's a great alternative to rice or pasta.

Whole-wheat flour: In recipes that call for all-purpose flour, replace half the amount with whole-wheat.

Whole-wheat pasta: Contains more than twice as much fiber as regular kinds.

Whole-wheat tortillas: Low-carb wrappers are a perfect bread substitute.

SAUCES, MARINADES & SPREADS

Applesauce (natural): Not only a healthy side but a great sub for fat in baking: Replace half the oil in a recipe with applesauce.

Hummus: Fantastic source of protein and fiber.

Salsa: Veggies in disguise!

Soy and/or teriyaki sauce (low-sodium): A low-cal way to add a lot of flavor.

Tomato sauce (no sugar added): Has lycopene, a cancer-fighting superhero.

FISH & POULTRY
(Canned or in a pouch)

Chicken: Most precooked canned chicken is made with lean breast meat.

Clams: An excellent source of important minerals and a classic linguine topping.

Crabmeat: Very low in calories. Mix with bread crumbs for a fast crab cake.

Salmon (wild): An omega-3 powerhouse ready for salads or sandwiches. The wild version contains fewer pollutants, like PCBs, than farmed.

Tuna (light, in water): Water-packed tuna has more omega-3 fatty acids than oil-packed. Avoid albacore tuna, which has a higher mercury content.

SOUPS

Bean and vegetable soups (canned or boxed, reduced-sodium, reduced-fat, predominantly broth-based): Great for dinner on the fly. Try low-fat cream soups as a sauce for chicken and rice.

Broth/stock (reduced-sodium): Beef, chicken, and vegetable. Use in place of water to add flavor to rice.

NUTS & NUT BUTTERS

Almond butter: A tasty alternative to peanut butter.

Almonds: These hunger-killing immune builders are a great protein boost.

Peanut butter: The classic sandwich spread also pairs well with apple slices, bananas, and celery sticks.

Sunflower seeds: Rich in vitamin E, these add crunch to salads, soups, and cereal.

Walnuts: Crush a few and throw them into salads, yogurt, and cereal.

FRUITS

Canned or jarred: Mandarin oranges, peaches, pineapple Avoid fruits packed in syrup. Toss into salads or plain yogurt, or snack on them straight up.

Fresh and/or dried: Apples, apricots, bananas, citrus fruits, grapes, raisins

Frozen: Berries (ALL), cherries, mangoes Blend with yogurt and ice for an instant smoothie.

VEGETABLES

Canned or jarred: Artichokes, corn, fire-roasted peppers, garlic (will last longer than fresh), olives (black or green), tomatoes (whole and diced), water chestnuts

Fresh: Beets, celery, onions, potatoes, shallots, sweet potatoes. All of these keep well for long periods.

Frozen: Asparagus, broccoli, Brussels sprouts, carrots, spinach, and mixes

LEGUMES

Canned, reduced-sodium: Black, cannellini, great northern, navy, pinto, and red beans; black-eyed peas; chickpeas; lentils. Excellent sources of protein and fiber. Rinse them off to reduce the sodium content, then wrap in whole-wheat tortillas or add to salads, soups, and pasta dishes.

Frozen: Green beans, soybeans (edamame)

EAT IT OR TOSS IT?

There's always going to be something of indeterminate age and origin in your kitchen, and you may be tempted to sniff, poke, and then taste it. But not so fast—you could be taking a risk you'll regret. Each year, 76 million Americans fall sick with foodborne illnesses and 5,000 die of them, estimates the Centers for Disease Control and Prevention. Many of those illnesses are a result of improper food handling at home, which includes eating food that has spent too much time on the refrigerator shelf. The fridge isn't the only problem spot, either. Food that's been in the freezer too long won't make you sick, but it certainly won't taste its best. And though canned and dried foods that are past their prime usually aren't a threat, they will lose nutritional value over time. (Eating food from a bulging can, however, could be potentially fatal because the swelling could signal bacterial contamination.)

"You can't count on sight or smell to tell you if food is safe or good to eat," says Elizabeth L. Andress, PhD, a food safety specialist at the University of Georgia. So skip the smell-prod-and-taste test, and follow our guide.

In the Fridge

If a few items in your refrigerator have been there since the last millennium, you're not alone. When Tennessee State University researchers peeked into the fridges in 210 homes, they found moldy, spoiled, or outdated foods inside 24 percent of them.

"Many consumers don't understand that while refrigeration slows bacterial growth, it doesn't stop it," says Janet B. Anderson, MS, RD, a clinical professor of nutrition and food sciences at Utah State University, who, when conducting a recent study, was horrified to find that 31 percent of respondents ate leftovers that were more than a week old.

The first step to ensuring the safety of your food supply is keeping track of when you purchased and opened each item. One easy way is to stash masking tape and a marking pen in the kitchen so you can label all edibles with "purchased on" and "opened on" dates. The next step is to pay close attention to the recommended storage times. Some refrigerated foods have expiration dates on their packages. But dating regulations vary from state to state, and many products come with no date at all. To avoid confusion—and possibly food poisoning—see "How Long Will It Last?" below.)

Next, remember that food lasts longer when it's stored properly. Nils Noren, former vice president of culinary and pastry arts at the French Culinary Institute, has three tips to help you store your food the right way.

1. Set your fridge temperature at just above freezing, around 34°F. That's cold enough to slow the growth of bacteria without freezing the food. In the Tennessee State study, an alarming 28 percent of the refrigerators were warmer than 40°F. (For less than $12, you can buy a refrigerator thermometer that will help you keep food at the optimal temperature.)

2. Put items with short shelf lives in the back. Milk, meat, fish, and eggs last longer in the back because that's where refrigerators are coldest—and that way they'll also be protected from a warm air blast every time you open the door.

3. Stash raw proteins on the lowest shelf so no meat juices can drip on other shelves and season your food with pathogens like *E. coli* and salmonella. And wipe down your fridge at least once a week with a disinfecting wipe or a clean cloth dipped in a solution of soap, water, and a little bleach.

In the Freezer

As long as food remains frozen, it will stay safe to eat. The flavor and texture, however, can deteriorate substantially over time, so you may want to think twice before serving your dinner guests that 2-year-old sirloin. Also keep in mind that freezing doesn't kill bacteria; it just puts them to sleep for a while. Once you thaw it out, follow the guidelines for refrigerated food.

Like refrigerator temperatures, freezer temperatures can vary. The recommended storage periods assume that your freezer is set at 0°F. For every 5-degree increase in temperature, you should cut storage time in half. An important caveat: If you have the type of refrigerator with a small freezer compartment inside (one that doesn't have its own exterior door), don't keep anything in it longer than a week because these freezers cannot maintain temperatures as low as 0°F.

In the Pantry

Because pasta, rice, and other dried foods don't contain enough moisture for bacteria to thrive, and canned food is airtight, pantry storage is also more a question of quality than safety. Toss any cans that are rusting, leaking, or bulging, and always put newly purchased items on the back of the shelf, so you use the oldest ones first. Then follow the rules below. (Unless otherwise noted, they apply to opened products that are kept in airtight containers after opening.)

No matter how fastidious you are, there's always going to be something that slips through your dating system or doesn't appear on any of the lists. In that case, remember this mantra: When in doubt, throw it out.

How Long Will It Last?

FRIDGE

Raw poultry and ground meat: Eat or freeze within 1 to 2 days

Leftovers: 3 to 4 days; with gravy, 1 to 2 days

Raw beef, pork, veal, and lamb: Eat or freeze within 3 to 5 days

Lunch meat: Opened, 3 to 5 days; unopened, 2 weeks

Hard cheese: Opened, 3 to 4 weeks; unopened, up to 6 months

Soft cheese: 1 week

Condiments: Up to 6 months

FREEZER

Ice cream: 2 to 4 months

Cooked meat: 3 to 4 months

Raw poultry, pork: Up to 12 months

Raw beef: Ground, 3 to 4 months; steaks and roasts, up to 12 months

Vegetables and fruits: Up to 12 months

PANTRY

Oils: Opened, 1 to 3 months; unopened, 6 months

Vanilla and other extracts: Opened, 12 months; unopened, 2 years

Spices and herbs: Herbs and ground spices, 6 months; whole spices, 2 years

Baking powder: 3 months

Baking soda, sugar, bouillon, pasta, rice: 12 months

Canned soups, stews, meats: Unopened, 2 to 5 years

Chapter 22

Shop Once, Eat for a Week

WITH A LITTLE FORETHOUGHT—AND THESE RECIPES—YOU CAN MAKE FIVE DAYS' WORTH OF MEALS FOR UNDER $50.

Your weekday schedule and your budget have a lot in common: It's tough to squeeze more out of either of 'em. Lucky for you, buying quality food that's both delicious and nutritious is easier—and less expensive—than you might think. There's no need to browse the food market every day, prep piles of ingredients, and create meals from scratch night after night. That's because this chapter is brimming with a game plan and five mouthwatering entrée recipes that will help trim your body and boost your health. Just head to the supermarket with our plan for a week's worth of simple, satisfying dinners and prepare to tighten your belt, in more ways than one.

Your Shopping List

PRODUCE

1 pint cherry or grape tomatoes

2 bell peppers (1 red, 1 green)

1 large Spanish onion

1 jalapeño chile pepper

1 package arugula

1 bunch broccoli rabe

1 bunch cilantro

1 head garlic

MEAT

1 whole chicken (3 to 3½ lb)

1 package (1 lb) hot Italian sausage

1 package (1 lb) smoked turkey sausage

1 lb skirt steak

GROCERY

2 whole-wheat sub or hero rolls (8")

1 can (14.5 oz) stewed tomatoes

1 can (28 oz) whole San Marzano tomatoes in juice

1 can (15.5 oz) black beans

1 small package (10 oz) corn tortillas

1 lb fettuccine

DAIRY

1 small container (8 oz) sour cream

PANTRY ITEMS
(always keep these in stock)

Kosher salt

Black peppercorns

Extra-virgin olive oil

A block of Parmesan cheese

Dijon mustard

Balsamic vinegar

Hot sauce

DAY 1

CHICKEN WITH ROASTED ONIONS, PEPPERS, AND TOMATOES

Why is Monday a great day to roast a chicken? It's all about smart time management. With the oven already fired up, you can knock out elements for four more dinners this week.

- 2 bell peppers (1 red, 1 green), ribs and seeds removed, cut into ¼" slices
- 1 large Spanish onion, cut into ¼" slices
- 1 pint cherry or grape tomatoes
- 2 Tbsp extra-virgin olive oil
- 2 tsp salt plus a pinch
- 1 tsp freshly ground black pepper
- 1 chicken (3 to 3½ lb), giblets removed, rinsed and patted dry
- 1 head garlic

1. Preheat oven to 450°F, with racks positioned in upper and lower third of oven. Place peppers and onion in baking pan. Add tomatoes, oil, 1 tsp of the salt, and ½ tsp of the pepper and toss.

2. Season chicken inside and out with remaining 1 tsp salt and ½ tsp pepper. Place chicken in separate baking pan.

3. Cut off top third of garlic head. Peel cloves from that top third and toss with vegetables. Sprinkle a pinch of salt over cut side of bottom part of garlic, wrap tightly in foil, and place on baking pan with chicken.

4. Place pan with chicken on lower rack and roast 15 minutes. Then place pan with vegetables on upper rack. Keep roasting until chicken is golden brown, skin pulls away from drumsticks, and vegetables are browned in spots, 25 to 30 minutes, switching pans halfway through.

5. Transfer chicken to cutting board and let stand 10 minutes. Transfer vegetables to chicken pan to soak up pan juices. Serve half of chicken with half of vegetables.

WRAP IT UP

For meals later in the week, refrigerate leftover chicken, vegetables, and roasted garlic, all in separate containers.

DAY 2

SMOKY & SPICY SAUSAGE HEROES

The only time-consuming part of making sausage sandwiches is roasting the onion and peppers. Luckily, you cooked them yesterday with the roast chicken. Look at you—a man with a plan!

- 1 Tbsp extra-virgin olive oil
- 1 lb smoked turkey sausage
- Reserved roasted pepper-onion mixture (about 1½ cups)
- 2 whole-wheat sub or hero rolls (8")
- ½ cup arugula
- Hot sauce

1. Heat oil in large heavy skillet over medium heat until it shimmers. Add sausage and cover. Cook, turning sausage occasionally, until browned and cooked through, 10 to 12 minutes.

2. Add pepper-onion mixture to skillet and cook until vegetables are hot, 1 to 2 minutes.

3. Split and toast rolls. Fill each with a piece of sausage, some pepper-onion mixture, and arugula. Add hot sauce to taste.

Shop Once, Eat for a Week

DAY 3

QUICK CHICKEN ADOBO AND BLACK BEAN TACOS

Make a superfast, spicy adobo sauce to flavor these chicken tacos. Using the leftover roast chicken from Monday's feast gives you time to sip a cerveza while the sauce is simmering.

- 1 bunch cilantro, stems and leaves separated
- 1 can (14.5 oz) stewed tomatoes
- 1 jalapeño chile pepper, stem and seeds removed (wear plastic gloves when handling)
- ½ reserved roast chicken (skin and bones removed), shredded
- Salt and freshly ground black pepper
- 1 can (15.5 oz) black beans, rinsed and drained
- 4 corn tortillas
- ½ cup sour cream

1. In blender or food processor, combine cilantro stems, tomatoes, and chile pepper. Blend or process until smooth. Transfer mixture to medium saucepan and bring to a boil over medium-high heat. Cook, stirring occasionally, until sauce is thickened and reduced by half, 8 to 10 minutes.

2. Remove adobo sauce from heat and stir in chicken. Season to taste with salt and pepper.

3. Heat beans in small skillet over medium heat, stirring and smashing beans with the back of a large spoon, until slightly thickened, 3 to 4 minutes. Season beans with salt and pepper.

4. In dry skillet, heat tortillas until warm and pliable. Assemble tacos with adobo chicken, beans, sour cream, and cilantro leaves.

DAY 4

SPICY SAUSAGE BOLOGNESE WITH FETTUCCINE AND BROCCOLI RABE

The roasted garlic you made earlier in the week adds subtle depth to this flavor-packed pasta sauce. The recipe makes enough to feed four, so ask a couple of friends to come over with a nice bottle of red.

- 1 can (28 oz) whole tomatoes in juice (preferably San Marzano)
- ½ head reserved roasted garlic, peeled
- 2 Tbsp extra-virgin olive oil
- 1 lb hot Italian sausage, casings removed
- ½ cup grated Parmesan cheese, plus more for topping
- 1 bunch broccoli rabe, trimmed
- 1 lb fettuccine

1. In blender or food processor, combine tomatoes and garlic. Blend or process until smooth.

2. Heat oil in large heavy skillet over medium-high heat until it shimmers. Add sausage and cook, stirring and breaking up lumps with spatula or wooden spoon, until it's well browned and cooked through, about 10 minutes.

3. Add pureed tomatoes to skillet and bring to a boil. Cook, stirring occasionally, until sauce has thickened, about 10 minutes. Stir in cheese and keep sauce warm.

4. Bring large pot of salted water to a boil and add broccoli rabe. Cook until crisp-tender, 6 to 8 minutes. Remove with tongs to colander, then add fettuccine to water. Cook until al dente and drain. Serve pasta topped with Bolognese sauce and extra cheese, with broccoli rabe on the side.

DAY 5

GRILLED MUSTARD-GARLIC SKIRT STEAK WITH ARUGULA

You've managed to cook incredible dinners every night this week without breaking a sweat. It's time to kick off the weekend with a well-deserved steak, topped with peppery arugula, Tuscan-style.

- ½ head reserved roasted garlic
- ½ tsp hot sauce
- 3½ tsp Dijon mustard
- 1 tsp salt
- ¾ tsp freshly ground black pepper
- 1 lb skirt steak
- 2 Tbsp extra-virgin olive oil
- 1 Tbsp balsamic vinegar
  Reserved arugula

1. Peel roasted garlic and use side of a knife to mash it into a paste. In small bowl, stir together garlic, hot sauce, 3 tsp of the mustard, ¾ tsp of the salt, and ½ tsp of the pepper. Rinse steak and pat dry, then rub garlic-mustard mixture all over it.

2. Preheat grill or grill pan to high. When hot, add steak and cook, flipping once, until grill marks appear and steak is medium rare, 4 to 6 minutes for thinner pieces and 6 to 8 minutes for thicker ones. Let steak rest 10 minutes, then slice.

3. Meanwhile, in small bowl whisk together oil, vinegar, and remaining ½ tsp mustard, ¼ tsp salt, and ¼ tsp pepper. Toss arugula with dressing and serve with steak.

BROWN-BAG IT
Not cooking for two? That's even better. Having leftovers means you're all set for tomorrow's lunch.

Chapter 23

Best Packaged Foods for Men

WHAT COULD BE BETTER TO ROUND OUT YOUR EATING TRANSFORMATION THAN THIS: A LIST OF THE BEST FOOD OPTIONS AVAILABLE TO YOU.

It's time to stop the grocery guesswork. Add these brand-name all-stars to your shopping list, and you won't need to scan labels or compare brands. We've sampled, tested, and rated hundreds of products to find the healthiest, tastiest foods for men. They'll help you fight fat, keep fit, and stay healthy.

How we named the winners: Within each category, we looked for foods with the fewest calories that delivered the most protein and fiber. We eliminated products that contained partially hydrogenated soybean oil, soy lecithin, and high-fructose corn syrup. Organic products were given preference over nonorganic. In categories with products of similar nutritional numbers, we conducted blind taste tests with the staff. And yes, that last part of the job was awesome.

BREADS AND GRAINS

1. BEST CEREAL

Kellogg's Fiber Plus Cinnamon Oat Crunch
Plenty of fiber and a good dose of soy-free protein.
Per ¾ cup: 110 calories, 3 g protein, 26 g carbs (9 g fiber), 1.5 g fat

2. BEST INSTANT OATMEAL

Quaker Organic Instant Oatmeal
Just one ingredient—organic oats. As it should be.
Per packet: 100 calories, 4 g protein, 19 g carbs (3 g fiber), 2 g fat

3. BEST STEEL-CUT OATS

Arrowhead Mills Organic Steel Cut Oats
High in fiber. Great flavor.
Per ¼ cup: 160 calories, 6 g protein, 27 g carbs (8 g fiber), 3 g fat

4. BEST GRANOLA

Nature's Path Organic Peanut Butter Granola
Because honestly, who doesn't love peanut butter?
Per ¾ cup: 260 calories, 7 g protein, 35 g carbs (4 g fiber), 11 g fat

5. BEST BAGEL

Rudi's Organic Bakery Honey Sweet Wheat
Hearty but with half the calories of its rivals—and loads more flavor. Top with #66.
Per bagel: 150 calories, 6 g protein, 32 g carbs (5 g fiber), 1 g fat

6. BEST ENGLISH MUFFIN

Rudi's Organic Bakery Whole Grain Wheat English Muffins
Top a split muffin with mustard, ham, and Swiss cheese and broil.
Per muffin: 130 calories, 5 g protein, 23 g carbs (3 g fiber), 1.5 g fat

7. BEST BURGER BUN

Martin's Famous Whole Wheat Potato Rolls
Toast, cut side down, in a dry pan over medium-high heat.
Per roll: 100 calories, 7 g protein, 17 g carbs (3 g fiber), 1.5 g fat

8. BEST HOT DOG ROLL

Martin's Famous Long Potato Rolls
They're soft but tough enough to handle a topping-heavy dog.
Per roll: 130 calories, 7 g protein, 25 g carbs (1 g fiber), 1.5 g fat

9. BEST WRAP

La Tortilla Factory EVOO Multi Grain SoftWraps
Use them as a base for hearty huevos rancheros.
Per tortilla: 100 calories, 9 g protein, 18 g carbs (12 g fiber), 3.5 g fat

10. BEST PIZZA CRUST

Rustic Crust Organic Pizza Originale
Whole grains give this crust a robust flavor.
Per ⅙ crust: 120 calories, 5 g protein, 25 g carbs (1 g fiber), 1.5 g fat

11. BEST PASTA

Bionaturae Organic Pasta, Whole Wheat Penne Rigate
A satisfying bite and a belly-filling dose of fiber.
Per 2 oz: 180 calories, 7 g protein, 35 g carbs (6 g fiber), 1.5 g fat

12. BEST QUICK-COOKING RICE

Uncle Ben's Ready Rice Whole Grain Brown
Just nuke it for 90 seconds.
Per cup: 190 calories, 5 g protein, 39 g carbs (3 g fiber), 3 g fat

13. BEST GRAIN

Nature's Earthly Choice Premium Organic Quinoa
This whole grain boasts fiber and complete protein.
Per ¼ cup cooked: 160 calories, 6 g protein, 28 g carbs (3 g fiber), 2.5 g fat

14. BEST FLOUR

King Arthur 100% Organic Unbleached White Whole Wheat
It's amazing for making a healthy DIY pizza crust or pasta.
Per ¼ cup: 100 calories, 4 g protein, 22 g carbs (4 g fiber), 0.5 g fat

15. BEST PITA

Thomas' Sahara 100% Whole Wheat Pita Pockets
Slip your next burger inside one of these.
Per pita: 140 calories, 7 g protein, 27 g carbs (4 g fiber), 1.5 g fat

16. BEST BREAD

Rudi's Organic Bakery Honey Sweet Whole Wheat Bread
Mild tasting but packed with fiber and protein.
Per slice: 100 calories, 4 g protein, 19 g carbs (3 g fiber), 1 g fat

DAIRY AND DELI

17. BEST MILK
Organic Valley Reduced Fat 2% Milk
Skip the skim. The fat in 2% milk helps you better absorb nutrients.
Per cup: 130 calories, 8 g protein, 13 g carbs, 5 g fat

18. BEST CHOCOLATE MILK
Organic Valley Reduced Fat 2% Chocolate Milk
Combine it with #113 for the best-tasting muscle fuel.
Per cup: 170 calories, 8 g protein, 24 g carbs, 5 g fat

19. BEST SHREDDED CHEESE
Horizon Organic Shredded Mexican Cheese
It tastes great melted, too.
Per ¼ cup: 110 calories, 7 g protein, 1 g carbs, 9 g fat

20. BEST SNACKING CHEESE
Sargento Natural Light String Cheese
Has none of the plastic taste of many string cheeses.
Per stick: 50 calories, 6 g protein, 1 g carbs, 2.5 g fat

21. BEST CREAM CHEESE
Kraft Philadelphia Whipped Cream Cheese
It has all the creaminess without excess calories.
Per 2 Tbsp: 60 calories, 1 g protein, 2 g carbs, 5 g fat

22. BEST COTTAGE CHEESE
Horizon Organic Regular Cottage Cheese
Pack in protein at breakfast with this instant side.
Per ½ cup: 120 calories, 14 g protein, 4 g carbs, 5 g fat

23. BEST BUTTER
Kerrygold Pure Irish Unsalted Butter
Sweet and fresh, this butter beats the rest. Just don't overdo it.
Per Tbsp: 100 calories, 11 g fat

24. BEST BUTTER SPREAD
Smart Balance Butter & Canola and EVOO Blend
Real butter gives this spread a delicious flavor foundation.
Per Tbsp: 100 calories, 11 g fat

25. BEST PLAIN YOGURT
Fage Total 2% Greek Yogurt
Our tasters loved its tang; gym rats will love its protein payload.
Per 7 oz: 150 calories, 20 g protein, 8 g carbs, 4 g fat

26. BEST FLAVORED YOGURT
Chobani Non-Fat Vanilla Greek Yogurt
No high-fructose corn syrup. All good.
Per 6 oz: 140 calories, 16 g protein, 17 g carbs

27. BEST PROBIOTIC YOGURT
La Yogurt Light Probiotic Strawberry Banana Blended Nonfat Yogurt
Some probiotic yogurts have a chemical aftertaste. This one goes down smooth.
Per 4 oz: 90 calories, 6 g protein, 15 g carbs

28. BEST EGGS
Eggland's Best Organic Eggs
Rich, buttery yolks are perfect for breakfast, lunch, or dinner.
Per large egg: 70 calories, 6 g protein, 4 g fat

29. BEST COLD CUTS
Applegate Organic Smoked Turkey Breast
This fresh-tasting lunch meat has no nasty additives or binders.
Per 2 oz: 50 calories, 12 g protein

FROZEN FOODS

30. BEST APPETIZER
Annie Chun's Organic Chicken & Vegetable Potstickers
Add to broth and top with scallions and a dash of #121.
Per 7 pieces: 220 calories, 14 g protein, 32 g carbs (2 g fiber), 3.5g fat

31. BEST BEEF ENTRÉE
Artisan Bistro Grass-Fed Beef with Mushroom Sauce
Grass-fed beef in the frozen aisle? Finally.
Per container: 350 calories, 23 g protein, 32 g carbs (4 g fiber), 13 g fat

32. BEST CHICKEN ENTRÉE
Kashi Lemongrass Coconut Chicken
It also contains red quinoa and plenty of vegetables.
Per container: 300 calories, 18 g protein, 38 g carbs (7 g fiber), 8 g fat

33. BEST FISH ENTRÉE

Artisan Bistro Wild Alaskan Salmon
A low-cost way to enjoy wild salmon.
Per patty: 280 calories, 18 g protein, 39 g carbs (4 g fiber), 6 g fat

34. BEST PASTA ENTRÉE

Kashi Pesto Pasta Primavera
This pesto-packed meal tastes great when you add chicken or shrimp.
Per meal: 290 calories, 11 g protein, 37 g carbs (7 g fiber), 11 g fat

35. BEST VEGETARIAN ENTRÉE

Amy's Cheese Enchilada Whole Meal
Top with cilantro, sour cream, and #59.
Per meal: 370 calories, 17 g protein, 41 g carbs (9 g fiber), 15 g fat

36. BEST PLAIN PIZZA

Evol. Four Cheese & Basil
A crisp crust and quality cheeses help this pie rise above the rest.
Per ½ pizza: 300 calories, 15 g protein, 34 g carbs (2 g fiber), 12 g fat

37. BEST BURRITO

Evol. Cilantro Lime Chicken Burrito
This fresh-tasting burrito is also packed with brown rice, Cheddar, and corn salsa.
Per burrito: 340 calories, 15 g protein, 49 g carbs (4 g fiber), 11 g fat

38. BEST VEGGIE BURGER

Amy's California Veggie Burger
Made with mushrooms, onions, and oats.
Per patty: 150 calories, 6 g protein, 21 g carbs (4 g fiber), 5 g fat

39. BEST FISH STICKS

Ian's Fish Sticks
Dip these lightly breaded fish sticks, made from wild-caught fish, in #62.
Per 6 sticks: 190 calories, 11 g protein, 24 g carbs (1 g fiber), 5 g fat

40. BEST FRENCH FRIES

Alexia Crinkle Cut Sweet Potato Fries
These crisp fries have a satisfying blend of sweet and salty, with a hit of pepper.
Per 12 pieces: 140 calories, 2 g protein, 22 g carbs (2 g fiber), 5 g fat

41. BEST BREAKFAST SANDWICH

Smart Ones Canadian Style Bacon English Muffin Sandwich
Pair one with a banana for a great breakfast.
Per sandwich: 210 calories, 13 g protein, 27 g carbs (2 g fiber), 6 g fat

42. BEST WAFFLE

Kashi 7 Grain Waffles
Apply liberal amounts of warmed #44 for maximum enjoyment.
Per 2 waffles: 150 calories, 4 g protein, 25 g carbs (7 g fiber), 5 g fat

43. BEST VEGETABLE

Woodstock Organic Frozen Broccoli Florets
This brand's fresh-tasting florets make a fast side for any protein.
Per cup: 60 calories, 2 g protein, 8 g carbs (4 g fiber)

44. BEST FRUIT

Cascadian Farm Organic Harvest Berries
Add a dose of flavor and antioxidants to your yogurt or smoothie.
Per cup: 60 calories, 1 g protein, 17 g carbs (4 g fiber)

45. BEST ICE CREAM

Breyers Natural Vanilla
Smooth, rich, and not too sweet—ideal as a cheat-meal
Per ½ cup: 130 calories, 3 g protein, 14 g carbs, 7 g fat

46. BEST FROZEN TREAT

Yasso Blueberry Frozen Greek Yogurt Bars
A creamy, low-calorie frozen dessert with protein? Yes, please.
Per bar: 80 calories, 6 g protein, 15 g carbs

47. BEST PIZZA WITH TOPPINGS

Evol. Chicken, Spinach & Ricotta
Bye-bye, delivery guy.
Per ½ pizza: 280 calories, 14 g protein, 36 g carbs (2 g fiber), 9 g fat

CANNED AND JARRED GOODS

48. BEST SOUP

Campbell's 100% Natural Chicken Tuscany
White beans and vegetables pump up this can's nutrients.
Per cup: 90 calories, 6 g protein, 12 g carbs (4 g fiber), 1.5 g fat

49. BEST CHILI

Eden Organic Black Bean & Quinoa Chili
Quinoa raises the protein content.
Per cup: 190 calories, 10 g protein, 35 g carbs (6 g fiber), 1.5 g fat

50. BEST REFRIED BEANS
Eden Organic Refried Pinto Beans, Lightly Salted
Heat and slather on a #9, top with #19, #117, and grilled #104.
Per ½ cup: 90 calories, 6 g protein, 19 g carbs (7 g fiber), 1 g fat

51. BEST CANNED BEANS
Eden Organic Garbanzo Beans
Add these fiber-packed, nutty beans to pasta sauce or toss them into a Greek salad.
Per ½ cup: 130 calories, 7 g protein, 23 g carbs (5 g fiber), 1 g fat

52. BEST CANNED TOMATOES
Cento Certified San Marzano Organic Peeled Tomatoes
A rich-tasting Italian variety that doesn't taste like the can.
Per ½ cup: 25 calories, 1 g protein, 5 g carbs (2 g fiber)

53. BEST OLIVES
Peloponnese Country Gourmet Mixed Olives
Eat as is or chop some up to spread on a hoagie.
Per oz: 60 calories, 2 g carbs, 6 g fat

54. BEST PICKLE
McClure's Garlic & Dill Spears
Taste one of these snappy, tangy pickles and you won't go back to those yellowish, flavor-free alternatives.
Per oz: 5 calories, 2 g carbs

55. BEST READY-TO-EAT TUNA
Wild Planet Wild Albacore Tuna
This brand boasts sustainably caught fish with high omega-3 levels and low mercury. Plus it tastes great in a sandwich.
Per 2 oz: 120 calories, 16 g protein, 6 g fat

56. BEST READY-TO-EAT SALMON
Wild Planet Wild Alaska Pink Salmon
Mix with #64, lemon juice, minced red onion, fresh dill, and salt and pepper for a spin on tuna salad.
Per 2 oz: 65 calories, 12 g protein, 1.5 g fat

SPREADS, DIPS, AND TOPPINGS

57. BEST BBQ SAUCE
Dinosaur Bar-B-Que Sensuous Slathering Sauce
This sauce has no corn syrup; it does have tomatoes, vinegar, brown sugar, and green pepper.
Per 2 Tbsp: 28 calories, 7 g carbs

58. BEST DIP
Sabra Cucumber & Dill Veggie Dip, Made with Greek Yogurt
Skip the ranch dressing and use this as a dip for broccoli, red bell peppers, or carrots.
Per 2 Tbsp: 35 calories, 2 g protein, 2 g carbs, 2.5 g fat

59. BEST GUACAMOLE
Wholly Guacamole Pico de Gallo Style Dip
The pico de gallo adds a slightly spicy salsa kick.
Per 2 Tbsp: 45 calories, 1 g protein, 2 g carbs (1 g fiber), 4 g fat

60. BEST HUMMUS
Athenos Original
Creamy and smooth, with just the right punch of garlic. Try it with carrots and celery.
Per 2 Tbsp: 50 calories, 1 g protein, 5 g carbs (<1 g fiber), 3 g fat

61. BEST JAM
Fiordifrutta Strawberry
One of the few organic jams on the market, it's made with wild strawberries and sweetened with apple juice.
Per Tbsp: 30 calories, 7 g carbs

62. BEST KETCHUP
Simply Heinz Tomato Ketchup
The bright, flavorful classic we love is now free of corn syrup. Mix some with #125 for an incredible dip for #40.
Per Tbsp: 20 calories, 5 g carbs

63. BEST MARINADE
World Harbors Jamaican Style Jerk Marinade and Sauce
The sweet and spicy tropical bite works well with chicken, beef, pork, and even shellfish.
Per Tbsp: 20 calories, 5 g carbs

64. BEST MAYONNAISE
Blue Plate Light Mayonnaise
This mayo has a lemony tang that pumps up the flavors of tuna or turkey sandwiches. And it's low in calories.
Per Tbsp: 50 calories, 1 g carbs, 5 g fat

65. BEST PANCAKE SYRUP
Spring Tree 100% Pure Grade A Dark Amber Maple Syrup
Real maple syrup. Nothing more needed. Just don't go crazy with the stuff.
Per Tbsp: 53 calories, 13 g carbs

66. BEST PEANUT BUTTER
Cream-Nut Natural Peanut Butter
Uniquely smooth and creamy, this jar houses an intense peanut flavor.
Per 2 Tbsp: 190 calories, 8 g protein, 6 g carbs (2 g fiber), 16 g fat

67. BEST SALAD DRESSING
Newman's Own Lite Honey Mustard Dressing
It works wonders as a marinade for chicken breasts.
Per 2 Tbsp: 70 calories, 7 g carbs, 4 g fat

68. BEST SALSA
Frontera Double Roasted Tomato Salsa
Stir this smoky salsa into a pan of scrambled eggs.
Per 2 Tbsp: 10 calories, 1 g carbs

69. BEST MUSTARD
Grey Poupon Country Dijon Mustard
Mustard seeds ratchet up the texture of this blend. Try it as a dip for #73.
Per Tbsp: 5 calories

70. BEST SANDWICH SPREAD
Cento Diced Hot Cherry Peppers
Spice up any sandwich with this chili-packed spread. It's especially good on Italian subs.
Per Tbsp: 5 calories, 1 g carbs

71. BEST STEAK SAUCE
Goodall's Irish Steak Sauce
Enhanced with apples and dates, it adds complexity to meat loaf, burgers, and steaks.
Per Tbsp: 15 calories, 4 g carbs

72. BEST TOMATO SAUCE
Amy's Organic Light in Sodium Tomato Basil Pasta Sauce
Perfectly sweetened.
Per ½ cup: 90 calories, 2 g protein, 11 g carbs (2 g fiber), 4.5 g fat

SNACKS

73. BEST PRETZEL
Newman's Own Organics High Protein Pretzels
Flour made from peas cranks up the protein content.
Per 22 pretzels: 120 calories, 5 g protein, 22 g carbs (4 g fiber), 1.5 g fat

74. BEST TORTILLA CHIP
Utz Organic Blue Corn Tortilla Chips
Our tasters said these chips had just the right levels of salt and crunch.
Per oz: 140 calories, 2 g protein, 19 g carbs (1 g fiber), 6 g fat

75. BEST CRACKER
Back to Nature Organic Stoneground Wheat Crackers
Great for scooping dips.
Per ½ oz: 70 calories, 1 g protein, 11 g carbs (1 g fiber), 2.5 g fat

76. BEST POPCORN
Newman's Own Organics Pop's Corn, Light Butter
It has a great flavor, without chemicals.
Per 3 cups: 112 calories, 3 g protein, 19 g carbs (3.5 g fiber), 3 g fat

77. BEST JERKY
Perky Jerky Ultra Premium Beef Jerky
This brand has no preservatives.
Per oz: 90 calories, 11 g protein, 6 g carbs, 2 g fat

78. BEST NUT
Planter's *Men's Health* NUT-rition Mix
Did you think any other kind would win? We helped make this stuff!
Per oz: 170 calories, 6 g protein, 5 g carbs (3 g fiber), 15 g fat

79. BEST NUT ALTERNATIVE
Woodstock Organic Pumpkin Seeds
Store a bag in your desk at work for a healthy midday snack.
Per ¼ cup: 180 calories, 9 g protein, 4 g carbs (3 g fiber), 14 g fat

80. BEST DRIED FRUIT
Sunsweet D'Noir Preservative Free Prunes
If you need to snack on something sweet, you might as well take in some antioxidants too.
Per 5 prunes: 100 calories, 1 g protein, 24 g carbs (3 g fiber)

81. BEST TRAIL MIX
Kopali Organics Superfood Mix
Lots of fiber and packed with mulberries, pistachios, cacao nibs, and goji berries.
Per ¼ cup: 120 calories, 4 g protein, 13 g carbs (4 g fiber), 6 g fat

82. BEST SNACK BAR
Larabar Peanut Butter Cookie
Just three simple ingredients: dates, peanuts, and sea salt.
Per bar: 220 calories, 7 g protein, 23 g carbs (4 g fiber), 12 g fat

83. BEST CHOCOLATE BAR
Green & Black's Organic Dark Chocolate 85%
Organic vanilla extract mellows the dark chocolate bite of this bar.
Per 1.4 oz: 250 calories, 4 g protein, 15 g carbs (4 g fiber), 20 g fat

84. BEST COOKIE
Kashi Chocolate Almond Butter Cookies
They contain whole grains and just the right amount of sweet.
Per cookie: 130 calories, 3 g protein, 19 g carbs (4 g fiber), 5 g fat

85. BEST POTATO CHIP
Boulder Canyon 60% Less Sodium Totally Natural Kettle Chips
You won't miss the salt.
Per 14 chips: 140 calories, 2 g protein, 17 g carbs (1 g fiber), 7 g fat

86. BEST SPICY SNACK
Hapi Sriracha Peas
Eat them straight up, or crush them and use as a spicy coating for baked chicken.
Per 28 g: 120 calories, 4 g protein, 19 g carbs (1 g fiber), 3 g fat

DRINKS

87. BEST BEER
Guinness Draught
This classic Irish stout is dark and rich, but never heavy on the gut—as long as you're drinking in moderation, of course.
Per 12 oz: 125 calories, 10 g carbs

88. BEST LOW-CALORIE BEER
Amstel Light
If you're looking to slim down without sacrificing bar nights, turn to this light lager. Despite its modest calorie count, it still carries decent flavor.
Per 12 oz: 95 calories, 5 g carbs

89. BEST CRAFT BEER
Abita Amber
This New Orleans lager boasts smooth, nuanced flavor without a heavy calorie load. Think of it as a craft upgrade from your favorite go-to American lager.
Per 12 oz: 128 calories, 10 g carbs

90. BEST BOTTLED SMOOTHIE
Bolthouse Farms Green Goodness
Most protein smoothies use soy—not a good idea for guys. Instead, blend your own with #25, and try this for a fast refuel.
Per 8 oz: 140 calories, 2 g protein, 33 g carbs, 2 g fiber

91. BEST BOTTLED TEA
Honest Tea Honey Green Tea
A favorite among *Men's Health* editors for its high antioxidant content, modest calorie count, and refreshing taste.
Per 17 oz: 70 calories, 18 g carbs

92. BEST BOTTLED WATER
Fiji
The cleanest tasting of the major brands, according to our well-hydrated tasters.
0 calories

93. BEST CAFFEINATED TEA BAGS
Tazo China Green Tips Tea
Brews up aromatic and fresh, not grassy like many supermarket green teas.
0 calories

94. BEST COFFEE BEANS
Starbucks Medium House Blend
These beans yield a cup with a deep but not bitter taste, with a hit of nuttiness on the finish.
0 calories

95. BEST FLAVORED WATER
Hint Mango-Grapefruit
This subtly fruity water doesn't have the funky chemical aftertaste of most other varieties we sampled.
0 calories

96. BEST FRUIT JUICE
Simply Grapefruit
Ounce for ounce, grapefruit juice contains fewer calories than orange juice. Tastes tart and refreshing, too.
Per 8 oz: 100 calories, 25 g carbs

97. BEST HERBAL TEA BAGS

Better Off Red Rooibos Tea
Wound up at bedtime? Brew a cup of this clean-tasting, caffeine-free tea.
0 calories

98. BEST INSTANT COFFEE

Starbucks VIA Ready Brew Colombia Coffee
Finally, on-the-go coffee that brews to barista standards with just a mug and some boiling water.
0 calories

99. BEST WHITE WINE UNDER $15

Joel Gott California Sauvignon Blanc 2011
Easy to say, easy to find, easy to enjoy. With flavors of apricot and lemon, this white lights up a meal.
Per 5 oz: about 128 calories

100. BEST RED WINE UNDER $15

Beronia Rioja Crianza 2008, Spain
The cherry and spice flavors in this smooth, robust red work with everything from chicken to steak.
Per 5 oz: about 127 calories

101. BEST SPORTS DRINK

Gatorade G2 Natural Berry
This low-calorie sports drink boasts sea salt and natural fruit flavors instead of fake ingredients.
Per 8 oz: 20 calories, 5 g carbs

102. BEST RECOVERY DRINK

Skratch Labs Exercise Hydration Mix
Dump and stir this powder into a glass of water to replenish your electrolytes after an intense cardio workout.
Per 16 oz: 80 calories, 20 g carbs

103. BEST VEGETABLE JUICE

R.W. Knudsen Family Very Veggie Low Sodium Organic Juice
Packed with organic tomatoes, celery, beets, and more.
Per 8 oz: 60 calories, 2 g protein, 12 g carbs, 3 g fiber

PROTEINS

104. BEST CHICKEN

Bell & Evans Organic Boneless Skinless Chicken Breasts
This company raises fresh-tasting organic birds that are juicy even without the skin.
Per 4 oz: 120 calories, 27 g protein, 1.5 g fat

105. BEST STEAK

Organic Prairie Premium Organic New York Strip Steak
Elevate your steak with this cut, which has just the right amount of delicious fat.
Per steak: 450 calories, 50 g protein, 28 g fat

106. BEST GROUND BEEF

Organic Prairie Organic Grass-Fed Ground Beef
Form into patties, sear to medium rare, and serve on a #7 with a swipe of #69.
Per 4 oz: 240 calories, 21 g protein, 17 g fat

107. BEST GROUND TURKEY

Shelton's Ground Turkey
This poultry purveyor pledges never to give antibiotics to its birds, and its turkey tastes great in homemade chili.
Per 4 oz: 170 calories, 21 g protein, 10 g fat

108. BEST BACON

Farmland Hickory Smoked Bacon
Our porked-out taste testers loved its balanced levels of salt and smoke.
Per 2 slices: 80 calories, 4 g protein, 7 g fat

109. BEST SAUSAGE

Al Fresco Spicy Jalapeño Chicken Sausage
Try one tucked inside a #8 and topped with #70. Beat the heat with a #89 on the side.
Per link: 130 calories, 14 g protein, 2 g carbs, 7 g fat

110. BEST HOT DOG

Applegate The Great Organic Uncured Beef Hot Dog
Year after year, this dog prevails for its savory snap and modest calorie count.
Per hot dog: 90 calories, 6 g protein, 7 g fat

111. BEST EXOTIC MEAT

Maple Leaf Farms Boneless Duck Breast Filet
Richer tasting than chicken. Give it a shot.
Per 4 oz: 210 calories, 16 g protein, 17 g fat

112. BEST CHOP

Organic Prairie Organic Bone-In Pork Chop
Cook it bone-in for added flavor, and accompany with a side of applesauce.
Per chop: 220 calories, 26 g protein, 13 g fat

113. BEST PROTEIN POWDER
Optimum Nutrition 100% Whey Gold Standard Double Rich Chocolate
A balanced workout-recovery fuel that you'll actually enjoy.
Per scoop: 120 calories, 24 g protein, 3 g carbs, 1 g fat

COOKING STAPLES

114. BEST BREAD CRUMBS
Wel-Pac Japanese Style Panko
Use this instead of regular bread crumbs to lighten meat loaf and to bread fish.
Per ½ cup: 110 calories, 4 g protein, 20 g carbs (1 g fiber), 1 g fat

115. BEST CANOLA OIL
Spectrum Organic Canola Oil
Light, neutral tasting, and free of genetically modified ingredients.
Per Tbsp: 120 calories, 14 g fat

116. BEST OLIVE OIL
California Olive Ranch Extra Virgin Olive Oil
This versatile, affordable oil is great for sautéing vegetables or drizzling on mozzarella, or as a base for salad dressings.
Per Tbsp: 120 calories, 14 g fat

117. BEST HOT SAUCE
Frank's RedHot Original Cayenne Pepper Sauce
Our tasters loved its slow burn and assertive vinegar kick.
0 calories

118. BEST LOW-SODIUM BROTH
Pacific Organic Free Range Low Sodium Chicken Broth
It's full of chicken flavor without the salt lick of sodium.
Per cup: 10 calories, 2 g protein, 1 g carbs

119. BEST PEPPER
Simply Organic Black Peppercorns
Pour these whole peppercorns into a grinder, crank, and you'll taste the difference—and move the pre-ground stuff to the back of your spice rack.
0 calories

120. BEST SALT
Diamond Crystal Kosher Salt
These coarse flakes are more intense than table salt, so you can get away with using less.
0 calories

121. BEST SOY SAUCE
La Choy Lite Soy Sauce
Taste testers liked its light flavor. Use this savory condiment to complement (not overpower) your next stir-fry.
Per Tbsp: 15 calories, 1 g protein, 2 g carbs

122. BEST VINEGAR
Newman's Own Organic Balsamic Vinegar
Mellow and not too sweet, this balsamic ranked as the most balanced in our taste tests. Try it drizzled over sliced strawberries.
Per Tbsp: 20 calories, 5 g carbs

123. BEST TERIYAKI SAUCE
Soy Vay Veri Veri Teriyaki
Fueled by real ginger and garlic, it works great as a flavoring for salmon, turkey burgers, or steak.
Per Tbsp: 35 calories, 6 g carbs, 1 g fat

124. BEST ALL-PURPOSE SPICE
Old Bay 30% Less Sodium Seasoning
Dust this spicy, not-too-salty mix on top of everything from corn to chicken to fish.
0 calories

125. BEST SECRET INGREDIENT
McCormick Smoked Paprika
Use a pinch of this Spanish spice to add richness to deviled eggs, chili, or even a bag of #76.
0 calories

Part 6

Tough Nutrition Questions... Answered

With all of the nutrition information constantly thrown at you—some of which can seem conflicting or contradictory—it's easy to get overwhelmed. To help ease your confusion, we rounded up the most frequently asked, or consistently perplexing, questions out there. That way, you can worry less about the nitty-gritty and focus on what's really important: Eating the best foods and getting the best results possible.

Is Gluten Free Worth a Shot?

AN INCREASING NUMBER OF TOP ATHLETES AND WEIGHT LOSS EXPERTS SWEAR THAT GLUTEN FREE IS THE WAY TO GO. BUT WILL GIVING UP WHEAT ULTIMATELY HELP OR HURT YOUR PERFORMANCE?

You've probably noticed an uptick in the number of products at your local grocery store bearing the label "gluten free." Once regarded strictly as a treatment for a chronic digestive disorder called celiac disease, a diet free of gluten—a protein found in wheat, barley, and rye—is now thought by some to be a remedy for everything from migraines to fatigue to weight gain. It's a trend that's been sweeping the nation over the last few years, and it doesn't look like it's going away anytime soon. In fact, sales of gluten-free products—from cupcakes to ketchup—grew nearly 30 percent a year from 2006 to 2010, according to the market research company Packaged Facts. And market research firm Mintel reported that 10 percent of new foods launched in 2010 featured a "gluten-free" claim, up from only 2 percent 5 years earlier.

But what exactly is gluten, and will giving it up ultimately help you lead a healthier, leaner, more energetic life?

THE BACKGROUND

Gluten is a surprisingly common, often beneficial, substance. It's what makes bread and other baked goods chewy and pizza dough stretchy, and is sometimes used as an additive to thicken soups, salad dressings, or sauces. But for people with celiac disease, says Alessio Fasano, MD, director of the University of Maryland Center for Celiac Research in Baltimore, eating gluten can trigger an immune response, causing a number of bad reactions like damage to the small intestine, poor nutrient absorption, diarrhea, abdominal pain, bloating, anemia, and fatigue.

Experts once thought this was a rare disorder, affecting only one in every 10,000 people. But a 2003 study in the *Archives of Internal Medicine* revealed that it's a much more common affliction: About one in 133 people suffer from the disease.

Even if you don't have celiac disease, gluten may still be bad for you, says Lara Field, MS, RD, a dietitian at the University of Chicago's Celiac Disease Center. A rising percentage of people in the United States consider themselves "gluten sensitive." "These people may have a food intolerance or experience many celiac-type symptoms after consuming foods that contain gluten," says Field. Some may have a form of wheat allergy. Fasano estimates that 20 million people are gluten sensitive.

THE HEALTH HYPE

A growing number of people are giving up gluten for reasons other than gluten sensitivity or celiac disease: They think gluten encourages weight gain and claim to feel more energetic when they don't consume it. Many advocates of this philosophy say that humans didn't evolve the ability to digest certain domesticated grains containing gluten and that avoiding gluten also leads to better absorption of nutrients.

For example, NFL quarterback Drew Brees won a Super Bowl while on a gluten-free diet. Cyclist Tom Danielson—a record-breaking member of the Garmin-Transitions team, who, like any competitive cyclist, burns and eats an immense number of calories and pays close attention to what seems to work—says his training and racing have improved since he and his teammates went gluten free. "After I started the diet, I had better results. I didn't feel as fatigued, and my recovery period was quicker," says Danielson, who puts in 6-plus hours during a typical training session. Allen Lim, PhD, a former exercise physiologist for Garmin-Transitions, agrees that going gluten free has helped his team perform at a higher level.

But, on the flip side, mainstream research still hasn't substantiated the claims of those who believe gluten is bad for everyone. "There is no strong scientific evidence to support the assertion that avoiding gluten leads to benefits for the general population," says Tricia Thompson, MS, RD, author of *The Gluten-Free Nutrition Guide* and the Web site glutenfreedietitian.com.

Still, going gluten-free *can* help you lose weight, but perhaps not for the reasons you think. "There's nothing magical about a gluten-free diet that's going to help you lose weight," says Mark DeMeo, MD, director of gastroenterology and nutrition at the Adult Celiac Disease Program at Rush University Medical Center in Chicago. Instead, adhering to a gluten-free diet helps you avoid highly refined and processed carbohydrates, like white bread, pastries, and beer. "Gluten itself probably isn't the reason you've packed on pounds," says Field. "Eating too many refined carbohydrates is what expands your waistline."

But this approach to weight loss can backfire, too, because gluten free doesn't mean fat free or calorie free. "You can buy gluten-free versions of practically every type of wheat-based food—pizza, pasta, cookies, you name it," says Thompson. But, adds Shelley Case, RD, author of *Gluten-Free Diet: A Comprehensive Resource Guide*, and a medical advisory board member for the Celiac Disease Foundation, "without gluten to bind food together, food manufacturers often use more fat and sugar to make the product more palatable." Plus, people might overindulge in gluten-free options because they seem like "safe" foods. Says Field: "People see 'gluten free' and think they can down an entire box of gluten-free cookies with no repercussions."

So even if you stick to a gluten-free diet, it can lead to weight gain. A 2006 study in the *American Journal of Gastroenterology* followed 188 people with celiac disease (half of whom were overweight or obese) on a gluten-free diet for 2 years and discovered that 81 percent of them gained weight.

YOUR BEST MOVE

If you think you may have symptoms of a gluten intolerance (see "Six Signs of Gluten Sensitivity" below), ask your doctor about scheduling a blood test to find out for sure.

If you're simply interested in losing weight, a gluten-free diet can work, but dealing with the diet's restrictions can be daunting. "You have to commit to a true lifestyle change, and that can be tough," says Edward Abramson, PhD, a professor emeritus of psychology at California State University at Chico and the author of *Emotional Eating*. "Men might be able to follow gluten free for a short time, but without a real medical need, they might have a rough time sticking to it."

Besides the hassle, you can end up with serious nutritional deficiencies. "Gluten free doesn't necessarily equal healthy, especially when people yank vitamin-enriched and whole-grain foods from their diets and replace them with gluten-free brownies," says Case. In fact, research suggests that those

Six Signs of Gluten Sensitivity

More than 2.5 million people may have celiac disease, yet only an estimated 150,000 have been diagnosed. That's because people can be asymptomatic for years, and the symptoms of celiac disease can also overlap with other medical problems, so it often confuses both patients and doctors. That said, if you think you might have a problem, don't ax gluten from your diet before being screened by a specialist. If you go off gluten entirely before having a test done, your results may come back negative even if you have the disease.

Celiac disease has hundreds of recognized symptoms, according to the Celiac Sprue Association, a nonprofit for those with the disease. Here are six common problems:

- Chronic diarrhea or constipation
- Unexplained weight loss
- Fatigue
- Infertility
- Abdominal pain and bloating
- Anemia

who forgo gluten may be more likely to miss out on important nutrients such as iron, B vitamins, and fiber.

Avoiding gluten takes constant monitoring—the same attention to detail you need to excel in your workouts. "I became more dedicated and took a more professional approach to my training when I went gluten free," Danielson says. "I couldn't get lazy and down whole pizzas and bowls of pasta. I had to focus on putting better food in my body, and this made me realize how much my eating habits off the bike affected my performance on it." Mindful eating is key. After all, "you don't need to go gluten free to avoid refined processed carbs," says Thompson.

This is where careful meal planning comes in, which may explain why some people feel so good when they go G free: They're eating real food instead of ultraprocessed packaged fare. "If you skip the gluten-free goodies and focus on fruits, vegetables, lean protein, dairy, and gluten-free grains like amaranth and quinoa, this can be a very healthy way of eating," says Marlisa Brown, RD, author of *Gluten-Free, Hassle Free*. "But you can't just wing it."

If you do give up gluten, use your new eating plan as a lens to reexamine your diet—and your life. "I don't know if it was directly tied to the food, but I found that by having to pay more attention to my daily diet, I became more focused on my cycling," says Danielson.

Do You Need More Salt?

MANY FOODS ARE PACKED WITH SODIUM, BUT AVOIDING IT MAY NOT BE THE ANSWER, EITHER.

Insidious health threat, innocent flavor enhancer, or essential nutrient? America has declared war on salt. And it's no surprise considering these hypertension stats: More than 20 percent of American men between 35 and 44 have high blood pressure. Even the Institute of Medicine is leaning on the government to set standards for sodium content in foods; and the American Heart Association, along with the City of New York and 30 other cities, is promoting a new National Salt Reduction Initiative. So should you enlist? It's a tough battle. "If people want to avoid salt, they really can't—not unless they skip processed, prepared, and restaurant foods," says Marion Nestle, PhD, MPH, a professor of nutrition, food studies, and public health at New York University and author of *Food Politics*. What's more, shedding the salt could do you more harm than good. Before you sign up to fight, tune out the hysteria and plunge into the latest nutrition intel.

THE BACKGROUND

Salt is essential to health. Your body can't make it, and your cells need it to function, says Aryan Aiyer, MD, visiting assistant professor of medicine at the Division of Cardiology at the University of Pittsburgh. In fact, the Institute of Medicine recommends consuming at least 3.8 grams of salt a day (just over ½ teaspoon), mainly for the sodium.

Sodium is an electrolyte, a humble member of that hyped class of minerals that help maintain muscle function and hydration; that's why sport drinks contain sodium. You're constantly losing sodium through sweat and urine, and if you don't replenish that sodium and water, your blood pressure may drop far enough to make you dizzy and light-headed. "Sodium acts like a sponge to help hold fluids in your blood," says Rikki Keen, MS, RD, an adjunct instructor of dietetics and nutrition at the University of Alaska. This is also a similar risk for people who chug too much water, which can lower their sodium levels so far that they develop hyponatremia, a potentially deadly condition more common among recreational exercisers than professional athletes, says Marie Spano, MS, RD, a sports nutritionist in Atlanta.

Another thing to consider: Common table salt is one of the biggest sources of iodine—a key component in healthy thyroid function—in your diet. The thyroid gland is often described as the thermostat of the human endocrine system. It regulates your body's use of energy, and creates and stores hormones that control everything from your metabolism to your growth rate. The essential chemical for all these functions is iodine. Without enough of this element pumping through your thyroid, you may begin to experience fatigue, depression, lethargy, cloudy thinking, and weight gain. Left untreated, an iodine deficiency may potentially cause thyroid cancer and, some doctors theorize, even heart disease.

What's more, the CDC notes that median iodine levels in the United States have dropped by almost 50 percent over the past 40 years. And a 2011 CDC study found that almost a quarter of American men should be considered iodine deficient.

On the other hand, more and more processed products are being loaded with salt, and that's not necessarily a good thing. Sure, salt makes food taste good. But that's not the only reason fast-food meals and processed foods are laced with it. For starters, people become hooked on the flavor profile of familiar products, says Howard Moskowitz, PhD, a food scientist and cofounder of the journal *Chemical Senses*. "They've become accustomed to this richer, deeper taste due to salt. Take out the salt, and people will complain and stop buying the product."

Salt also masks off-flavors created during the production of processed foods while acting as a preservative and improving texture and color. And let's face it, where else can a $600 billion industry find an ingredient that can do so much so cheaply? Whether or not salt itself is a help or hindrance for you, it can definitely run with a bad crowd.

Sneaky Sources of Salt

If you're looking to sidestep some of the processed sodium in your diet, look no further than the list below. These foods account for more than 40 percent of the total intake in our diets, according to the CDC. Eat more fresh food and check the labels of any prepared foods you bring home.

THE TOP 10 SOURCES

1. Breads and rolls
2. Cold cuts and cured meats
3. Pizza
4. Poultry (includes processed products)
5. Soups
6. Sandwiches
7. Cheese
8. Pasta dishes
9. Meat dishes
10. Savory snacks

THE HEALTH HYPE

If you have high blood pressure, you've probably been advised to cut back on salt. The mechanism seems clear: Sodium causes your blood to hold more water, so your heart has to pump harder, making your blood pressure rise. If your blood pressure is already high, that's a problem. (A high intake of salt can also be dangerous for people who are salt sensitive—that is, they have trouble excreting excess salt.)

But your body is constantly balancing the sodium on the outside of each cell and the potassium on the inside. A 2006 statement from the American Heart Association in the journal *Hypertension* revealed that an increase in potassium can lower blood pressure just as much as a decrease in sodium can. Even the Institute of Medicine doesn't deny this: "The sodium to potassium ratio is typically more closely associated with blood pressure than with intake of either substance alone."

Unfortunately, super-salty processed meals tend to crowd out our main dietary sources of potassium—fresh fruits and vegetables. Nutrition surveys reveal that younger men consume only about 60 to 70 percent of the recommended daily intake: 4,700 milligrams of potassium. Imagine the effect on our blood pressure levels if fast-food cashiers always asked, "You want broccoli with that?"

What if you're a healthy guy? The Institute of Medicine is adamant in recommending that people ages 14 and over consume no more than 1,500 milligrams of sodium a day—that is what is in about $2/3$ of a teaspoon of salt.

But even though the average American blows past that limit, consuming an average of 3,400 milligrams of sodium a day, some experts say that's not a problem for most men. "I don't know of any evidence that suggests that healthy men with normal blood pressure should reduce their sodium intake," says Michael Alderman, MD, a professor emeritus of medicine at Yeshiva University.

For starters, reducing the salt content of your diet could adversely affect your health, Alderman says. In a study review published in the *Journal of Hypertension*, people who reduced their sodium intake by about 1,000 milligrams experienced lower blood pressure but also higher heart rates and decreased insulin sensitivity, which can raise diabetes risk. Because of these effects, he says, we need clinical trials to determine whether lowering salt intake actually improves health outcomes in the general population.

And what about the effects that a low-salt diet has on your iodine levels? Theoretically, if all the people in the United States reduced their daily sodium intake to the recommended 1,500 milligrams, everyone would still consume plenty of iodine. This assumes, however, that most of the salt in our diets is the iodized kind that we shake onto our plates. But in fact, industry data suggests that more than 70 percent of what we swallow comes from processed foods and restaurant dishes—and almost none of that salt is iodized.

Even when we cook our meals at home, we often unwittingly deprive ourselves of the opportunity to ingest iodine, says Sara Blackburn, DSc, RD, a clinical associate professor of nutrition at Indiana University–Purdue University Indianapolis. "People watch and mimic chef demonstrations on TV food shows," she says. "More and more, those chefs are talking about the better flavors of kosher salt and the different forms of sea salt. Those sea salts just aren't good sources of iodine."

YOUR BEST MOVE

While a quarter of US men aren't consuming enough iodine, experts agree that Americans young and old have access to more than enough iodized salt to keep their thyroids healthy. The real issue is that most people aren't aware that a problem exists, says Purnendu Dasgupta, PhD, a professor of chemistry and biochemistry at the University of Texas at Arlington, who conducted a 2008 study of the iodine levels in table salt. Most people don't know how much iodine they're consuming or where it comes from.

Compounding the problem is that there isn't much more insight to be gleaned from the average MD. "You can't ask a doctor to check for iodine deficiency," Dasgupta says. The benchmark assessment for iodine is the urinary iodine concentration test (UIC), which determines how much of the element is lost in urine. With UIC, doctors either take a spot sample of urine or gather several samples over 24 hours. In either case, problems arise. "The spot-sample collection may not be representative of what will be passed in 24 hours," says Francis Tayie, PhD, an assistant professor of nutrition and dietetics at Central Michigan University. "And significant losses of iodine can occur during the 24-hour collection—both storage losses and collection losses." Furthermore, Dasgupta says, only a handful of labs nationwide actually perform UIC testing, due to the expense of preparing the samples. He and other researchers obtain their data and extrapolate iodine presence through spot urine samples taken from large groups and populations.

But even if an accurate test were readily available for individuals, Dasgupta says most people wouldn't think to ask their doctors for it. "The problem of iodine deficiency falls on deaf ears," he says. "No one seems to care." Blackburn agrees that public awareness is the key to a long-term solution, but she's more optimistic. She says she has started to see iodine added to multivitamins. She also points to research that's beginning to defuse the salt-hypertension scare by suggesting that high sodium intake is linked to high blood pressure only in people who are "salt sensitive," meaning they respond to salt by retaining fluid. And since the thyroid regulates metabolism, iodine is important in controlling body weight, which is a definite factor in hypertension.

The important thing, Blackburn says, is for people to know their own bodies and to be responsible for their health and that of their children. "It is concerning that over time people will not take in enough iodine in their diets," she says. "The yet-to-be-born may bear the consequences of our current good intentions."

That said, tossing some salt into your pasta water isn't likely to send your blood pressure soaring. That's because 77 percent of the sodium in the average diet comes from processed and restaurant foods, according to the Centers for Disease Control and Prevention. Only 12 percent of sodium is naturally occurring in foods, and, according to the CDC, just 5 percent of the sodium in the average diet comes from home cooking. So there's no need to ban salt from your house or buy an additive-laden salt substitute—especially since salt is an important seasoning and the only natural source of that basic taste, says Harold McGee, the author of *On Food and Cooking*. After all, our brains evolved to crave salt because it's necessary for survival, says Leslie Stein, PhD, director of science communications at the Monell Center in Philadelphia, which researches the senses of taste and smell. Salt creates a fuller mouthfeel when you eat while suppressing bitterness and releasing sweetness. In fact, without a decent hit of salt, many foods would taste flat, not flavorful. It's also essential in the chemistry of baking, says Stein.

The No-Sodium Option for Upping Your Iodine Intake

Until America's salt situation is straightened out, a multivitamin may be your best iodine insurance, says Angela Leung, MD, an assistant professor of medicine at Boston University School of Medicine. That's because many multis supply the proper dose—150 micrograms (mcg)—and contain additional thyroid-supporting nutrients, such as selenium. Before you buy, check the label for the words "potassium iodide," not "kelp." In a 2009 study, Leung found that the iodine amounts in 19 multis with kelp-derived iodine were off by at least 20 percent from their advertised amounts. "Kelp's iodine content depends on the seawater it grew in, so it can vary," she says. One more caution: Don't pop more than 150 mcg a day. Megadoses of iodine (1,100 mcg daily) may actually hurt your thyroid.

Chapter 26

Should You Take Probiotics?

RESEARCH INDICATES THAT THESE "HELPFUL BACTERIA" CAN EASE DIGESTIVE DISTRESS, BOOST YOUR IMMUNE SYSTEM, AND EVEN PROTECT AGAINST CERTAIN TYPES OF CANCERS. BUT ARE THEY WORTH THE HYPE?

If you believe the current buzz (and Jamie Lee Curtis), when it comes to the benefits probiotics have on your health, you may come to view these "healthy bacteria" as the key to solving the majority of your gastrointestinal problems—plus a host of others.

THE BACKGROUND

Walk down the dairy aisle of any grocery store and it's hard to miss the bevy of products whose labels proclaim the presence of probiotics or "good" bacteria. These naturally occurring microorganisms are often added to food, especially yogurt, and can be beneficial to your health. They're getting so common that they're turning up in everything from pizza to chocolate. They now tally $20 billion in global sales, expanding at 20 to 30 percent a year. If you're not already consuming them in some form, chances are you will be soon. Studies show that certain probiotics can help you fight colds, diarrhea, and more. But those aren't always the ones in your food. This chapter outlines what you need to know about finding the probiotics that are best for your body.

THE HEALTH HYPE

"Probiotics are the new vitamins," says Shekhar Challa, MD, a gastroenterologist in Topeka, Kansas, and author of *Probiotics for Dummies*. That's a bold statement, because probiotics are actually live microbes—specifically, beneficial bacteria that promote human health if consumed in large enough quantities. For germophobic Americans, it's a revolutionary concept.

But the 100 trillion microbes that live in your large intestine do dozens of good things for you. They process indigestible fibers and help keep bowel function regular. They produce a number of vitamins, including B_6, B_{12}, and K_2, and aid in the absorption of minerals such as iron, calcium, and magnesium. Equally important, they help fend off bad bacteria such as salmonella and *E. coli*, which can cause diarrhea and, in extreme cases, severe anemia, kidney failure, and death. "The intestines are a war zone, where beneficial and harmful bacteria are fighting to establish predominance," says A. Venket Rao, PhD, emeritus professor of nutritional sciences at the University of Toronto. The key is for the good guys to outnumber the bad. If you want to give them a competitive edge, a regular supply of probiotics can help.

The payoff can extend well beyond your gut, and your immune system is a prime beneficiary. In a Swedish study of 262 workers, those who took probiotics for 80 days were 42 percent less likely to take a sick day for an upper respiratory infection or gastrointestinal disease. Regular doses can help reduce urinary tract infections. If you're prone to allergies or eczema, probiotics may even help tamp down an overactive immune system. They accomplish all this by producing their own form of antibiotics, blocking pathogens from adhering to the gut, and spurring production of chemical messengers called cytokines, which communicate with the immune system throughout the body. Probiotics may even enhance your mood, thanks to a similar cross talk with the central nervous system.

YOUR BEST MOVE

So the conclusion is simple, right? Take probiotics. Unfortunately, it's not that easy. There are more than 3,000 species of good bacteria in your gut, and each has its own talents. The cultures you're consuming may not be the ones that reduce colds or fight diarrhea. And they have to be handled correctly so they aren't killed during processing or storage. "No more than 10 percent of products that claim to be probiotic have been proven in human trials," says Gregor Reid, PhD, chair of human microbiology and probiotics at the Lawson Health Research Institute in Ontario.

So how do you know which ones to pick? Mary Ellen Sanders, PhD, executive director of the International Scientific Association for Probiotics and Prebiotics, offers this four-step process to help you find the best ones.

Step 1:
Know the Names

There are three elements of a probiotic's name: the genus, species, and strain. The trouble is, most companies list only the genus and species of a strain. That's like a restaurant serving "fish" without telling you what kind it is. Not having enough information makes determining any health benefits a difficult task. You should choose products that include the full names of their probiotics. Chances are, more research is available about the benefits, which is why the food company chose to spotlight the strains it included.

Step 2:
Ignore the Usual Suspects

Don't be impressed by foods that list only *L. bulgaricus* and *S. thermophilus*. These organisms do help you digest lactose, but they mostly just help create yogurt. To be labeled a probiotic, an organism has to have a health benefit. *L. acidophilus* is also common. Some companies use studied strains of it as probiotics, but others use it only for flavor. Check the label for bacteria strains with proven health benefits, like these listed by consumerlab.com: *Lactobacillus GG, L. casei, L. reuteri,* and *Saccharomyces boulardii.*

Step 3:
Vet the Research

Bifidobacterium lactis DN-173 010 is found only in Dannon Activia—because Dannon developed it, studied it, and patented it. (Dannon claims this strain helps regulate your digestive system.) This is common: Many strains are studied primarily by the companies that developed them. Then those same companies promote the benefits. Watch for definite claims, like "clinically proven" or "scientifically proven"—Dannon had to scrap these claims in a 2010 settlement and replace them with less-certain phrases, like "clinical studies show."

Step 4:
Read the Label Closely

Questions about probiotics shouldn't stop you from eating yogurt, a good source of protein and calcium. Hey, if the live cultures have other health benefits, that's all the better. But probiotics are now being added to lots of unfermented foods, too, including cookies, pizza crust, coffee beans, and powdered smoothie mixes. Unless the label promises "live and active cultures," don't count on them—particularly in products that require heating, such as coffee and pizza. High temperatures are likely to destroy the bacteria. Chocolate, on the other hand, is one product in which added probiotics do well. Attune Foods makes three varieties with beneficial levels of tested strains. Find them in the dairy case at chains such as Safeway. Be wary of probiotic supplements: Many may have no proven benefits. Look for products with labels that list the full names of probiotics, the number of colony-forming units, and the scientifically studied benefits of each strain. Dosage and storage suggestions should also be included.

MORE WAYS TO BOOST THE BENEFITS OF PROBIOTICS

Be Cultured

The microbes that turn milk into yogurt and kefir are among the most beneficial, and they seem to thrive in dairy. "Milk contains compounds called oligosaccharides [complex carbohydrates] that the bacteria feed on," says Roger A. Clemens, DrPH, adjunct professor of pharmacology at the University of Southern California. Dairy products are also kept chilled, which is important for heat-sensitive organisms, and are only weakly acidic, another plus. (Bacteria can perish in the strongly acidic environment of the stomach, but dairy provides protection.) Just make sure the container says "live and active cultures." Dead bacteria won't help. The more reliable brands tell you which specific bacteria they contain.

Learn to Pickle

Microbes are responsible for fermentation, turning cabbage into sauerkraut, cucumbers into sour pickles, and soybeans into miso. For thousands of years, fermented foods have been staples of the human diet. But we eat far fewer of these foods today, and when we do, modern processing often kills off the good bacteria. "Stores can't have jars exploding on shelves when bacteria produce gas, so manufacturers pasteurize sauerkraut and pickles," says Sanders. "Unless you're pulling your pickles out of a crock in a deli or buying them from a small local producer who labels them 'raw fermented,' you're not getting live microbes."

For the best results, make your own, says Sandor Ellix Katz, author of *The Art of Fermentation*. For sauerkraut, slice cabbage thin, massage it in a bowl with 1 tablespoon of salt to draw out the water, and store it in the brine you've just created. Wait a week or more while it ferments. That's it! Just be sure to keep the kraut completely covered in the brine to prevent rotting caused by bad bacteria. Robyn Jasko, the author of *Homesweet Homegrown*, recommends a type of jar called Pickl-It (pickl-it.com), which has an airlock that keeps bad bacteria out and good bacteria in.

Eat Prebiotics

For colonies to thrive, you need to create favorable living conditions for them. One of the best ways to do that is to consume a diet rich in fruits and vegetables. "Processed foods contain preservatives, which are antimicrobial by definition," Reid says. By contrast, many natural whole foods include prebiotics, or foods that the good microbes themselves feed on—namely, insoluble fibers that people cannot digest but bacteria can. These fibers are in a variety of foods, including onions, bananas, asparagus, leeks, garlic, artichokes, wheat, oats, and soybeans. Prebiotics are being added to some packaged foods, too. Look for terms like inulin, FOS, GOS, or polydextrose on the ingredient list.

Chapter 27

Is Drinking Milk Risky?

MANY HEALTH ADVOCATES (INCLUDING US!) OFTEN CITE THE FAT-FIGHTING, MUSCLE-BUILDING BENEFITS OF COW'S MILK. BUT INCREASING CONCERNS ABOUT HORMONES AND ANTIBIOTICS ARE GIVING IT AN IFFY REP.

Does milk do your body good? Some experts say it's a health hazard. Others say it's the most nutritious food you can find.

"Milk is a deadly poison," according to the Dairy Education Board. In fact, if you peruse this special interest group's Web site, notmilk.com, you'll find dozens of articles about the purported evils of this popular beverage. One claim, for example, is that milk from cows contains cancer-causing hormones and that dairy industry dollars have kept this fact bottled up. All of which may leave you second-guessing your next sip.

However, an entirely separate school of thought says that most men thrive on milk, whether their goal is to lose fat or build muscle. So which side is correct? Or is there even a correct answer? We investigated all the claims—and the result? All your milk questions, answered.

THE BACKGROUND

The concern about the possible hazards of drinking milk stem from two primary concerns: hormones and antibiotics.

Here's the full story: In 1993 the FDA approved the use of recombinant bovine growth hormone (rBGH) in cattle. This practice resulted in greater milk production at less cost to the dairy farmer, a savings that has been passed on to you at your local supermarket. But it has also sparked much controversy, because rBGH boosts milk's concentration of insulin-like growth factor (IGF), a hormone that's been linked to cancer.

But unlike steroid hormones, which can be taken orally, rBGH and IGF must be injected to have any effect. That's because the process of digestion destroys these "protein" hormones. So drinking milk from hormone-treated cows doesn't transfer the active form of these chemicals to your body. However, there is one ethical downside to consider: It's not good for the cows. Canadian researchers discovered that cows given hormones are more likely to contract an udder infection called mastitis.

No one really knows what the effects antibiotics given to cows may have on your body. Some scientists argue that milk from cows given antibiotics leads to antibiotic resistance in humans, making these types of drugs less effective when you take them for an infection. But this finding has never been proved.

THE HEALTH HYPE

The jury's still out when it comes to the claim that milk helps burn fat. In a 6-month study, University of Tennessee researchers found that overweight people who downed three servings a day of calcium-rich dairy lost more belly fat than those who followed a similar diet minus two or more of the dairy servings. In addition, the researchers discovered that calcium supplements didn't work as well as milk. Why? They believe that while calcium may increase the rate at which your body burns fat, other active compounds in dairy (such as milk proteins) provide an additional fat-burning effect. Of course, the key to success is following a weight loss diet to begin with. After all, downing your dairy with a box of doughnuts is no way to torch your gut.

However, milk *is* a proven muscle builder. In fact, milk is one of the best muscle foods on the planet. You see, the protein in milk is about 80 percent casein and 20 percent whey. Both are high-quality proteins, but whey is known as a "fast protein" because it's quickly broken down into amino acids and absorbed into the bloodstream. That makes it a very good protein to consume after your workout. Casein, on the other hand, is digested more slowly. So it's ideal for providing your body with a steady supply of smaller amounts of protein for a longer period of time—like between meals or while you sleep. Since milk provides both, one big glass gives your body an ideal combination of muscle-building proteins.

Another hot button topic: The raw milk debate. Unpasteurized milk is rumored to be healthier. But is it? "We've seen an interest in raw milk in recent years as more consumers seek out more natural foods," says Sally Fallon Morell, president of the Weston A. Price Foundation, a nutrition education group in Washington, DC. Proponents claim that pasteurization, the process of heating milk to kill bacteria, destroys healthy nutrients. Some even say unpasteurized milk (available at some health food stores and dairies) can help prevent and treat certain health woes.

But there's limited research to back these claims, and some states have outlawed raw milk due to health risks. "Even on the cleanest farms, cows can carry disease-causing microorganisms," says Martin Wiedmann, PhD, a professor of food science at Cornell University. Between 1998 and 2008, the CDC reported 86 outbreaks of illness from raw milk consumption. Bottom line: Pasteurized milk is safest.

YOUR BEST MOVE

If you want to make milk a part of your daily diet, go for it. If you're uneasy about antibiotics or hormones, you can purchase antibiotic-free (and typically hormone-free, as well) milk from specialty grocers, such as Trader Joe's or Whole Foods, or select USDA-certified organic milk, which is available at most supermarkets.

As for what kind of milk to choose—skim, whole, or somewhere in between—this depends on your taste. While you've probably always been told to drink reduced-fat milk, the majority of scientific studies show that drinking whole milk actually improves cholesterol levels, just not as much as drinking a lower-fat variety does. One exception: Danish researchers found that men who consumed a diet rich in whole milk experienced a slight increase in LDL cholesterol (six points). However, it's worth noting that these men drank six 8-ounce glasses a day, an unusually high amount. Even so, their triglycerides—another marker of heart disease risk—decreased by 22 percent.

The bottom line: Drinking two to three glasses of milk a day lowers the likelihood of both heart attack and stroke, a finding confirmed by British scientists.

ARE YOU LACTOSE INTOLERANT?

If you believe milk upsets your stomach, perhaps you should try to prove it. In a study at the Veterans Administration Medical Center in Minneapolis, researchers found that people who described themselves as "severely lactose intolerant" responded no differently to 2 cups of milk than to a placebo beverage. Scientists think that people who've noticed discomfort after consuming dairy—abdominal cramps, bloating, or diarrhea—often eliminate it altogether, even though small amounts may not produce the same symptoms. Here's how to test yourself.

Step 1
Buy two types of milk: regular and lactose-free. Then ask a friend to pour each type into identical containers, labeling one A and the other B.

Step 2
For 1 week, drink 2 cups a day from container A on an empty stomach and avoid all other dairy. Record any symptoms of intestinal discomfort.

Step 3
Discontinue container A for at least 1 day.

Step 4
Repeat step 2, but drink from container B instead.

Step 5
Compare the results from each container.

No Difference?
You aren't lactose intolerant. However, if you tested positive, you can use these strategies for better digestion of dairy products.

1. Limit your milk intake to 1 cup at a time. And drink it with food, which slows the absorption of lactose and helps alleviate side effects.

2. Have more cheese. It contains very little lactose. (Hint: The fewer carbohydrates a dairy product has, the less lactose it contains.)

3. Try kefir. Ohio State University scientists found that this fermented milk beverage improves lactose digestion. Yogurt may provide similar benefits.

DAIRY-FREE MILKS AND THEIR BENEFITS

You've seen them on the shelf: milks made from rice, nuts, and yes, even hemp. Cow-free milk is no passing trend: The milk-alternatives market grew 12.5 percent in 2011, according to the Beverage Marketing Corporation. "While cow's milk contains nutrients such as calcium, vitamin D, and protein, people are turning to nondairy varieties because of allergies, lactose intolerance, and concerns about hormones and antibiotics," says Elisa Zied, RD, author of *Nutrition at Your Fingertips*. Some faux milks are more beneficial than good old moo juice and clock in at fewer calories (skim milk has 90 per 8-ounce glass), while others lack nutritional value or harbor hidden calories and sugar, particularly the vanilla- and chocolate-flavored ones. Consult this guide before you drink up.

Almond Milk
Almond Breeze Original
Per cup: 60 calories, 1 g protein, 8 g carbs (1 g fiber, 7 g sugars), 2.5 g fat (0 g sat), 150 mg sodium
Taste: Creamy, rich, and slightly nutty with a hint of sweetness
Pros: The least caloric of the bunch, it's fortified with vitamin E, a powerful antioxidant that fights UV damage, as well as calcium and vitamins A and D
Cons: While almonds are a good source of fiber and protein, the milk contains skimpy amounts of these nutrients (because the milk is made by grinding the nuts and mixing with water); almond milk is higher in sodium than other alternatives
Best in: Smoothies, coffee, and cereal

Hemp Milk
Tempt Original
Per cup: 100 calories, 2 g protein, 9 g carbs (0 g fiber, 6 g sugars), 6 g fat (0.5 g sat), 110 mg sodium
Taste: Nutty and earthy

Pros: Naturally rich in omega-3 fatty acids—wonder nutrients for your heart, brain, and mood; made with cannabis seeds, but won't get you high because it lacks significant THC (the psychoactive ingredient in marijuana)
Cons: Depending on the brand, you may gulp only 10 percent of your daily calcium needs; not a great source of protein
Best in: Mashed potatoes, muffins, and quick breads; a good stand-in for cow's milk in baked foods

Coconut Milk
So Delicious Coconut Milk Beverage Original
Per cup: 70 calories, 0 g protein, 8 g carbs (1 g fiber, 7 g sugars), 4.5 g fat (4 g sat), 15 mg sodium
Taste: Thick, creamy, and, well, coconut-y
Pros: Has the least amount of sodium and can be fairly low-cal—even some flavored kinds will cost you only 90 calories per serving—plus, most brands are fortified with half a day's worth of vitamin B_{12}, a brain-boosting nutrient
Cons: The majority of fat is saturated
Best in: Coffee, tea, pudding, smoothies, and oatmeal—it's a go-to thickener

Rice Milk
Rice Dream Enriched Original
Per cup: 120 calories, 1 g protein, 23 g carbs (0 g fiber, 10 g sugars), 2.5 g fat (0 g sat), 100 mg sodium
Taste: Light, watery, and sweet
Pros: The carbs, which provide fuel; a glass before or after a workout is also hydrating and a good source of electrolytes
Cons: The carbs—it has zero so you'll have to get that filling fiber from whole-grain carbs
Best in: Desserts, baked goods, pancakes, and French toast; complements indulgent foods

Soy Milk
Silk Original
Per cup: 90 calories, 6 g protein, 8 g carbs (1 g fiber, 6 g sugars), 3.5 g fat (0.5 g sat), 100 mg sodium
Taste: Faintly sweet; some varieties have a slight tofu flavor
Pros: Has almost as much protein as cow's milk, plus plant chemicals that may help inhibit absorption of cholesterol; it's often fortified, so shake the carton well since added calcium tends to settle at the bottom
Cons: Some studies suggest that overconsuming soy promotes breast cancer (keep consumption of soy protein to about 25 grams per day)
Best in: Creamy soups and salad dressings, sauces, casseroles, and other savory dishes; vanilla-flavored varieties are great in coffee or tea (or by the glass)

Chapter 28

How Important Are Antioxidants?

WE INVESTIGATED THESE WARRIORS OF THE HEALTH WORLD AND DISCOVERED HOW THEY PATROL EVERY PART OF YOUR BODY.

It's billed as an epic story of good versus evil—biology in comic-book form. The villains: free radicals, those nefarious DNA-attacking poisons of modern life. Our fearless defenders: antioxidants, poised to protect us from, well, everything, right? You've heard the claims:

    They cure cancer!

    They prevent aging!

    They supercharge your immune system!

But while we think we know what antioxidants do, few of us know what antioxidants actually are. And food manufacturers are fine with that: The less you know, the more likely you are to swallow the hype. "Antioxidants have a health aura around them," says Marion Nestle, PhD, MPH, a professor of nutrition, food studies, and public health at New York University and author of *Food Politics*. "They are supposed to fight something bad in your body. Who wouldn't want to consume more of a helper like that?"

There's no doubt that antioxidants can be good for you. But to maximize their benefit, we first have to strip away some assumptions.

THE BACKGROUND

Antioxidants are nutrients that are derived from natural sources. In fact, the entire plant kingdom—including beans, nuts, seeds, and grains—is awash in antioxidants, according to a study from the University of Scranton. That's because all plants produce antioxidants to fight against predators and UV rays, says Joe Vinson, PhD, a professor of chemistry at the University of Scranton in Pennsylvania. It's important to steer clear of refined grains, though; they've been stripped of most of their antioxidant benefits. Even meat, dairy products, and eggs contain some antioxidants, which mainly come from the nutrient-rich plants the animals fed on.

Antioxidants fight free radicals, which are unstable molecules in the body that can cause DNA mutation. Even though free radicals have been linked to serious conditions like heart disease, Parkinson's, and cancer, they aren't necessarily villains—they're byproducts of a basic metabolic process called oxidation. "They're absolutely essential to life," says Jeffrey Blumberg, PhD, director of the antioxidants lab at Tufts University. "For example, immune cells will shoot free radicals onto invading bacteria in order to kill them. They're an important part of the body's defenses."

THE HEALTH HYPE

Too many free radicals are harmful to your body. Pollutants, cigarette smoke, and sun overexposure can generate so many free radicals that your normal antioxidant defenses become overwhelmed, leaving you vulnerable to cell damage and disease. Some researchers also link free-radical oxidation with aging.

That's where antioxidants come in. "We need to make sure we have adequate antioxidant defenses to combat all the excess free radicals," says Blumberg.

Any molecule that protects your cells against oxidation is technically an antioxidant, says Vinson. "They're anti-oxidation." This includes familiar nutrients, like vitamins, as well as more unfamiliar types of antioxidants, like flavonoids and polyphenols—about 8,000 varieties in all.

But don't assume that all antioxidants operate the same way, Blumberg warns. "You can't say, 'Well, I'm not going to worry about taking in enough vitamin E, because I take lots of vitamin C.' All the vitamin C in the world won't substitute for vitamin E," says Blumberg. Some antioxidants excel at fighting certain types of free radicals (yep, there are different varieties of those, too), while others are effective only in specific parts of a cell. Still others can battle free radicals only under the right conditions.

"Think of antioxidants as an army," he says. "You need generals, lieutenants, corporals, privates, and others with specific duties. You can't fight an enemy with only generals." So how do you create an effective defense system in the battle for your life? By building a multi-pronged counteroffensive—er, diet.

Where To Find Antioxidants

Antioxidants are our nutritional best friends. But what foods are best to eat? Oxygen Radical Absorbance Capacity, or ORAC, is a method of measuring antioxidant capacities of different foods. The higher the score, the more antioxidant power a food has. Here's a sampling of foods to give you an idea of how they score—berries, legumes, and some vegetables come in high. Pure cocoa is the world champ. But other foods that are considered nutritious are low in antioxidants (see bananas and corn). That doesn't mean you shouldn't eat low-scoring foods, just don't assume you get antioxidant protection from them.

Per 100g Serving	ORAC Score*
Apple, red delicious, with skin	4,275
Artichokes, raw	6,552
Bananas, raw	879
Black beans, raw	8,040
Navy beans, raw	1,520
Blueberries	6,552
Broccoli, raw	1,362
Cocoa, dry, unsweetened	80,933
Corn, raw	728
Cranberries	9,584
Elderberries	14,697
Garlic, raw	5,346
Lentils, raw	7,282
Oranges, raw	1,819
Spinach, raw	1,515

*The amount shown is the ORAC score per 100 grams, according to the USDA (see usda.gov for a comprehensive ORAC food list).

YOUR BEST MOVE

If you eat a wide variety of fruits and vegetables, your diet is naturally rich in thousands of antioxidants. Studies suggest eating at least five servings of fruits and vegetables a day to reap the most health benefits. To get your fill without overloading on one particular food, branch out and try something new in the produce aisle. In a study, researchers at Colorado State University found that people who ate the widest variety of fruits and vegetables had the most DNA protection.

When possible, stick to whole foods. These days, it seems like antioxidant-fortified products are popping up everywhere—and can include anything from chocolate to soda. You can even chug an antioxidant-fortified version of Cherry 7UP. The FDA requires food manufacturers to list the variety of antioxidant in a product; that part is often in fine print. Look closely, and the label reveals that you're receiving a tiny helping of vitamin E. Perhaps "Cherry 7UP Vitamin E" didn't sound as impressive.

So, if you're relying on processed foods to supplement your antioxidant intake, you may be surprised to find that many processed foods have relatively small amounts of just one or two kinds. Since variety is critical, you probably aren't making up for lost ground. So ignore the hype—there's no research to prove that packaged products provide the same health benefits that whole foods do. Instead, focus on the ingredient list. If a food product contains mostly plant foods, it's likely to be rich in antioxidants.

So eat whole-grain foods, beans, nuts, and seeds regularly. When animals are on the menu, make sure they've been grass fed; meat and dairy products from these better-fed beasts have been shown to contain higher levels of antioxidants. Eggs from pastured hens also rank higher in antioxidants—look for them at farmers' markets.

Getting your antioxidants from foods, not supplements or other fortified products, is especially important if you're trying to lose weight. Exercising leads to more oxidation and an increase in free radicals. That's not a bad thing. "Since free-radical production is a normal response to exercise, taking a large dose of antioxidants right after a workout could interfere with the natural, beneficial response to exercise," says Alan Aragon, MS, a *Men's Health* nutrition advisor. The logic is unexpected but clear: Scientists speculate that the oxidative stress triggered by exercise promotes insulin sensitivity and weight loss, and possibly reduces your risk of diabetes.

Case in point: A German study found that when exercisers took antioxidant supplements (vitamins C and E), they weren't rewarded with the typical postexercise boost in insulin sensitivity. Also, a British study found that runners who took 1,000 milligrams of vitamin C daily for a week lost muscle strength. So much for that well-intentioned antioxidant-fortified recovery drink. Michael Ristow, MD, an author of the study and professor at the Energy Metabolism Laboratory in Zurich, speculates that other antioxidant supplements might have similar negative effects, though more study is needed.

Chapter 29

Is Sugar Toxic?

THERE'S NO DOUBT ABOUT IT, SUGAR IS A HUGE CONTRIBUTING FACTOR TO TODAY'S OBESITY CRISIS. BUT IT MAY NOT BE AS HORRIBLE AS MOST PEOPLE THINK IT IS.

Sugar caused the recession. Sugar makes your nipples grow. Sugar keyed your car. Sugar's crazy. Somebody should drop a safe on sugar. Well, maybe. It's true that sugar is insidious—diabolical, even—and hidden in countless processed foods. It certainly contributes to the obesity crisis. It makes people fat and diabetic. These claims are correct, to a limited and oversimplified extent. But sugar is only as big a bogeyman as you make it out to be.

THE BACKGROUND

The sugar in our bodies, glucose, is a fundamental fuel for body and brain, says David Levitsky, PhD, a professor of psychology and nutritional sciences at Cornell University. The health threat to the vast American public arises from a very personal level, Levitsky says: "It's that sugars taste good. Sweetened foods tend to make us overeat. And that threatens the energy balance in our bodies."

In the 1970s and 1980s, the average American's body weight increased in tandem with the food industry's use of high-fructose corn syrup (HFCS), a staple because it's cheap. But it's not a smoking gun. "This is a correlation, not a causation," says Levitsky.

"Obesity is about consuming too many calories," says Lillian Lien, MD, the medical director of inpatient diabetes management at the Duke University medical center. "It just so happens that a lot of overweight people have been drinking HFCS in sodas and eating foods that are high on the glycemic index—sweet snacks, white bread, and so forth. The calorie totals are huge, and the source just happens to be sugar-based."

THE HEALTH HYPE

Studies dating back decades show that eating too much fructose, a sugar found naturally in fruit and also added to processed foods, raises blood lipid levels. And while the relatively modest quantities in fruit shouldn't worry you, a University of Minnesota study shows that the large amounts of fructose we take in from processed foods may prove especially nasty: Men on high-fructose diets had 32 percent higher triglycerides than men on high-glucose diets.

Why? Your body can't metabolize a sweet snack as fast as you can eat it, says Levitsky. So your liver puts some of the snack's glucose into your bloodstream, or stores it for later use. But if your liver's tank is full, it packages the excess as triglycerides. The snack's fructose goes to your liver as well, but instead of being deposited into your bloodstream, it's stored as glycogen. Your liver can store about 90 to 100 grams of glycogen, so it converts the excess to fat (the triglycerides).

Too much sugar stresses your system. Doctors use the oral glucose tolerance test (OGTT) to diagnose prediabetes and diabetes. For an OGTT, you consume 75 grams of glucose to see how your system processes sugar. It's like a stress test—downing that kind of sugar load is not something you should normally do.

And yet a 24-ounce soda often contains more than 75 grams of sugar, most of it likely HFCS. Roughly half of that 75 grams is fructose, so that soda shock may be worse than the doctor's test is. "The way people eat and drink these days, unintentional stress tests probably happen quite often," says Lien.

Excess sugar can lead to other problems as well, including diabetes. Diabetes means your body can't clear glucose from your blood. And when glucose isn't processed quickly enough, it destroys tissue, Levitsky says. People with type 1 diabetes were born that way—sugar didn't cause their diabetes. But weight gain in children and adults can cause metabolic syndrome, which leads to type 2 diabetes.

"That's what diabetes is all about—being unable to eliminate glucose," says Levitsky. "The negative effect of eating a lot of sugar is a rise in glucose. A normal pancreas and normal insulin receptors can handle it, clear it out, or store it in some packaged form, like fat."

YOUR BEST MOVE

We can demonize food manufacturers because they produce crap with enough salt and sugar to make us eat more of it than we should—or even want to. But it comes down to how much we allow in our mouths. "A practical guide for anyone is weight," says Lien. "If your weight is under control, then your calorie intake across the board is reasonable. If your weight rises, it's not. That's more important than paying attention to any specific macronutrient."

By maintaining a healthy weight, most people can keep their triglycerides at acceptable levels. "If you're overweight or gaining weight, however, they'll accumulate and become a core predictor of heart disease and stroke," Levitsky says.

If you're one of those overweight people, you need to drop the pounds and watch your sugar intake. Research has shown for years that dropping 5 to 7 percent of your body weight can reduce your odds of developing diabetes. Your first step is to lay off sugary and starchy foods, beer, and sweet drinks. Your body wasn't built to handle all that sugar. Consider this: You'd have to eat four apples in order to ingest roughly the same amount of fructose in one large McDonald's Coke.

Overeating forces your pancreas to work overtime cranking out insulin to clear glucose. Eric Westman, MD, an obesity researcher at the Duke University medical center, says that in today's world, "it's certainly possible that the unprecedented increase in sugar and starch consumption leads to pancreatic burnout." But researchers can't be sure; everyone's body and diet are different, so generalization is iffy. One thing that is sure, Westman says, is that the rise in sugar consumption over the past 100 years is unprecedented.

Maybe you figure your body can process a big sugar load without damage. But that's like pointing to a man who smokes until he's 90 and dodges emphysema or cancer, Westman says. Why gamble?

Severe hyperglycemia (high blood sugar) can cause blurred vision, extreme thirst, and frequent urges to urinate. Hypoglycemia (low blood sugar) is easier to spot: You feel weak with cold sweats and anxiety, blurred vision, or tiredness a couple of hours after a sugar binge. Sound familiar? Ask about an OGTT, which is more accurate than the simpler fasting glucose blood test.

If you live large—big meals, lots of beer, little moderation—you may be shortening your life even if your weight is okay. Repeated blood-sugar spikes stress the organs that make up the metabolic engine of your body. That takes a toll.

And you might not notice. "People can live symptom free for years in a prediabetic state even though they've lost as much as 50 percent of their pancreatic function," says Lien. "And they don't even know it." People with prediabetes share the same health risks, especially for heart disease, that haunt people with full-blown diabetes.

The smartest sugar strategy is simple, yet difficult. Think about what you put in your mouth. Sugar is diabolical; it tastes great and is less filling. Back off on the high-impact glycemics: beer, sugary soft drinks and sport drinks, potatoes, pasta, baked goods, pancakes. "The less sugar stress you put on your system, the longer it will function properly," says Levitsky. But stop blaming sugar for all the world's problems. Even if it is diabolical.

STRAIGHT TALK ON SUGAR SUBSTITUTES

Once upon a time, sugar alternatives were heralded as the slim solution. But according to research presented at the American Diabetes Association Scientific Sessions in 2011, products that contain these sweeteners can be linked to an expanding waist size. One possible reason, says researcher Sharon Fowler, MPH: These pseudo sugars trick your body into some of the same responses that the real thing produces. But some sweeteners are better than others. See how five popular subs stack up:

Stevia

This powdered extract of the stevia plant is all natural and 200 to 400 times sweeter than sugar. (Brands include Stevia Extract In the Raw and PureVia.) Consult your doctor before using it if you have any kind of health condition, since it hasn't been studied extensively.

Saccharin

In the 1970s, animal studies prompted the National Toxicology Program to name it a likely carcinogen, but no such link was ever found in human studies, so saccharin was eventually declared safe. Try to use no more than four packets a day, though. Your body can't digest it, so too much can lead to stomach issues.

Sucralose
Zero calories and 600 times sweeter than sugar, sucralose is considered by many nutritionists to be among the safest of the subs. It is derived from real sugar, not from chemical additives, and has been heavily studied, says Kristin Kirkpatrick, MS, RD, of Cleveland Clinic's wellness manager.

Aspartame
About 200 times sweeter than sugar, aspartame (used in packaged foods and sold under the brands NutraSweet and Equal) was once thought to be linked to cancer, but the FDA maintains it's not a health risk.

Agave
This naturally sweet plant syrup can be up to 90 percent fructose—more than HFCS—and has 20 calories per teaspoon. But it's 25 percent sweeter than sugar, so you might not use as much, and it blends well in liquids like coffee.

What Are the Best Supplements for Men?

THE SUPPLEMENTS IN THIS CHAPTER HAVE PROVEN HEALTH BENEFITS, AND WE'VE LISTED NATURAL SOURCES OF THESE NUTRIENTS, TOO.

If you condensed a recent meal down to a few pills, would they be tiny dynamos or the nutritional equivalent of Tic Tacs? If you're like most men, what's on your plate falls somewhere in between. "If men start to favor certain foods, they may develop nutritional blind spots as a result," says Kristie Lancaster, PhD, an associate professor of nutrition at New York University. This can be a problem, because your body needs a basic roster of vitamins and minerals to run properly. If your regular diet comes up short, you may need a multivitamin to reach this nutritional baseline.

But to boost your health, you need to consider moving beyond a multi by folding in some less common elements. The right supplements can help your heart, sharpen your immune system, and even improve your sex life. But the wrong ones can be ineffective or even harmful. "You run into problems because most men are 'prescribing' these things themselves," says Tod Cooperman, MD, president of ConsumerLab.com, an independent tester of health and nutritional products. "Don't take supplements with abandon. They should be used carefully, because taking in too much of certain nutrients can cause problems."

We consulted with top doctors, reviewed the latest research, and waded through marketers' claims to bring you 18 of the best supplements for men and the problems they address. Use our guide—along with advice from your own doctor, since many supplements can interact with other medications—to fine-tune your strategy.

Important Tip

If you're on aspirin therapy, check with your doctor before taking supplements. For example, pairing aspirin with vitamin E or niacin may increase your risk of stomach bleeding and exacerbate stomach pain, a review published in *Annals of Pharmacotherapy* reports. Aspirin can also worsen side effects from vitamin C, such as nausea and stomach damage.

STARTING POINT: THE BEST MULTIVITAMIN

Don't be fooled by the ingredient overload on multivitamin labels. "Manufacturers may throw in a little something sexy—say, lutein or lycopene—to flesh out the list, but it's rarely enough to be worthwhile," Cooperman says. Go for a conservative multi, such as Target Men's Daily Multivitamin or Centrum Ultra Men's Multivitamin. These nail the essentials in case your diet falls short. Of course, ultimately you want to amend your diet so you can ditch the multis altogether.

PROBLEM: BRAIN DRAIN
Solution: ACETYL-L-CARNITINE

This amino acid converts fats to energy and boosts antioxidant activity in the body. In supplement form, it may protect gray matter from stress caused by alcohol and aging. And in a study, people who received 1,000 milligrams of acetyl-L-carnitine a day saw relief from mild chronic depression.
Dose: 1,000 mg/day*
Natural sources: Red meat, dairy products

PROBLEM: ERECTILE DYSFUNCTION
Solution: KOREAN RED PANAX GINSENG

Sixty percent of men with erectile dysfunction who took this supplement noticed improvement, according to a 2002 Korean study. The herb may also protect your heart—in a Canadian study, a daily dose reduced arterial stiffness.
Dose: 900 mg, up to three times a day*
Natural source: Korean ginseng root

PROBLEM: HIGH BLOOD PRESSURE
Solution: COENZYME Q-10

CoQ-10 can lower your blood pressure while boosting your levels of ECso D, an enzyme thought to protect blood vessels from damage. CoQ-10 may improve sperm quality, according to Italian researchers. Japanese researchers found it can increase fat burning during exercise.

Dose: 30 to 200 mg/day*
Natural sources: Meat, fish, eggs, broccoli

PROBLEM: BONE WEAKNESS
Solution: VITAMIN D

Vitamin D is a hormone that helps your bones absorb calcium. That's a critical benefit, but there are other compelling reasons to take it, Cooperman says. For instance, vitamin D has been linked to reduced levels of depression, reduced risk of colorectal cancer, and less chance of a heart attack.

Dose: 1,000 IU/day*
Natural sources: Sunshine, fortified milk

PROBLEM: HEART DISEASE
Solution: FISH OIL

Loaded with the essential omega-3 fatty acids EPA and DHA, fish oil can reduce triglycerides, boost HDL cholesterol, and lower blood pressure. But your heart isn't the only beneficiary: The healthy fats may also reduce inflammation and improve cognitive performance, and may lower your risk of colon and prostate cancers.

Dose: At least 500 mg DHA and 500 mg EPA daily*
Natural sources: Salmon, tuna, or other fatty fish

* The doses shown here have been used in studies, but your doctor can recommend an appropriate dose for you.

PROBLEM: MIGRAINES
Solution: MAGNESIUM

A drop in magnesium can be a major headache. "Blood vessels in your brain constrict, and receptors in the feel-good chemical serotonin malfunction," says Alexander Mauskop, MD, director of the New York Headache Center. Result: a migraine. The mineral also might help regulate blood pressure and could ward off stroke and diabetes.

Dose: 250 mg/day, plus the magnesium in your diet*
Natural sources: Leafy greens, whole grains, pumpkin seeds, coffee, nuts

PROBLEM: DIABETES
Solution: PSYLLIUM HUSK

This fiber is more than a colon cleanser. In a Finnish study, the addition of psyllium to meals reduced participants' blood sugar and insulin response. Paired with protein, it was also shown to suppress ghrelin, a hormone that makes you hungry. Psyllium is one of five

---

Weight Loss Wonder Drugs?

Not a chance. "You can take any combination of weight loss supplements, but without diet and exercise, you won't manage your weight," says David Katz, MD, MPH, a *Men's Health* weight loss advisor.

Alli
It offers no weight loss advantage over diet modification, notes a Durham, North Carolina, VA Medical Center study. Plus, eating more than 15 grams of fat in a meal while on Alli may result in diarrhea.

Hydroxycut
An older version was shown by University of Southern California researchers to cause liver damage. No trials have confirmed the safety or effectiveness of the newest blend.

Mega-T
Research shows that EGCG, the primary antioxidant in green tea, can boost fat burning, but at doses nearly four times the amount in Mega-T Green Tea.

soluble fibers approved by the FDA for lowering LDL cholesterol.
Dose: 20 to 35 g/day, divided and taken with at least 8 oz liquid
Natural sources: Some fortified cereal grains

PROBLEM: DIGESTIVE UPSET
Solution: PROBIOTICS

Probiotics are healthy bacteria that crowd out the disease-causing bad bacteria in your gut. Some can reduce diarrhea caused by certain infections, antibiotics, irritable bowel syndrome, and chemotherapy, Cooperman notes. The encapsulated good guys may also boost your immune function.
Dose: 1 capsule (with at least 1 billion bacteria) a day*
Natural sources: Yogurt, kefir, and other dairy products

PROBLEM: LOW ENDURANCE
Solution: QUERCETIN

Want to extend your cardio session? People who didn't exercise regularly but took 500 milligrams of this antioxidant twice a day for a week were able to bicycle 13 percent longer than the placebo group, a University of South Carolina study found. It may also help reduce the oxidation of LDL particles and reduce blood-vessel constriction.
Dose: Up to 500 mg, twice a day*
Natural sources: Red wine, parsley, grapefruit, onions, and apples

PROBLEM: POOR MEMORY
Solution: PYCNOGENOL

This supplement's antioxidants fight free-radical stress in your brain and stop the degradation of nitric oxide, which helps preserve neural connections. According to an Australian study, it improved memory in elderly people. Pycnogenol also supports better

Fallen SUPPLEMENT Stars

Manufacturers regularly unveil life-changing supplements that consumers flock to.

Then science catches up to the claims. Make sure you move these recent flops from your cabinet to the trash can.

Flaxseed Oil
Original claim: Helps lower cholesterol and fights heart disease.
New science: Flaxseed oil's omega-3s are delivered as ALA (alpha-linoleic acid), which your body struggles to convert to the usable forms—EPA and DHA. Worse, Australian researchers found that flaxseed oil can increase free radicals in your body, potentially causing inflammation.

Ginkgo Biloba
Original claim: Improves memory and attention.
New science: Long-term use of ginkgo biloba was no more effective than a placebo for mental acuity in older people, according to a University of Pittsburgh clinical trial.

St. John's Wort
Original claim: Beats the blues as well as antidepressants do, minus the side effects.
New science: Your mood may improve, but potentially at the cost of rendering other prescription meds less effective. Clinical trials show that this herb interferes with roughly 12 classes of drugs, including antianxiety meds, statins, and certain antibiotics.

Valerian
Original claim: Helps treat insomnia.
New science: It's a placebo. According to a Spanish review, valerian may improve your perceived quality of sleep but does little to actually enhance it.

bloodflow, which helps fight joint pain and reduce muscle cramps.
Dose: 150 mg/day*
Natural source: Pine bark (extract)

PROBLEM: JOINT PAIN
Solution: GLUCOSAMINE

Glucosamine, a building block of cartilage, can relieve pain and inflammation in joints, explains Nicholas DiNubile, MD, an orthopedic surgeon. One study found glucosamine is more effective than acetaminophen (aka Tylenol) at relieving symptoms of knee osteoarthritis, often caused in younger men by joint injury.
Dose: 1,500 mg/day*
Natural sources: Crustacean shells

PROBLEM: INJURY
Solution: VITAMIN C

Sixty percent of adult men don't get enough vitamin C in their diets, according to an *American Journal of Clinical Nutrition* study. Vitamin C helps protect your cells from the tissue-damaging free radicals produced by exercise. It also helps heal wounds, and it's key to production of the collagen found in ligaments and tendons.
Dose: Up to 1,000 mg/day in spaced doses*
Natural sources: Citrus fruits, sweet peppers, broccoli, kale, Brussels sprouts

PROBLEM: EXTRA BODY FAT
Solution: EGCG (FROM GREEN TEA EXTRACT)

Men who took green tea extract burned 17 percent more fat after moderate exercise than those taking placebos, according to one study. EGCG, the most active antioxidant in green tea, is thought to prolong exercise-induced boosts in metabolism. It has also been shown to help prevent cancer and can improve heart health.
Dose: 890 mg/day green tea extract (containing 340 mg of EGCG)*
Natural source: Green tea

PROBLEM: PROSTATE-CANCER RISK
Solution: LYCOPENE

Found in tomatoes, this potent antioxidant may reduce your risk of prostate cancer, according to a University of Illinois study review. The researchers say it may work by altering hormone metabolism and by causing cancer cells to self-destruct.
Dose: 15 to 20 mg/day*
Natural sources: Fresh or cooked tomatoes and other red/pink fruits

PROBLEM: CHOLESTEROL
Solution: RED YEAST RICE

It contains lovastatin—a prescription statin—as well as other compounds that may help manage cholesterol. In an *Annals of Internal Medicine* study, patients who took red yeast rice during a 12-week diet and exercise program cut their LDL by 27 percent, compared with 6 percent for those who only dieted and exercised.
Dose: 600 mg, 3 times a day* (consult your doctor if you're on heart meds)
Natural sources: Red yeast rice, some types of sake, red rice vinegar

PROBLEM: CANCER RISK
Solution: RESVERATROL

You can't stop the clock, but you can slow it down. This chemical, found in the skin of grapes, seems to interact directly with genes that regulate aging, says Katz. Resveratrol has been shown to promote DNA repair in animals, enhance bloodflow to people's brains, and halt the growth of prostate cancer and colon cancer cells.
No dosage recommendations
Natural sources: Red wine, red grape juice

PROBLEM: DEPRESSION
Solution: SAMe

Talk about head-to-toe relief: A synthetic form of a dietary amino acid, SAMe has been found to treat depression as effectively as prescription antidepressants, according to Canadian researchers. It has also been shown to reduce joint pain and inflammation, and may aid cartilage repair.

Dose: 600 to 1,600 mg/day, depending on the condition*

Natural sources: Made in your body, possibly after eating meats, greens, and oranges

PROBLEM: ENLARGED PROSTATE
Solution: SAW PALMETTO

As you age, your risk rises for benign prostatic hyperplasia (BPH), a condition that makes you trickle at the toilet. Saw palmetto may help restore the flow. In a Korean study, men taking 320 milligrams of saw palmetto daily saw their BPH symptoms decrease by 50 percent after 1 year.

Dose: 320 mg/day*

Natural source: Saw palmetto berries

If Your Diet Pill Works... It's Bad for You

So say leading doctors, who warn that the Wild West of online weight loss supplements is an increasingly risky place. Here's what you must know to protect yourself against the new crop of hazardous drugs.

"Dietary supplements may represent the next big drug safety catastrophe," says Steven Nissen, MD, a cardiologist at the Cleveland Clinic. "We don't know exactly what most supplements contain, so we don't know if they're actually safe." More and more, weight loss products—along with supplements that purport to treat sexual dysfunction or enhance athletic performance— are being "adulterated" with potentially dangerous ingredients by their manufacturers. "Originally, the makers would throw in something like caffeine to give you a kick," says Cooperman. "Now they're adding in compounds you find in prescription drugs without including that information on their labels."

Special Section

The other thing consumers don't realize is that adulterated products can be far riskier than prescription diet pills. That's because, in the virtually unregulated world of weight loss supplements, there's no way to know definitively what you're getting, how much, or what it can do to you.

In recent years, the FDA has gone after more than 70 tainted weight loss products—many with names like Slim Burn, 24 Hours Diet, and Natural Model—after finding that they had been adulterated with undeclared stimulants, diuretics, and antidepressants, often in amounts exceeding the maximum recommended dosages at which such drugs can be prescribed.

Sometimes the additives aren't legal even with a prescription. For example, one supplement targeted by the FDA contained fenproporex, a stimulant not approved in the United States because it can cause arrhythmia and possibly even sudden death.

In addition, these products often are not effective for the conditions for which they're advertised and may divert patients from legitimate medications, according to Nissen. If they do seem to be making a difference, that may be cause for concern, too. "If a weight loss supplement is working, it could be due to a stimulant whose safety is unproven," says Arthur Agatston, MD, a cardiologist and developer of the South Beach Diet. "Even if you lose weight, you may have unpleasant, even dangerous cardiac side effects."

WHY THE RULES DON'T WORK

"People who are overweight or obese are desperate to lose weight and vulnerable to snake oil salesmen pitching weight loss products," says Nissen. "Sadly, action may not get taken until there is a high-profile death." Dangerous products often slide under the radar until there's a disaster because, although the FDA is nominally charged with the safety of supplements, its ability to police them is limited by the size of the industry, the scope of the FDA's other duties, and the fact that the agency is not empowered to subject supplements to the same kind of scrutiny it gives to drugs—especially before they go on the market.

"The reality is that we are lacking resources in terms of authority, manpower, and money," admits Siobhan DeLancey, an FDA spokesperson. With an already tight budget, "we allocate our funds to best protect the public health, focusing on issues like food-borne illnesses that are causing serious illness and death."

The problem would be significant even if the FDA were better equipped. Expert estimates of the number of products range from 40,000 to nearly 75,000 products, including everything from vitamin C to sketchy weight loss drugs. Supplement makers are required to register with the FDA—and Steve Mister, president and CEO of the Council for Responsible Nutrition, asserts that all legitimate ones who make safe products do. But the agency concedes that there are so many it can't keep track of them all. And makers of adulterated supplements may not register at all. "Anyone can set up a Web page and put a US address on it," DeLancey says. "This is a group of individuals that's willfully operating outside the law."

Cracking down on supplements' fraudulent and exaggerated advertising is the responsibility of the Federal Trade Commission. But again, resources are scant. "When you have thousands of products and hundreds of thousands of advertisements, and you can look at only a dozen or so cases a year, then it is virtually an unregulated area," says Richard Cleland, an assistant director in the FTC's Division of Advertising Practices.

Over the years, several bills have been proposed in Congress to give the FDA more power to take action against the offenders. So far, none has made it out of committee and been passed. Until that happens, it's up to you to keep yourself safe.

HOW TO PROTECT YOURSELF
Be a Cautious Consumer
If, with your doctor's okay, you take a supplement such as fish oil or calcium, look for a seal on the bottle from NSF International, the United States Pharmacopeial Convention, or ConsumerLab.com. Note that these companies are paid by supplement makers to evaluate their products for safety, purity, and ingredient list accuracy. They don't run lengthy patient trials to ensure that the product works, but at least you know it won't be adulterated.

Speak Out about Side Effects
If you've taken a supplement and experienced unexpected symptoms, the FDA urges you to report the problem to MedWatch, its Safety Information and Adverse Event Reporting Program at www.fda.gov/Safety/MedWatch/default.htm or by phone at (800) 332-1088. Even a few such reports can help the FDA determine where to target its efforts to best effect.

Say No to Diet Supplements
"There's no diet supplement or drug that I know of that's safe and effective long term," says Agatston. What's more, according to Nissen, even if you do lose weight by using a drug or supplement, research suggests that once you stop taking the product, you will gain back the weight and may be at greater risk of a heart attack or stroke. Both physicians recommend a healthy diet and regular exercise as the only sustainable way to lose weight and stay healthy.

Chapter 31

Are You Getting Enough Fiber?

FIBER DOES MORE THAN JUST KEEP YOU FULL LONGER.

You hear the advice constantly: You need fiber. It's crucial to your health. Fine, but how much fiber, and how crucial is it?

Let's start with the basics. Fiber is a type of carbohydrate that makes up the structural material in the leaves, stems, and roots of plants. But unlike sugar and starch—the other two kinds of carbs—fiber stays intact until it nears the end of your digestive system. This, it seems, is what makes fiber beneficial, and why you've probably heard you can't eat enough of it. Now read on to separate the facts from the fiction.

THE BACKGROUND

There are two basic types of fiber, with different functions. Insoluble fiber is found in wheat bran, nuts, and many vegetables. Its structure is thick and rough, and it won't dissolve in water, so it zips through your digestive tract and increases stool bulk. Soluble fiber is found in oats, beans, barley, and some fruits. It dissolves in water to form a gel-like material in your digestive tract. This allows it to slow the absorption of sugar into your bloodstream. What's more, soluble fiber, when eaten regularly, has been shown to slightly lower LDL (bad) cholesterol levels.

Regardless of the type, fiber is essentially composed of a bundle of sugar molecules. These molecules are held together by chemical bonds that your body has trouble breaking. In fact, your small intestine can't break down soluble or insoluble fiber; both types just go right through you. That's why some experts say fiber doesn't provide any calories. However, this claim isn't entirely accurate. In your large intestine, soluble fiber's molecules are converted to short-chain fatty acids, which do provide a few calories. A gram of regular carbohydrates has about 4 calories, as does a gram of soluble fiber, according to the FDA. (Insoluble fiber has essentially zero calories.)

THE HEALTH HYPE

Fiber's few calories are more than offset by its weight control benefits. The conclusion of a review published in the journal *Nutrition* is clear: People who add fiber to their diets lose more weight than those who don't. Fiber requires extra chewing and slows the absorption of nutrients in your gut, so your body is tricked into thinking you've eaten enough, says review author Joanne Slavin, PhD, RD. And some fibers may also stimulate CCK, an appetite-suppressing hormone in the gut.

Although fiber usually shows up in natural sources—fresh fruits and vegetables are prime sources—fiber is showing up in everything these days, including yogurt, grape juice, and artificial sweetener. If this seems impossible, remember that these are molecules; you don't have to see or feel fiber for it to be present. Scientists now have a new class of fiber they refer to as "functional" fiber, meaning it's created and added to processed foods. "You can make fiber from bacteria or from yeast," says Slavin. "And as long as you prove that it can lower cholesterol or feed the good bacteria in your gut or increase stool weight, it's fiber."

What's more, in 2007, the FDA declared that a substance called polydextrose can be called fiber. Polydextrose is made from glucose, sorbitol (a sugar alcohol), and citric acid. It's what puts the fiber in that sugary cereal you love. Polydextrose received FDA approval because it mimics some attributes of dietary fiber: It isn't absorbed in the small intestine, and it increases stool weight. Polydextrose mainly bulks up foods so they're not as high in calories.

But foods with added fiber don't necessarily provide the benefits you might expect. Inulin, for example, a soluble fiber extracted from chicory root, can be found in products like Fiber One bars. In addition to boosting fiber content, it's also commonly used to replace fat. Inulin is known as a prebiotic, which means it promotes the growth of healthy bacteria in your gut. That's good, of course. "But," says Slavin, "inulin doesn't have the same cholesterol-lowering effect as the fiber found in oat bran." And there's no research to prove that polydextrose is as beneficial as the fiber found in whole foods.

Some research also suggests that fiber can be beneficial in warding off colon cancer. This idea arose in the 1960s when it was noted that fiber-scarfing Ugandans rarely developed colon cancer. But over five decades later, it still hasn't been proven.

In 1999, Harvard researchers found no link between dietary fiber intake and colon cancer. But a European study that tracked more than a half million people correlated a high-fiber diet with up to a 40 percent reduced risk of colorectal cancer. Then a 2005 review in the *Journal of the American Medical Association* found that people who ate the same amount of fiber as those in the European study didn't experience any benefit. The American Institute for Cancer Research calls protection "probable." This controversy aside, high-fiber diets are associated with preventing many chronic diseases, so it's smart to boost your intake.

And eating whole grains may lower your risk of high blood pressure, according to a Harvard School of Public Health study. The fiber in grains produces by-products that may reduce damage to your arteries and help prevent hypertension, says study coauthor Eric Rimm, ScD. The effect is synergistic: While fiber may be the nutrient most beneficial to blood pressure, Rimm says, its effect is enhanced by a food's antioxidants, vitamins, and minerals, most notably potassium.

YOUR BEST MOVE

The Institute of Medicine recommends eating 38 grams of fiber per day. Scientists there crunched data from three studies and squeezed out the number 38 in 2005. It equals 9 apples or 12 bowls of instant oatmeal. (Most people eat about 15 grams of fiber daily.) The studies found a correlation between high fiber intake and lower incidence of heart disease. But none of the high-fiber-eating groups in those studies averaged as high as 38 grams, and, in fact, people saw maximum benefits with a daily gram intake averaging from the high 20s to the low 30s. Also, it's worth noting that these studies don't show cause and effect, and that unless you're taking a supplement, it's hard for even those who eat the healthiest of diets to consume 38 grams of fiber. It's fine to shoot for that amount, but you're certainly not failing if you don't meet it.

A simple strategy for getting the fiber you need: Eat sensibly. Favor whole, unprocessed foods. Make sure the carbs you eat are fiber rich—this means produce, legumes, and whole grains—to help slow the absorption of sugar into your bloodstream. "The more carbohydrates you eat, the more fiber becomes important to help minimize the wide fluctuations in blood sugar levels," says Jeffrey Volek, PhD, RD, a nutrition and exercise researcher at the University of Connecticut.

Smart Sources of Fiber

Get your fill of fiber—even on a low-carb diet—with these nutritious suggestions. Your top choice: Chow on fresh veggies and nuts. "There can be more than 2 to 3 grams of fiber in a half cup of low-carb vegetables, including cooked spinach, broccoli, and Brussels sprouts," says Keri Glassman, RD, the founder of nutritiouslife.com. "Sprinkle peanuts, almonds, or walnuts on dishes for an extra boost of fiber plus healthy fats." If you're not a fan of greens, try fiber-fortified products like Dannon Activia with Fiber yogurt, La Tortilla Factory organic whole-wheat wraps, and Silk Plus Fiber soy milk.

Chapter 32

Do You Have a D-Ficiency?

HERE'S HOW TO TELL IF YOU'RE GETTING ENOUGH VITAMIN D AND WHAT TO DO IF YOU'RE NOT.

Could this common nutrient be the antidote to an overweight America? Explore the surprising benefits of a vitamin that's hiding in plain sight.

"In the past decade, there's been an explosion of research on vitamin D," says Anthony Norman, PhD, a professor emeritus of biochemistry at the University of California at Riverside.

Not all of that research began as an investigation of this vital mineral. In one study, at the University of Minnesota, Shalamar Sibley, MD, was examining how calorie reduction might affect hormone pathways. On a hunch, she decided to test one more variable: vitamin D. "Researchers have been tracking the relationship between low vitamin D and obesity," says Sibley. "So I wondered if people's baseline vitamin D levels would predict their ability to lose weight when cutting calories."

Her hunch paid off big time. People with adequate vitamin D levels at the start of the study tended to lose more weight than those with low levels, even though everyone reduced their calorie intake equally. In fact, even a minuscule increase in a key D precursor caused the study participants to incinerate an additional half pound of flab.

Sibley's study is just the latest indication that vitamin D could be our special ops agent in the war against body fat. For example, another study at Laval University in Quebec City found that people who consumed more dietary vitamin D had less belly fat than people who ate less.

Are You Getting Enough D?

If any of the following describes you, you might be deficient in vitamin D. To find out for sure, ask your doctor for a 25-hydroxy vitamin D test. You want to clock in above 40 nanograms per milliliter.

You're in middle age or older.
The older you are, the harder it is for your skin to make D. In a Boston University study, 36 percent of men and women under age 30 were D deficient by the end of winter. That rate jumped to 42 percent for people over 50.

You're a person of color.
The melanin pigment in your skin acts as a natural sunscreen, helping block UVB rays. The darker your skin (or the deeper your tan), the higher your natural SPF and the more sunlight your skin requires to make D.

Your body mass index is over 30.
Being obese increases your vitamin D needs by two to five times. Calculate your body mass index at nhlbisupport.com/bmi. Have a BMI over 30 but don't think you're fat? Ask for a skin fold test at your gym.

You're a northerner.
Imagine a line running from Los Angeles to Atlanta and then to the Atlantic coast. If you live north of that line, there's not enough sunlight for your skin to make adequate D between November and March, says Holick.

THE BACKGROUND

What's the big deal about D? Although you get some of it naturally from drinking milk or by being exposed to sunlight, these amounts aren't nearly enough. As a result, more than a third of American men are deficient in the nutrient—even young, healthy men who live in sunny states. And more than 50 percent of American men have suboptimal levels.

"Vitamin D deficiency is one of the most commonly unrecognized medical conditions," says Michael F. Holick, MD, PhD, a professor of medicine at Boston University School of Medicine and author of *The Vitamin D Solution*. "And that deficiency negatively affects every cell in your body, including your fat cells."

One reason vitamin D has flown under the research radar for so long is because it's more than just a vitamin—it's also a hormone, one that plays a role in a remarkable range of body processes. "In the past 20 years, we've found D receptors on up to 40 different tissues, including the heart, pancreas, muscles, immune-system cells, and brain," says Norman. He should know, having discovered the vitamin D receptor on intestinal cells back in 1969.

THE HEALTH HYPE

Think of vitamin D as your body's multitasking marvel. Heart disease? Adequate D might be equal to exercise in its ability to ward off this number one killer of men. Blood pressure? D helps keep it down. Diabetes? Studies show that D can combat this, too. Now add to this list the potential to ward off memory loss, certain cancers (including prostate), and even the common cold, and it should come as no surprise that D may also help solve the riddle of your expanding middle.

When you have adequate vitamin D levels, your body releases more leptin, the hormone that conveys a "we're full, stop eating" message to your brain. Conversely, less D means less leptin and more frequent visits to the all-you-can-eat buffet. In fact, an Australian study showed that people who ate a breakfast high in D and calcium (a mineral that works hand in hand with D) blunted their appetites for the next 24 hours. Vitamin D deficiency is also linked to insulin resistance, which leads to hunger and overeating, says Liz Applegate, PhD, director of sports nutrition at the University of California, Davis, and author of *Eat Smart, Play Hard*.

Vitamin D can also help you store less fat. When you have enough of this key nutrient in your bloodstream, fat cells slow their efforts to make and store fat, says Holick. But when your D is low, levels of parathyroid hormone (PTH) and a second hormone, calcitrol, rise, and that's bad: High levels of these hormones turn your body into a fat miser, encouraging it to hoard fat instead of burning it, says Michael B. Zemel, PhD, director of the Nutrition Institute at the University of Tennessee. In fact, a Norwegian study found that elevated PTH levels increased a man's risk of becoming overweight by 40 percent.

And while enough D can help you lose lard all over, it's particularly helpful for the pounds above your belt. Studies at the University of Minnesota and Laval University found that D triggers weight loss primarily in the belly. One explanation: The nutrient may work with calcium to reduce production of cortisol, a stress hormone that causes you to store belly fat, says Zemel.

One of Zemel's studies found that a diet high in dairy (which means plenty of calcium and vitamin D) helped people lose 70 percent more weight than a diet with the same number of calories but without high levels of those nutrients. What's more, a German study showed that high levels of vitamin D actually increased the benefits of weight loss, improving cardiovascular risk markers like triglycerides.

YOUR BEST MOVE

You might think that because you can get vitamin D from sunlight, all you need to do to ramp up your reserves is spend more time outside. Unfortunately, this isn't entirely true. When sunlight hits your skin, your body's built-in vitamin D factory kicks into operation, producing a form of the nutrient that lasts twice as long in your bloodstream as when you consume it through food or a supplement. The problem, of course, is a little thing called skin cancer: In order to manufacture enough D, you'd need about 10 minutes in the sun during the peak hours of 10 a.m. to 3 p.m. without sunscreen, says Holick.

Even if you could take cancer out of the equation, the amount of sunlight-derived D your body can produce depends on your location. People who live north of the equator probably make only 10 to 20 percent as much D in April as they do in June. And come December, a northerner's skin can produce hardly any D, says Holick. Even living in a sunny city is no guarantee of adequate natural D. Air pollution filters UVB rays, so less of them are able to reach your skin. That's one reason folks who live in Los Angeles and Atlanta tend to be deficient despite their sunny locations.

To increase your intake, supplementing is a good idea. In fact, the Institute of Medicine recently unveiled a new D recommendation for food and/or supplements: 600 international units (IU) a day. But even that might not be enough. "The Institute of Medicine is extremely cautious," says Norman. "Its guidelines are based on what it considers good for bone health, but that doesn't address what's needed to benefit the immune system, pancreas, muscles, heart, and brain." Instead, Norman argues that men may need a 1,000 to 2,000 IU supplement plus a D-rich diet. Turns out, this view is shared by a group of experts in all things hormonal: The Endocrine Society recently released a revised recommendation of 1,500 to 2,000 IU a day for good health.

Still, even that elevated recommendation is just a starting point. If you're overweight (that is, if your body mass index, or BMI, is over 25), you probably need more D. Body fat traps vitamin D in a Georges St-Pierre–style choke hold, preventing it from being used in your body. And the heavier you are, the more D is trapped and the less is available in your bloodstream. According to Holick, obese people (those with BMIs above 30) require two to five times the vitamin D that lean people need—a dosage that should be monitored by a doctor, of course. It's less clear how much vitamin D you need if you are overweight but not obese, but somewhere between 2,000 and 4,000 IU is a safe bet, says Holick.

The other problem with trying to ingest all that D from a handful of pills is that you may not reap the fat-burning benefits you were hoping for. "Dietary sources of D usually contain complementary nutrients that also contribute to weight loss," says Holick. Bottom line: A supplement is just that. To get your D naturally, try the vitamin-packed meal plan here and fill up on the D-rich foods listed on page 248.

FOR MORE D, COOK THIS

Superdose yourself with more than 1,400 IU by eating this dinner.

Grilled Wild Salmon
- 900 IU

Lightly brush 6-ounce fillets with olive oil and sprinkle them with salt and pepper. Grill them, skin side down, for about 5 minutes. Then flip them and grill until the flesh flakes when you prod the centers with a fork, 3 to 5 minutes.

Dill-Yogurt Sauce
- 30 IU

Serve the salmon with this quick yogurt sauce. A batch serves four. Mix 1 cup vitamin D–fortified plain yogurt with half a cucumber (grated), 1 tablespoon lemon juice, 2 teaspoons chopped fresh dill, 1 minced garlic clove, and salt and pepper to taste.

Balsamic-Glazed Mushrooms and Onions
- 400 IU

You won't find a lot of vitamin D in most produce—except Monterey Mushrooms, a brand of specialty mushrooms that have been exposed to UVB light. Use them in this easy side. On a baking sheet, toss 3 ounces sliced mushrooms and ½ cup sliced onions with olive oil and good-quality balsamic vinegar. Roast at 350°F until the mushrooms are lightly browned and glazed, about 40 minutes, stirring occasionally. Toss with chopped parsley.

And for Dessert, Berry Smoothie
- 120 IU

In a blender, puree a handful of berries with a cup of D-fortified yogurt or kefir. Pour into a bowl, top with more berries, and add cinnamon, which works along with D to help control blood sugar and insulin response.

MEET THE VITAMIN D FAMILY

Fatty Fish

- 900 IU in a 6-oz serving of wild sockeye salmon
- Wild salmon might be more expensive, but it's packed with more vitamin D.

You can do better than bland white fish like flounder. Fatty varieties, such as salmon and mackerel, contain up to four times the vitamin D of lean fish. What's more, these oily options also offer higher levels of omega-3 fatty acids—and omega-3s act in concert with vitamin D to promote weight loss and inhibit cancer-cell growth. "Of course you get the added benefit of appetite-suppressing protein, too," says Christopher Mohr, PhD, RD, a personal nutrition consultant in Louisville, Kentucky.

Supercharge your D: Choose wild, not farm-raised, salmon. A Boston University study found that farmed salmon has just 25 percent of the D of its wild cousins. Wild salmon derive their D from eating nutrient-rich plankton; farmed fish eat feed pellets, which are low in D.

Dairy

- 117 IU in an 8-oz serving of 1% milk
- Skip skim milk—your body needs some fat to absorb the vitamin D in dairy.

Most milk products boast calcium as well as vitamin D, and you've already read about how calcium helps reduce levels of fat-storage hormones. Dairy is also rich in the amino acid leucine, which helps stimulate muscle growth and fat burning. The D and leucine may be why dairy sources of calcium are twice as effective as calcium supplements at promoting weight loss, says Zemel.

Supercharge your D: Choose D-fortified dairy products. All milk is fortified with 100 IU of vitamin D per serving, but yogurt and other dairy foods are hit or miss. Some yogurt brands are fortified with as much as 30 percent of the daily value per 6-ounce serving, while others aren't fortified at all. This is also true of cereal, orange juice, and other fortified foods. Check labels to make the best choices.

Eggs

- 160 IU in 2 large omega-3 eggs
- One more reason not to skip the yolks: They're rich in vitamin D.

Like fatty fish, eggs contain omega-3s and protein as well as vitamin D. Small wonder that eating an egg at breakfast can improve weight loss by 65 percent and reduce appetite throughout the day, according to two Saint Louis University studies.

Supercharge your D: Pick omega-enriched eggs, not conventional eggs. Eggland's Best eggs, for example, are higher in omega-3s and also contain double the D.

Other Foods with D

Beef liver, cooked, 3.5 oz: 40 IU

D-fortified yogurt, 6 oz (with 20% of the daily value): 80 IU

D-fortified orange juice, 1 cup (amount of added D varies): 100 IU

Tuna canned in water, drained, 3 oz: 154 IU

Sardines canned in oil, drained, 3 oz: 164 IU

Mackerel, cooked, 3 oz: 388 IU

Wild mushrooms, 3 oz: 400 IU

Chapter 33

Does Organic Really Matter?

IN MANY CASES, GOING GREEN CAN GIVE YOU AN EDGE WHEN IT COMES TO NUTRITION. READ ON FOR ALL THE FACTS.

Nutrition decisions can mean the difference between suffering and soaring. While it's easy enough to fuel your workouts with whole grains, good fats, and protein, it's sometimes hard to swallow the cost of ensuring those nutrients are organic. So when a Stanford University report made headlines in 2012 by declaring organic produce no more nutritious than conventional, you may have considered the matter settled. Not so fast. There are plenty of health and environmental reasons that organic is a wiser choice, says Monica Reinagel, a board-certified licensed nutritionist in Baltimore. Here are a few.

THE BACKGROUND

These days the shelves are packed with products bearing the USDA round green "Organic" label—and a heftier price tag. Something about the word *organic* automatically implies a pure, healthy, overall better-for-you product. But is that really true?

The consensus among doctors, scientists, nutritionists, and chefs, it seems, is that some organic foods are worth the extra money because they've been proven safer, tastier, and more nutritious than the conventionally grown kinds. But they won't make you thin or guarantee good health for life. Others you can leave on the shelf; even though they may be slightly better for you, they're not so much better that they're worth paying extra for.

THE HEALTH HYPE

When you wheel past the organic section of the produce aisle, no doubt you start thinking a little harder about those tomatoes you picked up a few paces back. Suddenly all nonorganic fruits and vegetables seem tainted by horrible, bug-killing chemicals, and you can't help but wonder what all those foreign substances are doing to your body.

The Stanford study reported that organic produce is 30 percent less likely to contain pesticide residue—chemicals that cling to food after spraying—than conventionally grown plants. "Scientists don't yet know the long-term health consequences of chronic pesticide exposure in adults," says Marisa Bunning, PhD, assistant professor of food safety at Colorado State University. But they do know that kids with high levels of pesticide residues are almost twice as likely to have ADHD, and women exposed during pregnancy give birth to babies who have lower IQ

What's the Difference Between "Organic" and "Natural" on Food Labels?

Both words sell a greener eating experience, but only "organic" delivers the full grocery cart of nutritional goods. For a food to bear the USDA Organic logo, it must meet strict criteria, including no synthetic ingredients, no petroleum-based fertilizers, no synthetic pesticides, and no genetic modification. In the case of meat, poultry, and eggs, animals should have been fed 100 percent organic feed.

The bar is a lot lower for the word "natural." The FDA requires only that these foods contain no added color, artificial flavors, or synthetic substances. "'Natural' is a marketing gimmick," says Marion Nestle, PhD, MPH, a professor of nutrition, food studies, and public health at New York University and author of *Food Politics*. "Food companies have always used 'natural' to market products, but its use increased after the USDA passed its organic standards in 2002. The word 'natural' should serve as a warning for you to scan the ingredient label."

Be especially wary of natural ice cream, cereals, and fruit snacks, which often contain chemically processed ingredients, such as corn syrup, alkalized cocoa, partially hydrogenated soybean oil, vanillin, and maltodextrin. What's more, foods labeled "natural" are allowed to have genetically modified ingredients and to be grown using pesticides; and meat, fish, and poultry bearing that label can be raised with growth hormones and antibiotics.

scores by the time they start school. Research has also shown that farmers frequently exposed to pesticides have higher rates of chronic bronchitis and certain types of cancers, including lung, prostate, stomach, and brain, the National Cancer Institute reports.

What's more, chemicals from pesticides and fertilizer can make their way into the H_2O you guzzle. A 2011 study found that water runoff from conventional farms more frequently exceeds the legal limit for nitrate concentrations in drinking water compared with water from organic farms, which don't use chemical pesticides. Excess nitrate exposure can contribute to respiratory conditions, thyroid disorders, and cancer, according to the EPA.

Another often-cited concern: The hormones and antibiotics factor. Organic advocates say that organic meat, dairy, and eggs are healthier than the regular varieties because of what they don't contain—namely, the hormones and antibiotics given to conventionally raised livestock.

The practice of using antibiotics to fatten up livestock has contributed to the rise of antibiotic-resistant bacteria, dangerous superbugs that are difficult to treat in humans. The Stanford review found that livestock raised using nonorganic methods are 33 percent more likely to contain antibiotic-resistant bacteria.

And no less important, there's the taste test. Think of a juicy, tender organic tomato, rich in color and flavor. It's way tastier than your average pale tomato. Most conventional produce is picked before ripening so it can survive the trip on a semi to a supermarket across the country. Most organic food is grown locally and available only in season, so it travels less and has more time to develop flavor on the vine. What's more, organic farmers frequently grow "heirloom" versions of tomatoes and other crops that have been bred for taste, not toughness.

Likewise, organic chicken is much less rubbery than your run-of-the-mill bird, thanks to higher-quality feed and extra room to roam. And if you've ever done a side-by-side comparison of organic and nonorganic milk, you know that, at the same fat content, the former can taste fuller and richer. Experts say this difference is due to the varied diet of most organically raised cows: Eating grass in addition to standard feed boosts their milk's flavor.

Improved taste is why more and more chefs—and consumer foodies—are cooking with organic ingredients. Organic food still accounts for only 2 percent of the food industry, but sales are shooting up at a rate of 16 percent a year. "Most of the time, organic foods are grown with more care, and you can really taste that," says Akasha Richmond, author of *Hollywood Dish* and chef at Akasha, her Culver City, California, restaurant. "Fruit in particular—there's a huge difference. The taste is much richer, much deeper, much cleaner."

So what's the problem? The cost concern. While there's huge variation in how much more organic foods cost than their conventionally grown counterparts, you'll wind up paying around 50 percent more, on average. And that can be a problem. Even though Richmond loves buying organic for her family, "If it's too expensive, I won't," she says. To keep costs down, she shops for organic fruits and vegetables only when they're in season and therefore cheaper.

YOUR BEST MOVE

Some foods deserve the splurge—others don't. Take a look at this list of fruits, vegetables, meats, and dairy before you make your next grocery run.

WORTH IT

Fruits

These fruits are particularly easy for pesticides to penetrate, according to a study by the Environmental Working Group. And organic versions are higher in vitamins, minerals, and other nutrients.

- Apples
- Pears
- Grapes
- Raspberries
- Peaches
- Strawberries
- Cherries
- Nectarines (imported)
- Blueberries (domestic)

Vegetables

When grown conventionally, these veggies soak up more chemicals than most. The organic versions are also more nutritious.

- Sweet corn
- Potatoes
- Celery
- Bell peppers
- Cucumbers
- Lettuce
- Spinach

Meats

Though the price difference between organic and regular meats may be steep, the argument for buying meat organically is one of the strongest. You'll avoid antibiotics, which can encourage the growth of antibiotic-resistant bacteria in you.

- Ground beef
- Pork
- Chicken

Dairy

Organic dairy has up to five times the levels of conjugated linoleic acid, a compound that has been shown to help weight loss. Bonus: There are relatively few organic milk farms, so their products are pasteurized at superhigh temperatures to stay fresh during transport—which means they can last in your fridge for up to 6 weeks without spoiling.

- Yogurt
- Cheese
- Milk

NOT WORTH IT

Organic versions of these foods may be slightly better for you, but not enough to justify the higher price.

Fruit

- Papayas
- Pineapples
- Bananas
- Mangoes
- Kiwifruits

Vegetables

- Cauliflower
- Avocados
- Snow peas
- Broccoli
- Asparagus

Chapter 34

Is Your Cooking Oil Killing You?

TO PROTECT YOUR BODY, EASE YOUR MIND, AND PLEASE YOUR PALATE, FOLLOW THESE RULES.

They called it Formula 47, after the total cost in cents of a burger, fries, and shake, circa 1960. Formula 47 was a blend of rendered beef fat and vegetable oil, which, when used to fry shoestring slices of Russet Burbank potatoes, imparted a flavor so rich and appetizing that it helped the restaurant selling the fries to become the world's dominant fast-food chain: McDonald's. But that story turned into a cautionary tale whose lessons extend into every man's kitchen.

THE BACKGROUND

Health advocates blamed Formula 47 fries for raising customers' cholesterol, so the Golden Arches switched to what people assumed was healthier—100 percent vegetable oil. The new oils were good fats that had been altered—hydrogenated—for flavor retention and longer shelf life. But that made them even more damaging to cardiovascular health than the saturated fats had been thought to be.

Some public health experts now blame the trans fats in hydrogenated oils for tens of thousands of premature deaths. According to a study review by the Harvard School of Public Health, trans fats may increase your risk of a host of chronic diseases and also promote weight gain. So McDonald's and others have once again reformulated their frying medium, using vegetable-oil blends that are free of trans fats.

In short, oils aren't as simple as they seem. Like McDonald's, if you cook with the wrong oil, you may be sabotaging your health.

THE HEALTH HYPE

Corn, soybean, and other vegetable oils have high levels of omega-6s. These polyunsaturated fats aren't bad when they're balanced with plenty of omega-3 fatty acids, like the ones found in fish. But that often isn't the case in the typical American diet. "We now consume 20 to 1 omega-6s to omega-3s," says Jonny Bowden, PhD, author of *The 150 Healthiest Foods on Earth*. "Our inflammatory factory is overstaffed, and our anti-inflammatory factory is understaffed."

A high intake of omega-6 fats relative to omega-3 fats increases inflammation, which may increase your risk of heart disease, diabetes, and cancer, according to a 2008 review of studies by the Center for Genetics, Nutrition and Health. There are plenty of other choices.

Experts say the most nutritious way to go is with a few different cooking oils to help balance your intake of omega-3 and omega-6 polyunsaturated fats, as well as saturated and monounsaturated fats. "That's what most of the world has done. Old Mediterranean cultures had olive oil on salad, fish at night, and then cow or goat butter or cheese, and they were more or less accidentally coming up with the one-to-one-to-one ratio," says K.C. Hayes, PhD, a fats researcher at Brandeis University.

YOUR BEST MOVE

Here's an easy way to balance your diet: Match fats to the cuisine you're cooking. Making homemade spaghetti sauce? Use a drizzle of olive oil to sauté the onions. Try coconut or peanut oil when you're whipping up an Asian stir-fry. Start a French-style omelet by melting a pat of butter. The greater the variety of non-hydrogenated fats you incorporate into your diet, the better. A moderate intake of all types of non-hydrogenated fat is best, according to the American Heart Association.

Wait, did we just say butter? Yes, it's okay to use butter. "The health scare surrounding saturated fat and cholesterol was overblown," says Walter Willett, MD, chairman of the Department of Nutrition at Harvard University. A 2010 review of 21 studies, published in *The American Journal of Clinical Nutrition*, found no conclusive evidence that dietary saturated fat is associated with an increased risk of coronary heart disease, stroke, or cardiovascular disease. According to a review in the *European Journal of Nutrition*, a diet high in fat from dairy products like butter may raise levels of large HDL cholesterol, which is considered relatively harmless, while having no effect on levels of potentially harmful small LDL cholesterol.

Margarine, the once-sainted substitute, usually contains at least 80 percent vegetable oil, and that oil often contains trans fats. Butter also has trace amounts of naturally occurring trans fats, but not enough to cause concern. The point is that you can use butter; just don't go overboard, a caution that applies to any fat. Try whipped butter on your toast—you'll take in about a third less calories. Butter is known to be an excellent source of conjugated linoleic acid, which may be a cancer-fighting nutrient, according to Ohio State scientists.

That doesn't mean you want to kick traditionally healthy oils, like canola oil and olive oil, out of your kitchen. Just know that butter and other non-hydrogenated natural fats are not as bad as nutritionists once thought them to be. But there's one caveat.

Oils typically contain 100 to 125 calories per tablespoon—all of them from fat—so use sparingly. Cook smart. Usually 1 tablespoon of any oil is enough to coat the pan you're using. Any more is overkill.

At the supermarket, limiting dangerous fats is easy: Check labels to find products without partially or fully hydrogenated oils or trans fats. At restaurants, it's a little harder. Only California has a statewide ban on serving trans fat in restaurants. For a list of pending and enacted trans fats legislation in your state, go to ncsl.org and search "trans fat and menu labeling." Most fast-food chains are banning trans fats on their own, but without legislation, your primary defense is asking your restaurant kitchen directly. Or even better, use the info below to cook healthier, tastier meals at home.

WHICH OIL TO USE WHEN

Most cooking oils are better than solid fats because they're lower in artery-jamming saturated fats and brimming with antioxidants. That said, you have to choose the right oil for the job.

Besides the health perks, two big factors come into play: flavor and smoke point. If you have any doubts that oil affects taste, try baking cupcakes with extra-virgin olive. And the smoke point—the temp at which oil burns and then sets off your fire alarm—is crucial. The higher the smoke point (which ranges from 225°F for flaxseed to 490°F for rice bran), the more heat it can take. Stick this cheat sheet to your fridge and you'll pick the optimal oil every time.

Extra-Virgin Olive Oil
Food/Technique: Dipping bread; coating pasta. "Extra-virgin" means olives have gone through the press only once (versus at least twice for the regular kind), so the oil retains more of the fruit's deep, earthy taste—ideal for bread and pasta.
Health Benefits: Minimal processing may allow more of the olive's antioxidants—including heart-protecting polyphenols—to make it to your table.

Olive Oil
Food/Technique: Sautéing, grilling, pasta sauce. Heat kills extra-virgin's richer flavor, so basic olive oil (sometimes labeled "pure") does the trick for cooking. (You'll burn a lot less cash, too—a gallon of extra-virgin costs almost twice as much.) Medium smoke point (375°F) means worry-free sautéing and grilling. Thick consistency allows seasonings to stick to meats and vegetables.
Health Benefits: High in monounsaturated fats and antioxidants, such as oleuropein, which help prevent LDL (bad) cholesterol from clogging your arteries.

Canola Oil
Food/Technique: Baking, broiling. Light flavor is undetectable in baked goods. High smoke point (460°F) can withstand a hotter-than-hell oven.
Health Benefits: Very low in sat fats; also a good source of ALA.

Grapeseed Oil
Food/Technique: Pan-frying. Light, mild, fruity flavor adds a little zing. High smoke point (400°F) is perfect for the frying pan.
Health Benefits: A good source of vitamin E, beta-carotene, and sterols, which block the absorption of cholesterol.

Rice Bran Oil
Food/Technique: Deep-frying, stir-frying. Neutral flavor won't hijack food's natural taste. Superhigh smoke point (490°F) permits deep-frying without turning your kitchen ceiling black.
Health Benefits: Contains tocopherol, oryzanol, and tocotrienol—three vitamin E–related antioxidants that have been shown to inhibit skin cancer cells.

What's in Your Food?

Appendices

If you grow a tomato, pick it when it's ripe and slap a slice on your sandwich, you know you're getting tomato goodness. But do you know what you're really getting? Down to the last calorie? Probably not. And what about the scary stuff food manufacturers put in your snack food? Don't want to think about it? Well, you should—and we've made it easy. In the next three sections, we show you what's in the most common foods. It's not all bad. It's not all good. But knowing what you're eating will go a long way toward helping you make better eating choices.

Appendix A

Your Glossary of the Good, Bad, and Ugly in Your Food

One glance at a nutrition label and you can see how food truly is a science. You can also see how the food industry sometimes kidnaps real ingredients and replaces them with science experiments. Some substances are naturally wonderful (the B vitamin group, for example) and some are just creepy (Yellow Dye #5). But few of us know what the average food label is telling us. Yeah, we get serving size and calories. And yeah, a food with 75 percent of your recommended daily intake of vitamin D is probably a good thing. But what does vitamin D do for you? Not sure? It's crucial, and the answer is in here.

As with every chapter in this book, our goal is to educate you about what you're eating. There is good and bad in food. And frankly, not all additives are evil. Some are actually nutritious. After reading this chapter, you'll know exactly what's in the foods you eat, whether that food's as natural as a fresh fig or as artificial as a tub of icing.

The information herein is broken down into three sections: vitamins (naturally occurring good stuff in foods), minerals (naturally occurring good stuff in foods—and rocks), and food additives (unnaturally occurring stuff—good and bad—in too many foods).

For vitamins and minerals, we give you definitions, what they do for you, and which whole foods pack the biggest doses of them. And while a multivitamin may help make up for any dietary shortcomings, more and more research suggests that popping one just doesn't deliver the same health payload as vitamins and minerals in their natural state. And substituting natural sources for supplements means you're not getting the benefits of the fiber, healthy fats, and micronutrients found in fruits, vegetables, dairy, and meats.

We won't be referring you to any food additive sources, though. Sorry. For a lot of them, it's bad enough that they're out there at all. But after reading up on what they are and how they're used, you'll never look at an ingredients label the same way again. And that, friends, is a good thing.

The Yolk's on You!

Ordering an egg-white-omelet to fend off heart disease? Better think twice: A USDA study found that choline—a vitamin found primarily in egg yolks—lowers levels of homocysteine in the blood by 8 percent, which improves blood flow and lowers heart disease risk.

VITAMINS

Betaine
Betaine is best known for its power to lower homocysteine levels in the blood. Increased amounts of homocysteine, an amino acid, can cause symptoms such as extreme tiredness, osteoporosis, or blood clots. It's also linked to higher risk of major illnesses such as heart disease and stroke.
Natural Source: eggs.

Choline
Choline is the memory vitamin. Studies have shown that college students given 3 to 4 grams of choline 1 hour before taking memory tests scored higher than those who didn't receive the supplements. "We believe choline increases the release of acetylcholine, a neurotransmitter that helps your brain store and recall information," says Steven Zeisel, MD, PhD, a professor of nutrition at the University of North Carolina. Although studies have used supplements, Zeisel says that eating foods that are naturally rich in choline should do the trick just as well.
Natural Sources: eggs and milk.

Vitamin A
A is essential for a strong immune system. USDA researchers found that an increased intake of vitamin A boosted germ-killing cells by 8 percent. Because vitamin A can build up to toxic levels in the body with too much supplementation, experts recommend avoiding vitamin A supplements and getting what you need through diet (and, at most, a simple multivitamin daily).
Natural Sources: carrots, sweet potatoes, and mangoes.

Vitamin B

THIAMIN (B_1)

The B vitamin thiamin takes a hit from a night of heavy drinking. Consuming large amounts of alcohol makes you use it faster but absorb it more slowly. The result: You end up with a deficit of a vitamin essential to normal neurological functioning. This may explain phenomena such as beer goggles and Mel Gibson's answering machine messages.

Natural Sources: beef, pork, and pasta.

RIBOFLAVIN (B_2)

Riboflavin, or B_2, helps with oxygen absorption and the production of red blood cells. A Belgian study also found that high doses reduce the length and frequency of migraines.

Natural Sources: dairy products.

NIACIN (B_3)

At high doses, niacin, or B_3, can lower LDL (bad) cholesterol by 5 percent, cut triglycerides by 20 percent, and boost HDL (good) cholesterol by 15 percent. However, side effects include a dangerous rise in glucose levels in diabetics (so consult your doctor).

Natural Sources: poultry, fish, whole grains. Medication note: May increase some of the side effects of statins and reduce the effects of diabetes medications.

PANTOTHENIC ACID (B_5)

Pantothenic acid helps us process proteins, carbs, and fats. Some experts recommend B_5 as an anti-stress/pro-sleep supplement. According to Ron Klatz, MD, president of the American Academy of Anti-Aging Medicine, a B_5 supplement before bed could be your antidote to too much cortisol, the stress hormone that surges in middle-age men. If that doesn't help, ask your doctor about taking some Bayer with your B; aspirin may also help lower cortisol production.

Natural sources: It's present in most foods, though good natural sources are legumes, meats, eggs, broccoli, and avocado.

B_6

B_6 is needed for more than 100 enzymes involved in protein metabolism. It is also essential for red blood cell metabolism—it helps the body make hemoglobin and increases the amount of oxygen carried by hemoglobin. Your nervous and immune systems also need B_6 to function efficiently.

Natural Sources: potatoes, bananas, chicken, and oatmeal.

FOLATE OR FOLIC ACID (B_9)

Folic acid will help keep your bloodstream streaming. A Harvard study showed that men taking the most folic acid were 30 percent less likely to suffer a stroke than those taking the least. Credit folic acid's ability to dissolve homocysteine—a compound linked to heart disease.

Natural sources: spinach and broccoli.

B_{12}

B_{12} is vital to the production of myelin, the fatty sheath that insulates nerve fibers, keeping electrical impulses moving through the body as they should. Because of this important function, a whole host of problems can arise when B_{12} is in short supply: memory loss, fatigue, loss of balance, decreased reflexes, impaired touch or pain perception, numbness and tingling in the arms and legs, and noise-induced hearing loss. Researchers have discovered that a deficiency raises blood levels of homocysteine (shortages of folate and vitamin B_6 can do the same). Unless you're vegan and avoid all animal products, it's easy to get adequate amounts of vitamin B_{12} from food sources because you need so little of it.

Natural sources: Seafood is a terrific natural source: clams, herring, salmon, and tuna. So is ham. Vegans should look for B_{12}-fortified products or take a supplement.

The Folate Factor

Many researchers and doctors now believe that folate is the nutrient that best reveals how healthy your diet is. If folate levels are low, chances are your diet needs tweaking. Cruciferous vegetables are a great source (also, see the Folate entry on this page).

Vitamin C

While vitamin C can't cure a cold, there's evidence it can shorten the sniffles by a day. The C may also stand for "calm"—University of Alabama researchers found that it may help halt the secretion of stress hormones. And scurvy? Clears it right up.

Natural Sources: citrus fruit, tomatoes, and bell peppers.

Vitamin D

Vitamin D is responsible for getting the important bones builders—calcium and phosphorus—to the places in the body where they can help bone grow in children and re-mineralize in adults. It does this first by making certain that these minerals are absorbed in the intestines, second by bringing calcium from bones into the blood, and third by helping the kidneys reabsorb the two minerals.

While your body manufactures vitamin D in response to sunlight, it's important to get plenty of it, especially as you get older. After evaluating the calcium and vitamin D status of elderly people who were entering nursing homes, researchers determined that most had low vitamin D levels and that nearly 85 percent had symptoms of osteoporosis. There is mounting evidence that vitamin D deficiency in elderly people is a silent epidemic that results in bone loss and fractures.

Natural Sources: dairy. One cup of 1 percent D-fortified milk contains 100 IU (25 percent of your daily value). Fish like herring, salmon, and sardines are good sources. Also, spend 10 to 20 minutes in the sun every day.

Vitamin E

E is tough on cancer, especially when it's paired with selenium. Research shows that this antioxidant may reduce your risk of prostate cancer by up to 53 percent and bladder cancer by almost half.

Natural Sources: vegetable oils and leafy green vegetables. Note: Too much E may increase the effects of blood thinners or reverse the effects of statins.

Vitamin K

Vitamin K keeps paper cuts from being fatal. It's also key for liver function. Taiwanese researchers have found that a synthetic form of vitamin K stopped the spread of liver cancer in lab tests.

Natural sources: leafy green vegetables.

Vitamin K Is Special

One of the keys to a long life is preserving your insulin sensitivity—meaning your body doesn't produce wild swings in blood sugar after you eat, a condition that leads to diabetes. Recent research from Tufts University found that vitamin K helps keep insulin levels in check. The researchers recommend eating five or more servings a week of cruciferous or dark leafy vegetables.

MINERALS

Calcium
As the overachiever of minerals, calcium builds bones, helps with weight loss, and possibly decreases the risk of colon cancer. And a study published in the *American Journal of Medicine* found that 1,000 mg of supplemental calcium can increase HDL (good) cholesterol by 7 percent.
Natural Sources: dairy products, broccoli, and kale.

Copper
Copper is multitalented. It's an antioxidant, is active in nerve function and bone growth, and also helps the body burn sugar.
Natural Sources: oysters, beans, nuts, and whole grains.

Iron
Most of the body's iron is found in hemoglobin, helping the body transport oxygen. Women may face iron deficiencies because of their menstrual cycles, but for men it's better to lift this metal than swallow too much of it. If you take a multivitamin, find one that's iron-free: There may be a link between high iron levels and heart disease.
Natural sources: Eat meat and you're probably iron-fortified enough.

Magnesium
A drop in magnesium can be a major headache. "Blood vessels in your brain constrict, and receptors for the feel-good chemical serotonin malfunction," says Alexander Mauskop, MD, director of the New York Headache Center. Result: a migraine. The mineral also might help regulate blood pressure and could ward off stroke and diabetes.
Natural Sources: leafy greens, whole grains, coffee, and nuts.

Manganese
Manganese is an underrated nutritional superstar. It's crucial in digestion and metabolism, helping the body process cholesterol, carbs, and protein. It's also a potent antioxidant.
Natural Sources: pineapple, brown rice, spinach, beans, oatmeal, and leafy greens.

Phosphorus
Phosphorus is found in every cell in your body, but it's best known for helping you form bones and teeth. It also helps keep your kidneys humming and regulates heartbeat. In general, if you're eating enough protein and calcium, you're eating enough phosphorus.
Natural Sources: meat and milk.

Potassium
Research shows that most Americans come up 1,000 mg short on daily potassium intake. The consequences: elevated blood pressure and muscle cramps. Get it from your diet—potassium supplements can build up in the body and damage the heart.
Natural Sources: almonds, bananas, spinach.

Selenium
Men need selenium to produce sperm, but it's also like kryptonite to cancer. Harvard researchers found that men with the highest levels of this mineral had a 48 percent lower risk of advanced prostate cancer. It may also ward off lung cancer. If you use a supplement, go for 200 mcg from selenium yeast daily.
Natural Sources: Brazil nuts and meat. Note: May reduce the effectiveness of statins (talk to your doctor).

Sodium
Sodium hides in processed foods, put there by food companies to preserve products that would otherwise go bad, or to make bland or bitter food taste better, or maybe just to appeal to our craving for the stuff. Current recommended daily intake is 1,500 milligrams with

an upper limit of 2,300 mg. American men generally eat more than 4,000 mg sodium a day, and it's easy to take in 7,000 without trying. You do need a little bit—about 200 mg a day—to keep fluids in balance. Excessive sodium is now linked to illnesses such as stomach cancer and kidney stones. Too much can also make the body excrete calcium, threatening bone density and strength.

We also know for certain that sodium raises blood pressure. Roughly 20 percent of American adults have higher-than-optimal BP. Reducing intake by just 300 mg (about two slices of Cheddar) drops systolic pressure (the first number) by 2 to 4 points, and diastolic by 1 to 2 points, a British study shows.

Natural Sources: Sodium is added to food, so you control what you eat and how much.

Zinc

An antioxidant, zinc improves your lipid profile and blood circulation, which for men is crucial to erectile function. It may be especially important for testosterone and sperm production, and it's vital for the functioning of proteins, enzymes, and hormones. Because heavy alcohol use depletes zinc, it's critical for those who drink regularly.

Natural Sources: oysters, king crab, lobster, meat, and poultry.

The Muscle Mineral

Researchers at the Department of Agriculture's Human Nutrition Research Center on Aging, at Tufts University, found that foods rich in potassium help preserve lean muscle mass. After studying 384 volunteers for 3 years, they found that those whose diets were rich in potassium (getting more than 3,540 milligrams a day) preserved 3.6 more pounds of lean tissue than those with half the potassium intake. That almost offsets the 4.4 pounds of lean tissue that is typically lost each decade as we age.

FOOD ADDITIVES

Acesulfame potassium (Acesulfame-K)

A calorie-free artificial sweetener that's 200 times sweeter than sugar, it is often used with other artificial sweeteners to mask a bitter aftertaste. It's found in more than 5,000 food products worldwide, including diet soft drinks and no-sugar-added ice cream. Although the FDA has approved it for use in most foods, many health experts and food industry insiders claim that the decision was based on flawed tests. Animal studies have linked the chemical to lung and breast tumors and thyroid problems.

Alpha-tocopherol

The form of vitamin E most commonly added to foods and most readily absorbed and stored in the body. It is an essential nutrient that helps prevent oxidative damage to the cells and plays a crucial role in cell communication, skin health, and disease prevention. It's found in meats, foods with added fats, and foods that boast vitamin E health claims. Also occurs naturally in seeds, nuts, leafy vegetables, and vegetable oils. In the amount added to foods, tocopherols pose no apparent health risks, but highly concentrated supplements might bring on toxicity symptoms such as cramps, weakness, and double vision.

Artificial flavoring

Denotes any of hundreds of allowable chemicals such as butyl alcohol, isobutyric acid, and phenylacetaldehyde dimethyl acetal. The exact chemicals used in flavoring are the proprietary information of food manufacturers, which use these compounds to imitate specific fruits, butter, spices, and so on. They're in thousands of highly processed foods, such as cereals, fruit snacks, beverages, and cookies. The FDA has approved every item on the list of allowable chemicals, but because food marketers can hide their specific ingredients behind a blanket term, there is no way for consumers to pinpoint the cause of a reaction they might have had.

Ascorbic acid

The chemical name for water-soluble vitamin C. You'll find it in juices and fruit products, meat, cereals, and other foods with vitamin C health claims. Although vitamin C isn't associated with any known risks, it is often added to junk foods to make them appear healthy.

Aspartame

A near-zero-calorie artificial sweetener made by combining two amino acids with methanol. Most commonly used in diet soft drinks, aspartame is 180 times sweeter than sugar. It's in more than 6,000 grocery items, including diet sodas, yogurts, and the tabletop sweeteners NutraSweet and Equal. In the past 30 years, the FDA has received thousands of consumer complaints, mostly concerning neurological symptoms such as headaches, dizziness, memory loss, and, in rare cases, epileptic seizures. Many studies have shown aspartame to be completely harmless, while others indicate that the additive might be responsible for a range of cancers.

BHA and BHT (butylated hydroxyanisole and butylated hydroxytoluene)

These are petroleum-derived antioxidants used to preserve fats and oils. You'll find them added into products such as beer, crackers, cereals, butter, and foods with added fats. Of the two, BHA is considered the most troublesome. Studies have shown it to cause cancer in the fore-stomachs of rats, mice, and hamsters. The Department of Health and Human Services classifies the preservative as "reasonably anticipated to be a human carcinogen."

Blue #1 (brilliant blue) and Blue #2 (indigotine)

Synthetic dyes that can be used alone or combined with other dyes to make different colors. They're use in blue, purple, and green foods, such as beverages, cereals, candy, and icing. Both dyes have been loosely linked to cancers in animal studies, and the Center for Science in the Public Interest recommends that they be avoided.

Brown rice syrup

A natural sweetener about half as sweet as sugar. It is obtained by using enzymes to break down the starches in cooked rice. It's used in protein bars and organic and natural foods. Brown rice sugar has a lower glycemic index than table sugar, which means it provides an easier ride for your blood sugar.

Carrageenan

A thickener, stabilizer, and emulsifier extracted from red seaweed, it is found in jellies and jams, ice cream, yogurt, and whipped topping. Although it's technically natural, in animal studies, carrageenan has been shown to cause ulcers, colon inflammation, and digestive cancers. While these results seem limited to degraded carrageenan—a class that has been treated with heat and chemicals—a University of Iowa study concluded that even undegraded carrageenan could become degraded in the human digestive system.

> ### Did You Know. . .
> The Nutrition Labeling and Education Act of 1990 absolves restaurants of all nutritional liability to the American public. Under that legislation, no fast-food or chain restaurants are required to provide calorie, fat, or sodium information for any of their menu items unless they describe the items as "low sodium" or "low fat."

Casein
A milk protein used to thicken and whiten foods. It often appears by the names "sodium caseinate" or "calcium caseinate." It is a good source of amino acids and is found in protein bars and shakes, and in sherbet, ice cream, and other frozen desserts. Although casein is a byproduct of milk, the FDA allows it and its derivatives—sodium calcium caseinates—to be used in "nondairy" and "dairy-free" creamers. Most lactose intolerants can handle casein, but those with broader milk allergies might experience reactions.

Cochineal extract (or carmine)
A pigment extracted from the dried eggs and bodies of the female Dactylopius coccus, a beetle-like insect that preys on cactus plants. It is added to food for its dark crimson color and is used in artificial crabmeat, fruit juices, frozen-fruit snacks, candy, and yogurt. Carmine is the refined coloring, while cochineal extract comprises about 90 percent insect-body fragments. Although the FDA receives fewer than one adverse-reaction report a year, some organizations are asking for a mandatory warning label to accompany cochineal-colored foods. Vegetarians, they say, should be forewarned about the insect juices.

Corn syrup
A liquid sweetener and food thickener made by allowing enzymes to break cornstarches into smaller sugars. USDA subsidies to the corn industry make it cheap and abundant, placing it among the most ubiquitous ingredients in grocery food products—including breads, soup, sauces, frozen dinners, and frozen treats. Corn syrup provides no nutritional value other than calories. In moderation, it poses no specific threat, other than an expanded waistline.

Dextrose
A corn-derived caloric sweetener. Like corn syrup, dextrose contributes to the American habit of more than 200 calories of corn sweeteners per day via bread, cookies, and crackers. As with other sugars, dextrose is safe in moderate amounts.

Erythorbic acid
A compound similar to ascorbic acid, but with no apparent nutritional value of its own. It is added to nitrite-containing meats to disrupt the formation of cancer-causing nitrosamines and is used in deli meats, hot dogs, and sausages. Erythorbic acid poses no risks, though it may improve the body's ability to absorb iron, which is not an entirely positive quality for men. They should limit their iron intake because of the mineral's link to cardiovascular problems.

Evaporated cane juice
A sweetener derived from sugarcane, the same plant used to make refined table sugar. It's also known as "crystallized cane juice," "cane juice," or "cane sugar." Because it's subject to less processing than table sugar, evaporated cane juice retains slightly more nutrients from the grassy sugar cane. You'll find it in yogurt, soy milk, protein bars, granola, cereal, chicken sausages, and other natural or organic foods. Although pristine sugars are often used to replace ordinary sugars in "healthier" foods, the actual nutritional difference between the sugars is minuscule. Both should be consumed in moderation.

Fully hydrogenated vegetable oil
Extremely hard, waxlike fat made by forcing as much hydrogen as possible onto the carbon

---

Think About Your Last Meal
British scientists found that people who thought about their last meal before snacking ate 30 percent fewer calories than those who didn't stop to think. The theory: Remembering what you had for lunch might remind you of how satiating the food was, which then makes you less likely to binge on your afternoon snack.

backbone of fat molecules. (Yes, this is actually in your supermarket, being sold as an ingredient in food.) To obtain a manageable consistency, food manufacturers will often blend the hard fat with unhydrogenated liquid fats, the result of which is called interesterified fat (below). It's used in baked goods, doughnuts, frozen meals, and tub margarine. In theory, fully hydrogenated oils, as opposed to partially hydrogenated oils, should contain zero trans fat. In practice, however, the process of hydrogenation isn't completely perfect, which means that some trans fat will inevitably occur in small amounts, as will an increased concentration of saturated fat.

Guar gum

A thickening, emulsifying, and stabilizing agent made from ground guar beans. The legume, also known as a cluster bean, is of Indian origin, but small amounts are grown domestically. Guar gum is used in pastry fillings, ice cream, and sauces. It's a great example of a food additive that actually enhances the food's nutritional value: Guar is a good source of soluble fiber and might even improve insulin sensitivity. One Italian study suggested that partially hydrolyzed guar gum might have probiotic properties that make it useful in treating patients with irritable bowel syndrome.

High-fructose corn syrup (HFCS)

A corn-derived sweetener representing more than 40 percent of all caloric sweeteners in the supermarket. The liquid sweetener is created by a complex process that involves breaking down cornstarch with enzymes, and the result is a roughly 50/50 mix of fructose and glucose. Although about two-thirds of the HFCS consumed in the U.S. is in beverages, it can be found in every grocery aisle in products such as ice cream, chips, cookies, cereals, bread, ketchup, jam, canned fruits, yogurt, barbecue sauce, frozen dinners, and so on.

Since around 1980, the U.S. obesity rate has risen proportionately to the increase in HFCS, and Americans are now consuming at least 200 calories of the sweetener each day. Some researchers argue that the body metabolizes HFCS differently, making it easier to store as fat, but this theory has not been proved. What is known is that in some people, fructose can interfere with the body's ability to process leptin, a hormone that tells us when we're full.

Hydrogenated vegetable oil

See fully hydrogenated vegetable oil.

Hydrolyzed vegetable protein

A flavor enhancer created when heat and chemicals are used to break down a vegetable—most often soy—into its component amino acids. It allows food manufacturers to achieve stronger flavors from fewer ingredients and is used in canned soups and chili, frozen dinners, and beef- and chicken-flavored products. One effect of hydrolyzing proteins is the creation of MSG, or monosodium glutamate. When MSG in food is the result of hydrolyzed protein, the FDA does not require it to be listed on the packaging.

Interesterified fat

A semi-soft fat created by chemically blending fully hydrogenated and nonhydrogenated oils. It was developed in response to the public demand for an alternative to trans fats, because fully hydrogenated fats are supposedly free of trans fatty acids. You'll find it in pastries, pies, margarine, frozen dinners, and canned soups. Testing on these fats has not been extensive, but the early evidence doesn't look promising. A study by Malaysian researchers showed that a 4-week diet of 12 percent interesterified fats increased the ratio of LDL to HDL cholesterol. Furthermore, this study showed an increase in blood glucose levels and a decrease in insulin response.

> **Did You Know...**
>
> According to the Cornell Cooperative Extension, 70 percent of all the food we buy at the supermarket is genetically altered in some way. The FDA does not require foods to be labeled as such.

Inulin
Naturally occurring plant fiber in fruits and vegetables that is added to foods to boost the fiber in or help the texture of low-fat foods. Most of the inulin in the food supply is extracted from chicory root or synthesized from sucrose. It's in smoothies, meal-replacement bars, and processed foods trying to gain legitimacy among healthy eaters. Like other fibers, inulin can help stabilize blood sugar, improve bowel functions, and help the body absorb nutrients such as calcium (good) and iron (not so good).

Lecithin
A naturally occurring emulsifier and antioxidant that retards the rancidity of fats. The two major sources for lecithin as an additive are egg yolks and soybeans, and it's used in pastries, ice cream, and margarine. Lecithin is an excellent source of choline and inositol—compounds that help cells and nerves communicate and play a role in breaking down fats and cholesterol.

Maltodextrin
A caloric sweetener and flavor enhancer made from rice, potatoes, or, more commonly, cornstarch. Through treatment with enzymes and acids, it can be converted into a fiber and thickening agent and you'll find it in canned fruit, instant pudding, sauces, dressings, and chocolates. Like other sugars, maltodextrin has the potential to raise blood glucose and insulin levels.

Maltose (malt sugar)
A caloric sweetener that's about a third as sweet as honey. It occurs naturally in some grains, but as an additive it is usually derived from corn. Food manufacturers like it because it prolongs shelf life and inhibits bacterial growth. It's used in cereal grains, nuts and seeds, sports beverages, deli meats, and poultry products. Maltose poses no threats other than those associated with other sugars.

Mannitol
A sugar alcohol that's 70 percent as sweet as sugar. It provides fewer calories and has a less drastic effect on blood sugar. You'll find it in sugar-free candy, low-calorie and diet foods, and chewing gum. Because sugar alcohols are not fully digested, they can cause intestinal discomfort, gas, bloating, flatulence, and diarrhea.

Modified food starch
An indefinite term describing a starch that has been manipulated in a nonspecific way. The starches can be derived from corn, wheat, potato, or rice, and they are then modified to change their response to heat or cold, improve their texture, and create more efficient emulsifiers, among other reasons. You'll see modified food starch in most highly processed foods, low-calorie and diet foods, pastries, cookies, and frozen meals. The starches themselves appear safe, but the nondisclosure of the chemicals used in processing causes some nutritionists to question their effects on health, especially of infants.

Mono- and diglycerides
Fats added to foods to bind liquids with fats. They occur naturally in foods and constitute about 1 percent of normal food fats. They're in peanut butter, ice cream, margarine, baked goods, and whipped topping. Aside from being a source of fat, the glycerides themselves pose no serious health threats.

Monosodium glutamate (MSG)
The salt of the amino acid glutamic acid, used to enhance the savory quality of foods. MSG alone has little flavor, and exactly how it enhances other foods is unknown. It's used in chili, soup, and foods with chicken or beef flavoring. Studies have shown that MSG injected into mice causes brain-cell damage, but the FDA believes these results are not typical for humans. The FDA receives dozens of reaction complaints each year for nausea, headaches, chest pains, and weakness.

Neotame
The newest addition to the FDA-approved artificial sweeteners. It's chemically similar to aspartame and at least 8,000 times sweeter than sugar. It was approved in 2002, and its use is not yet widespread, though it's used in Clabber Girl Sugar Replacer, Domino Pure D'Lite, and Hostess 100-Calorie Packs. Neotame is the second artificial sweetener to be deemed safe by the Center for Science in the Public Interest (the first was sucralose). It's considered more stable than aspartame, and because it's 40 times sweeter, it can be used in much smaller concentrations.

Olestra
A synthetic fat created by Procter & Gamble and sold under the name Olean. It has a zero-calorie impact and is not absorbed as it passes though the digestive system. It's used in light chips and crackers. But it's hardly a perfect solution for those trying to cut calories: In even moderate doses, Olestra can cause diarrhea, intestinal cramps, and flatulence. Studies show that it impairs the body's ability to absorb fat-soluble vitamins and vital carotenoids such as beta-carotene, lycopene, lutein, and zeaxanthin.

Oligofructose
See inulin.

What About Iodine?
Your thyroid gland requires iodine to produce the hormones T3 and T4, both of which help control how efficiently you burn calories. That means insufficient iodine may cause you to gain weight and feel fatigued.

The shortfall: Since iodized salt is an important source of the element, you might assume you're swimming in the stuff. But when University of Texas at Arlington researchers tested 88 samples of table salt, they found that half contained less than the FDA-recommended amount of iodine. And you're not making up the difference with all the salt hiding in processed foods—US manufacturers aren't required to use iodized salt. The result is that we've been sliding toward iodine deficiency since the 1970s.

Hit the mark: Sprinkling more salt on top of an already sodium-packed diet isn't a great idea, but iodine can also be found in several nearly sodium-free sources: milk, eggs, and yogurt. Animal feed is fortified with the element, meaning it travels from cows and chickens to your breakfast table.

Partially hydrogenated vegetable oil

A manufactured fat created by forcing hydrogen gas into vegetable fats under extremely high pressure, an unintended effect of which is the creation of trans fatty acids. Food manufacturers like this fat because of its low cost and long shelf life. It's used in margarine, pastries, frozen foods, cakes, cookies, crackers, soups, and nondairy creamers. Cardiologists, on the other hand, hate it: Trans fat has been shown to contribute to heart disease more so than saturated fats. While most health organizations recommend keeping trans fat consumption as low as possible (no more than 2 to 2.5 grams daily for an average American), a loophole in the FDA's labeling requirements allows marketers to add as much as 0.49 grams per serving and still claim zero in their nutrition facts. That means you could eat four servings of "trans-fat-free" packaged goods and still approach your daily allotment. Progressive jurisdictions such as New York City, California, and Boston have approved legislation to phase trans fat out of restaurants, and pressure from watchdog groups might eventually lead to a full ban on the dangerous oil.

Pectin

A carbohydrate that occurs naturally in many fruits and vegetables, used to thicken and stabilize foods. You'll find it in jellies and jams, sauces, pie fillings, smoothies, and shakes. Pectin is a source of dietary fiber and might help to lower cholesterol.

Polysorbates

A class of chemicals usually derived from animal fats and used primarily as emulsifiers, much like mono- and diglycerides. Polysorbates are found in cakes, icing, bread mixes, ice cream, and pickles. Polysorbates allow otherwise fat-soluble vitamins to dissolve in water, an odd trait that seems to have a benign effect.

Propyl gallate

An antioxidant used often in conjunction with BHA and BHT to retard the rancidity of fats. It's found in mayonnaise, margarine, oils, dried meats, pork sausage, and other fatty foods. Rat studies in the early 1980s linked propyl gallate to brain cancer. Although these studies don't provide sound evidence, it is advisable to avoid this chemical when possible.

Red #3 (erythrosine) and Red #40 (allura red)

Food dyes that are orange-red and cherry red, respectively. Red #40 is the most widely used food dye in America. Red dyes are used in fruit cocktail, candy, chocolate cake, cereal, beverages, pastries, maraschino cherries, and fruit snacks. The FDA has proposed a ban on Red #3 in the past, but so far the agency has been unsuccessful in implementing it. After the dye was inextricably linked to thyroid tumors in rat studies, the FDA managed to have the liquid form of the dye removed from external drugs and cosmetics.

Saccharin

An artificial sweetener that's 300 to 500 times sweeter than sugar. Discovered in 1879, it's the oldest of the five FDA-approved artificial sweeteners. It's used in diet foods, chewing gum, toothpaste, beverages, sugar-free candy, and Sweet'N Low. Rat studies in the early 1970s showed saccharin to cause bladder cancer, and the FDA, reacting to these studies, enacted a mandatory warning label to be printed on every saccharin-containing product. The label was removed after 20 years, but the question over saccharin's safety was never resolved. More recent studies show that rats on saccharin-rich diets gain more weight than those on high-sugar diets.

Sodium ascorbate
See ascorbic acid.

Sodium caseinate
See casein.

Sodium nitrite and sodium nitrate
Preservatives used to prevent bacterial growth and maintain the pinkish color of meats and fish. They're used in bacon, sausage, hot dogs, and cured, canned, and packaged meats. Under certain conditions, sodium nitrite and nitrate react with amino acids to form cancer-causing chemicals called nitrosamines.

Sorbitol
A sugar alcohol that occurs naturally in some fruits. It's about 60 percent as sweet as sugar and used to both sweeten and thicken. You'll find it added to dried fruit, chewing gum, and reduced-sugar candy. Your body digests sorbitol slower than sugars, which makes it a better choice for diabetics, but it can cause intestinal discomfort and diarrhea.

Soy lecithin
See lecithin.

Sucralose
A zero-calorie artificial sweetener made by joining chlorine particles and sugar molecules. It's 600 times sweeter than sugar and largely celebrated as the least damaging of the artificial sweeteners. It's use in sugar-free foods, pudding, beverages, some diet sodas, and Splenda. After reviewing more than 110 human and animal studies, the FDA concluded that use of sucralose does not cause cancer. The sweetener is one of only three artificial sweeteners deemed safe by the Center for Science in the Public Interest.

Tartrazine
See Yellow #5.

Vegetable shortening
See partially hydrogenated vegetable oil.

Yellow #5 (tartrazine) and Yellow #6 (sunset yellow)
The second and third most common food colorings, respectively. They're used in cereal, pudding, bread mixes, beverages, chips, cookies, and condiments. Several studies have linked both dyes to learning and concentration disorders in children. One study found that mice fed high doses of sunset yellow had trouble swimming straight and righting themselves in water. Despite these results, the FDA does not view these as serious risks to humans.

Xanthan gum
An extremely common emulsifier and thickener made from glucose in a reaction requiring a slimy bacteria called Xanthomonas campestris—the same bacterial strain that appears as black rot on cruciferous vegetables such as broccoli. It's used in whipped topping, dressings, marinades, custard, and pie filling. Xanthan gum isn't associated with any adverse effects.

Xylitol
A sugar alcohol that occurs naturally in strawberries, mushrooms, and other fruits and vegetables. It is most commonly extracted from the pulp of the birch tree and is used in sugar-free candy, yogurt, and beverages. Unlike real sugar, sugar alcohols don't encourage cavity-causing bacteria. They do have a laxative effect, though, so heavy ingestion might cause intestinal discomfort or gas.

Appendix B

Nutritional Values of Common Foods

EATING HIGHER AMOUNTS OF PROTEIN IS NECESSARY TO BUILD MUSCLE, BUT ALSO BE AWARE WHERE YOU CAN ADD IN THE VALUABLE MICRONUTRIENTS FOUND IN WHOLE GRAINS, FRUITS, VEGETABLES, AND OTHER FOODS.

It might seem easier to ensure your daily value of nutrients by popping a multivitamin instead of eating a balanced diet. But there are two problems with nutrition that comes in a plastic container: First, multivitamins have no fiber, so this critical nutrient is missing if all you do is pop a pill for protection. Second, foods are loaded with plenty of nutrients beyond the standard vitamins C and E—and the importance of many of these nutrients, called phytochemicals, is only now being understood. "In a balanced diet, there are thousands of antioxidants. In pill form, you're just getting a few out of the thousands," says Edgar Miller, MD, PhD, of Johns Hopkins University in Baltimore.

To see how nutritionally complete your diet is, refer to the following chart for each food's vitamin and mineral values, and tally your total intake. If you come up short of the Recommended Dietary Allowances (RDAs) for men and women, don't worry. Just eat more foods high in whatever vitamins or minerals you're lacking, and take a multivitamin/mineral supplement each day.

	VITAMIN A (MCG)	VITAMIN B₁ (THIAMIN) (MG)	VITAMIN B₆ (MG)	VITAMIN B₉ (FOLATE) (MCG)	VITAMIN C (MG)
RDA (MEN/WOMEN)	**900/700**	**1.2/1.1**	**1.3/1.3**	**400/400**	**95/75**
Almonds (1 ounce)	0	0.05	0.03	11	0
Apple (1 medium)	8	0.02	0.06	4	6
Apricot (1)	67	0.01	0.02	3	3.50
Artichoke (1 medium)	0	0.10	0.15	87	15
Asparagus (1 medium spear)	12	0.02	0.01	8	1
Avocado (1)	122	0.20	0.60	124	16
Bacon (3 slices)	0	0.08	0.07	0.40	0
Bagel (4")	0	0.15	0.05	20	0
Banana (1 medium)	7	0.04	0.40	24	10
Beans, baked (1 cup)	13	0.40	0.34	61	8
Beans, black (1 cup cooked)	1	0.40	0.12	256	0
Beans, kidney (1 cup cooked)	0	0.28	0.21	230	2
Beans, lima (½ cup cooked)	32	0.12	0.16	22	9
Beans, navy (1 cup cooked)	0.36	0.40	0.30	255	1.64
Beans, pinto (1 cup cooked)	0	0.17	0.16	294	1.37
Beans, refried (1 cup)	0	0.07	0.36	28	15
Beans, white (1 cup cooked)	0	0.20	0.17	145	0
Beef, ground lean (3 ounces)	0	0.06	0.24	7	0
Beer (12 ounces)	0	0.02	0.18	21	0
Beets (½ cup)	3	0.02	0.05	74	3
Blueberries (1 pint)	17	0.11	0.15	17	28
Bran, wheat (1 cup)	0	0.14	0.35	14	0
Bread, rye (1 slice)	0.26	0.14	0.02	35	0.13
Bread, white (1 slice)	0	0.11	0.02	28	0
Bread, whole grain (1 slice)	0	0.11	0.10	30	0.08
Breakfast sandwich, fast-food (bacon, egg, and cheese)	0	0.53	0.16	73	2
Brussels sprouts (½ cup)	60	0.08	0.14	47	48

VITAMIN E (MG)	CALCIUM (MG)	MAGNESIUM (MG)	POTASSIUM (MG)	SELENIUM (MG)	ZINC (MG)	CALORIES
15/15	1,000/1,000	420/320	4,700/4,700	55/55	11/8	-
6	71	86	180	0	1	170
0.25	8	7	148	0	0.06	80
0.30	5	3.50	90	0.03	0.07	20
0.24	56	77	474	0.26	0.60	25
0.18	4	2	32	0.37	0.10	5
3	22	78	1,204	0.80	0.84	276
0.06	2	6	107	12	0.70	110
0.04	16	26	90	28	1	247
0.12	6	32	422	1	0.20	110
1.35	127	81	752	12	4	239
0.14	46	120	610	2	1.90	240
0.05	62	74	717	2	1.80	260
0.12	27	63	485	1.70	0.70	229
0.73	127	107	670	11	1.90	255
1.61	72	70	495	19	1.70	245
0	88	83	675	3	3	240
1.74	161	113	1,004	2.30	2.50	249
0.15	7	19	265	0	4	185
0	18	21	89	2.50	0.04	153
0.03	111	16	221	0.5	0.24	29
1.65	17	17	223	0.3	0.50	165
0.54	26	220	426	28	3	120
0.11	23	13	53	10	0.36	83
0.06	38	6	25	4.30	0.20	67
0.09	24	14	53	8	0.30	65
0.60	160	24	211	36.0	2	441
0.34	28	16	247	1.17	0.26	28

	VITAMIN A (MCG)	VITAMIN B₁ (THIAMIN) (MG)	VITAMIN B₆ (MG)	VITAMIN B₉ (FOLATE) (MCG)	VITAMIN C (MG)
RDA (MEN/WOMEN)	**900/700**	**1.2/1.1**	**1.3/1.3**	**400/400**	**95/75**
Cake, coffee (1 piece)	20	0.10	0.03	27	0.11
Cake, frosted (1 piece)	10	0.01	0.02	7	0.04
Canadian bacon (2 slices)	0	0.40	0.20	2	0
Candy, nonchocolate (1 package)	0	0	0	0	0
Cantaloupe (1 medium wedge)	345	0.04	0.07	21	37
Carrot (1)	734	0.04	0.08	12	4
Cauliflower (1 cup)	2	0.06	0.22	57	46
Celery (1 cup, strips)	55	0.03	0.10	45	4
Cereal, whole grain, with raisins (½ cup)	3	0.16	0.10	22	0.55
Cheddar cheese (1 slice)	75	0.01	0.2	5	0
Chef's salad with no dressing (1½ cups)	146	0.40	0.40	101	16
Cherries, sweet, raw (1 cup)	30	0.07	0.05	5.80	10
Chicken, skinless (½ breast)	4	0.04	0.32	2	0.71
Chickpeas (1 cup cooked)	4	0.19	0.22	282	2
Chili with beans (1 cup)	87	0.12	0.30	59	4
Chips, potato, light (1 ounce)	0	0.05	0.22	8	3.40
Chocolate (1.45 ounces)	20	0.05	0.01	5	0
Cinnamon bun (1)	0	0.12	0	17	0.06
Citrus fruits and frozen concentrate juices (12 ounces)	7	0.17	0.30	31	324
Clams, fried (¾ cup)	101	0.11	0.07	41	11.25
Coffee (1 cup)	0	0	0	5	0
Collards (1 cup cooked)	0.08	0.8	0.24	177	35
Cookie, chocolate chip (1)	0.04	0.01	0.01	0.90	0
Corn (1 cup)	0.26	0.06	0.16	115	12
Cottage cheese, low-fat (1 cup)	25	0.05	0.15	27	0
Crackers (12)	0	0.17	0	0	0
Cranberry juice cocktail (1 cup)	1	0.02	0.05	0	90

VITAMIN E (MG)	CALCIUM (MG)	MAGNESIUM (MG)	POTASSIUM (MG)	SELENIUM (MG)	ZINC (MG)	CALORIES
15/15	1,000/1,000	420/320	4,700/4,700	55/55	11/8	-
0.11	76	10	63	9	0.25	180
0	18	14	84	1.40	0.30	239
0.16	5	10	181	11	0.80	137
0	0	0	0	0	0	230
0.05	9	12	272	0.40	0.18	24
0.40	20	7	195	0.06	0.15	35
0.08	22	15	303	0.60	0.30	25
0.33	50	14	322	0.50	0.16	17
0.40	33	70	207	10	1	195
0.08	204	8	28	4	0.90	114
0	235	49	401	37	3	267
0.20	21	16	325	0.90	0.09	90
0.08	6.50	16	150	11	0.50	130
0.60	80	79	477	6	2.50	269
1.46	120	115	934	3	5	220
0.62	10	18	285	2	0.17	142
0.83	78	26	153	2	0.83	230
0.48	10	3.60	19	5	0.10	418
0.24	85	68	1,336	1	0.41	186
0	71	16	366	33	1.60	560
0.05	2	5	114	0	0.02	2
1.67	266	38	220	1	0.50	61
0.26	2.50	3	14	0	0.06	63
0.15	8	44	343	1.54	1.36	120
0.02	138	11	194	20	.86	180
0	28	12	48	2.40	0.20	155
0	8	5	46	0	0.18	137

	VITAMIN A (MCG)	VITAMIN B$_1$ (THIAMIN) (MG)	VITAMIN B$_6$ (MG)	VITAMIN B$_9$ (FOLATE) (MCG)	VITAMIN C (MG)
RDA (MEN/WOMEN)	**900/700**	**1.2/1.1**	**1.3/1.3**	**400/400**	**95/75**
Cream cheese (1 tablespoon)	53	0	0	2	0
Cucumber with peel (½ cup)	10	0.01	0.02	7	2.76
Doughnut (1)	17	0.10	0.03	24	0.09
Egg, whole (1 large)	84	0.03	0.06	22	0
Eggplant (1 cup)	4	0.08	0.09	14	1
English muffin, whole wheat (1)	0.09	0.25	0.05	36	0
Fig bar cookies (2 bars)	3	0.05	0.02	11	0.10
Fish, white (1 fillet)	60	0.26	0.50	26	0
French fries (10)	0	0.07	0.16	8	6
Fruit, dried (1 ounce)	208	0.01	0.05	1.10	1
Fruit juice, unsweetened (1 cup)	0	0.02	0.06	35	40
Garlic (1 clove)	0	0	0.04	0.09	0.90
Graham cracker (1 large rectangular piece)	0	0.03	0.01	6	0
Granola bar (1)	2	0.06	0.02	6	0.22
Grape juice (1 cup)	1	0.07	0.16	8	0.25
Ham (1 slice)	0	0.20	0.10	1	0
Hamburger, fast-food, with condiments and vegetables (1)	4	0.30	0.12	5	2
Hot dog, fast-food (1)	0	0.44	0.09	85	0.09
Ice cream (1 serving)	6	0.03	0.04	11	0.46
Jam or preserves (1 tablespoon)	0.20	0.0	0	2	2
Kale (1 cup)	955	0.07	0.11	18	33
Ketchup (1 tablespoon)	7	0	0.02	2	2
Kiwifruit (1 medium)	3	0.02	0.07	19	70
Lasagna, meat (7 ounces)	61	0.19	0.20	16	12
Lentils (1 cup cooked)	4.75	0.33	0.35	358	0.22
Lettuce, iceberg (1 cup)	8	0.02	0.03	31	2
Lettuce, romaine (½ cup)	81	0.02	0.02	38	7
Liver, beef (3 ounces)	8,042	0.16	0.86	215	1.62

VITAMIN E (MG)	CALCIUM (MG)	MAGNESIUM (MG)	POTASSIUM (MG)	SELENIUM (MG)	ZINC (MG)	CALORIES
15/15	**1,000/1,000**	**420/320**	**4,700/4,700**	**55/55**	**11/8**	**-**
0.04	12	1	17	0.40	0.10	51
0	7	6	75	0	0.10	8
0.90	21	9	60	4	0.30	230
0.50	25	5	63	15	0.50	74
0.40	6	11	122	0.10	0.12	35
0.26	101	21	106	17	0.61	134
0.21	20	9	66	1	0.12	111
0.39	51	65	625	25	2	168
0.12	4	11	211	0.20	0.20	100
0.31	11.82	11.13	226	0	0.14	69
0.20	160	9	154	0	0.20	117
0	5	0.75	12	0.40	0	4
0	3	4	19	1	0.10	59
0.05	15	24	82	4	0.50	117
0.62	23	25	334	0.25	0.13	154
0.32	2	5	94	6	0.50	30
0	126	23	251	20	2	512
.10	108	27	190	29	2	242
0	72	19	164	1.65	0.40	133
0	4	0.80	15	.40	0	56
1	180	23	417	1.17	0.23	39
0.20	3	3	57	0.04	0	15
1	26	13	237	0.15	0.10	50
0.94	220	41	372	28	3	318
2.97	37	71	731	5.54	2.51	230
0.02	11	4	84	0.28	0.10	8
0.04	9	4	69	0.10	0.06	5
0.43	5	18	300	31	4.50	162

Appendix B

	VITAMIN A (MCG)	VITAMIN B₁ (THIAMIN) (MG)	VITAMIN B₆ (MG)	VITAMIN B₉ (FOLATE) (MCG)	VITAMIN C (MG)
RDA (MEN/WOMEN)	900/700	1.2/1.1	1.3/1.3	400/400	95/75
Lunchmeat, salami (3 slices)	0	0.10	0.08	0.34	0
Macaroni and cheese (8 ounces)	48	0.25	0	0	0
Meat loaf (1 slice)	20	0.10	0.14	12	0.62
Melon, honeydew (1 cup)	5	0.07	0.16	34	32
Milk, fat-free (1 cup)	5	0.10	0.10	12	2
Milk, soy (1 cup)	0	0.15	0.16	40	0
Muffin, blueberry (1)	13	0.10	0.01	42	0.63
Mushrooms (1 cup sliced)	0	0.09	0.10	12	2
Nachos with cheese (6-8)	170	0.20	0.20	12	1
Nectarine (1)	23	0.05	0.03	7	7
Oatmeal (1 cup)	0.12	0.12	0.10	13	0
Olives (1 tablespoon)	1.70	0	0	0	0
Onion rings (10 medium)	0.98	0.10	0.07	64	0.68
Oyster (1 medium)	4.20	0.01	0.01	1.40	0.51
Pancakes (2)	7.60	0.16	0.07	28	0.15
Pasta with red sauce (4.5 ounces)	0	0.13	0.10	4	6
Peach (1 medium)	15	0.02	0.02	4	6
Peanut butter (2 tablespoons)	0	0.03	0.15	24	0
Peanuts (1 ounce)	0	0.12	0.07	41	0
Pear (1 medium)	1.60	0.02	0.05	12	7
Pepper, chile, raw (½ pepper)	21.6	0.03	0.23	10.35	65
Peppers, sweet (10 strips)	78	0.04	0.13	13	70
Pie, apple (1 piece)	37	0.03	0.04	32	4
Pizza, cheese (1 slice)	74	0.20	0.04	35	1
Pizza, vegetable (1 slice)	58	0.40	0.50	116	79
Plum (1)	21	0.03	0.05	1.45	6
Popcorn (1 cup)	0.80	0.02	0.02	2	0
Pork (3 ounces)	0	0.80	0.30	3	0
Potatoes, mashed (1 cup)	8.40	0.20	0.50	17	13
Potato salad (1 cup)	2.93	0.20	0.40	19	19

VITAMIN E (MG)	CALCIUM (MG)	MAGNESIUM (MG)	POTASSIUM (MG)	SELENIUM (MG)	ZINC (MG)	CALORIES
15/15	1,000/1,000	420/320	4,700/4,700	55/55	11/8	-
0.05	1.34	2.86	63	4	0.54	150
0	102	0	111	0	0	415
0.10	43	22	295	0	4	231
0.04	11	18	403	1.24	0.15	61
0.10	301	27	406	5	1	83
0	80	60	440	3	0.90	100
0.47	32	9	70	6	0.30	158
0.10	5	10	355	8	0.70	15
0	311	63	196	18	2	296
1	8	12	273	0	0.23	70
0.26	19	51	175	0	1.43	150
0.14	7	0.30	0.67	0.08	0	10
0.39	86	19	152	3	0.41	370
0.12	6	7	22	9	13	41
0.65	96	15	133	10	0.30	173
1.40	41	13	207	11	0.66	216
0.70	6	9	186	0.10	0.17	70
.0	12	51	214	2	1	190
.2	15	50	186	2	1	165
.20	15	12	198	0.17	0.17	100
.30	6	10	145	0.20	0.12	2
0.36	7	6.46	105	0	0	5
1.78	13	8	76	1	0.20	296
0	117	16	113	13	1	272
2	189	65	548	23	2	170
0	3	5	114	0.30	0.07	40
0	1	11	24	0.80	0.30	31
0.20	6	15	253	14	2	191
0.04	46	38	621	2	0.60	201
0.14	14	36	551	10	0.60	358

	VITAMIN A (MCG)	VITAMIN B₁ (THIAMIN) (MG)	VITAMIN B₆ (MG)	VITAMIN B₉ (FOLATE) (MCG)	VITAMIN C (MG)
RDA (MEN/WOMEN)	900/700	1.2/1.1	1.3/1.3	400/400	95/75
Potpie, chicken	256	0.30	0.20	41	2
Pretzels (10 twists)	0	0.30	0.07	103	0
Raisins (1.5 ounces)	0	0.05	0.08	1.28	2.30
Raspberries (10)	0.38	0.01	0.01	4	5
Rice, brown (1 cup)	0	0.20	0.30	8	0
Rice, white (1 cup)	0	0.03	0.15	5	0
Ricotta cheese, part skim (½ cup)	132	0.03	0.02	16	0
Salad dressing, light Italian (1 tablespoon)	0	0	0	0	0
Salmon (3 ounces)	9.84	0.20	0.71	22	0
Salsa (½ cup)	44	0.05	0.16	21	18
Sauerkraut (1 cup)	1.42	0.03	0.18	34	21
Sausage (1 link)	0	0.05	0.01	0.26	0
Shrimp (4 large)	0	0.01	0.03	0.77	0.48
Soft drink with caffeine (12 ounces)	0	0	0	0	0
Soup, cream of chicken (1 cup)	179	0.07	0.07	7	1.24
Soup, tomato (1 cup)	29.28	0.09	0.11	15	66
Soybeans (1 cup cooked)	14	0.47	0.10	200	31
Spaghetti with meatballs (1½ cups)	46	0.38	0.43	101	24
Spareribs (3 ounces)	1.91	0.26	0.22	3	0
Spinach (1 cup)	140	0.02	0.06	58	8
Steak (different cuts)	0	0.10	0.30	6	0
Strawberries (1 cup)	1.66	0.03	0.09	40	97
Submarine sandwich	71	1	0.10	87	12
Sunflower seeds (¼ cup)	6	0	0.28	82	0.50
Sweet potato (1)	350	0.09	0.25	9	19
Taco salad (1.5 cups)	71	0.10	0.20	83	4
Toaster pastry (1)	148	0.20	0.20	15	0
Tofu (4 ounces)	4.96	0.10	0.06	19	0
Tomato (1 medium)	26	0.02	0.05	9	8
Tuna salad (1 cup)	49	0.06	0.17	16	5

VITAMIN E (MG)	CALCIUM (MG)	MAGNESIUM (MG)	POTASSIUM (MG)	SELENIUM (MG)	ZINC (MG)	CALORIES
15/15	1,000/1,000	420/320	4,700/4,700	55/55	11/8	-
4	33	24	256	0.70	1	484
0.21	22	21	88	3	0.50	229
0.30	12	13	350	0.26	0.08	127
0.17	5	4	28	0.04	0.08	10
0.06	20	84	84	19	1	216
0.06	16	19	55	12	0.80	205
0.09	337	19	155	21	1.70	171
0	0	0	2	0.20	0	26
0.95	11	28	475	35	0.60	175
1.53	39	17	275	0.50	0.30	41
0.14	43	18	241	0.90	0.30	45
0.03	1.30	1.56	25	1.87	0.24	125
0	9	7	40	9	0.30	22
0	10	3	3	0.34	0	154
0.25	181	17	272	8	0.67	225
2	12	7	263	0.50	0.24	180
0.02	261	108	970	3	1.64	298
4	138	66	718	39	5	545
0.20	30	15	204	24	3	338
0.60	30	24	167	0.30	0.16	10
0.11	4	19	250	12	3.26	217
0.50	27	22	253	1	0.20	46
0	189	68	394	31	2.60	386
12	42	127	248	21.42	1.82	205
1.42	41	27	348	0.30	0.30	103
192	51	416	4	3	0	279
0.90	17	12	57	6.30	0.30	204
0.01	434	37	150	11	1	75
0.33	6	7	146	0	0.11	35
2	35	39	365	84	1	383

Appendix B **283**

	VITAMIN A (MCG)	VITAMIN B₁ (THIAMIN) (MG)	VITAMIN B₆ (MG)	VITAMIN B₉ (FOLATE) (MCG)	VITAMIN C (MG)
RDA (MEN/WOMEN)	900/700	1.2/1.1	1.3/1.3	400/400	95/75
Turkey, skinless (½ breast)	0	0.16	2.26	31	0
Vegetable juice (1 cup)	188	0.10	0.30	51	67
Walnuts (1 cup)	37	0.27	0.70	82	4
Watermelon (1 wedge)	104	0.20	0.40	6	31
Wheat germ (½ cup)	0	0.20	0.40	81	0
Whey protein powder (2 teaspoons)	0	0	0	0	0
Wine, red (3.5 ounces)	0	0	0.03	2	0
Wine, white (3.5 ounces)	0	0	0.01	0	0
Yogurt, low-fat (8 ounces)	2	0.10	0.09	24	1.70

VITAMIN E (MG)	CALCIUM (MG)	MAGNESIUM (MG)	POTASSIUM (MG)	SELENIUM (MG)	ZINC (MG)	CALORIES
15/15	1,000/1,000	420/320	4,700/4,700	55/55	11/8	-
0.30	39	109	1,142	95	5	413
12	26	27	467	1	0.50	50
0	73	253	655	21	4.28	654
0.40	41	31	479	0.30	0.20	86
0	27	275	166	91	14	104
0	0	0	260	0	0	21
0	8	13	111	0.20	0.10	88
0	9	10	80	0.20	0.07	86
0	415	37	497	11	1.88	193

Appendix C

Glycemic Loads for Selected Foods

How to use this chart: The numbers in this chart represent the glycemic loads (GLs) of common foods. The GL is the product of a food's glycemic index and the amount of carbohydrates available per serving. Essentially, the GL estimates the projected elevation in blood glucose caused by eating a particular food. The higher a food's GL, the more likely it is to raise your blood sugar, and the higher it will likely be in calories and carbs. Try to focus on foods with a GL of 19 or less and shoot for a total GL of less than 120 per day if you decide to count.

Food	Value	Food	Value
Peanuts	1	Cheese tortellini	10
Low-fat yogurt, artificially sweetened	2	Frozen waffles	10
Carrots	3	Honey	10
Grapefruit	3	Lima beans, frozen	10
Green peas	3	Low-fat yogurt, sweetened with sugar	10
Fat-free milk	4	Pinto beans	10
Pear	4	White bread	10
Watermelon	4	Bran Chex cereal	11
Beets	5	Apple juice	12
Orange	5	Banana	12
Peach	5	Kaiser roll	12
Plum	5	Orange juice	12
Apple	6	Saltine crackers	12
Kiwifruit	6	Bran flakes	13
Tomato soup	6	Oatmeal	13
Baked beans	7	Graham crackers	14
Chickpeas, canned	7	Special K cereal	14
Grapes	7	Vanilla wafers	14
Pineapple	7	Bran muffin	15
Whole-wheat bread	7	Cheerios cereal	15
Popcorn	8	French bread	15
Soy milk	8	Grape-Nuts cereal	15
Taco shells	8	Mashed potatoes	15
All-Bran cereal	9	Shredded Wheat cereal	15
Grapefruit juice	9	Bread stuffing mix	16
Hamburger bun	9	Cheese pizza	16
Kidney beans, canned	9	Whole-wheat spaghetti	16
Lentil soup	9	Black bean soup	17
Oatmeal cookies	9	Blueberry muffin	17
Sweet corn	9	Corn chips	17
American rye bread	10	Doughnut	17

Grape-Nuts Flakes cereal	17
Instant oatmeal	17
Rice cakes	17
Sweet potato	17
Total cereal	17
Brown rice	18
Fettuccine	18
Angel food cake	19
Cornflakes cereal	21
French fries	22
Jelly beans	22
Macaroni	22
Rice Krispies cereal	22
Couscous	23
Linguine	23
Long-grain rice	23
White rice	23
Bagel	25
Baked potato	26
Spaghetti	27
Raisins	28
Macaroni and cheese	32
Instant rice	36

Index

Underscored page references indicate boxed text.

A

Abdominal fat, 5, 215, 245–46
Acesulfame potassium, 264
Acetylcholine, 260
Acetyl-l-carnitine, 230
Addictive foods, <u>75</u>, 90–91
Additives, list of, 264–69
Advertising. *See* Marketing
Agave, 227
Aging, 30, 221
Agricultural subsidies, 144
Airport foods, tips for, 46
Alcoholic beverages, 19, 30, 63, <u>147</u>, 194
Allergies
  to milk, 266
  probiotics and, 210
  to wheat, 8, 200
Alli, <u>231</u>
Allura red (dye), 270
Almond butter, 54, 177
Almond milk, 217
Almonds, 16, 177, <u>274–75</u>
Alpha-linoleic acid, <u>232</u>
Alpha-tocopherol, 264
American cheese, 50
American flavors, for side dishes, 87

Animal products
  antibiotics/hormones in, 214, <u>250</u>, 251
  as protein source, 9
Anthocyanins, 29, 133
Antibiotics, in animal products, 214, <u>250</u>, 251
Antioxidants
  about, 220–22, 273
  sources of, 124, 133, 147, 220–21, <u>221</u>, 233, 255
Appetite
  imagery and, 47–48, <u>75</u>, 93–94
  liquid calories and, 58
  neurology of, 83, 90–94, <u>266</u>
  saturated fat role, 91
  stimulants, 63
Apple juice, <u>147</u>
Apples, 17, 144, <u>221</u>, <u>274–75</u>, <u>288</u>
Applesauce, 176
Apricots, <u>274–75</u>
Arabica coffee, 60
Arctic char, 52
Artichokes, 151, <u>221</u>, <u>274–75</u>
Artificial flavorings, 264–65
Artificial sweeteners
  about, 226–27, 264, 265, 269, 270
  in energy foods, 120

  pitfalls of, 14
  in sodas, 63
Arugula, 18
Ascorbic acid, 265
Asian flavors, for side dishes, 87
Asparagus, 151, <u>274–75</u>
Aspartame, 14, 227, 265
Aspirin therapy, <u>230</u>
Avocados, 16, 46, 144, 151, <u>274–75</u>

B

Bacon, 194, <u>274–75</u>
Bagels, 188, <u>274–75</u>, <u>289</u>
Balsamic vinegar, 176
Bananas, 128, <u>137</u>, <u>221</u>, <u>274–75</u>, <u>288</u>
Barley, 119
BBQ sauce, 191
Beans
  antioxidants in, <u>221</u>
  canned, 29, 177, 191
  glycemic loads, <u>288</u>
  green, 152
  as protein source, 126
  RDA information, <u>274–75</u>
Bed-and-breakfasts, 47

291

Beef
  grass-fed, 28–29
  liver, 248
  packaged, recommendations, 189–90, 193, 194
  RDA information, 274–75, 278–79, 282–83
  serving recommendations, 17
Beer, 19, 147, 274–75
Beets, 274–75, 288
Bell peppers, 151
Belly fat. *See* Abdominal fat
Beta-alanine supplements, 135
Betaine, 260
Beverages. *See also* Smoothies; Water
  alcohol, 19, 30, 63, 147, 194
  recommendations regarding, 19, 58–62, 193
  satiety and, 58
BHA/BHT, 265
Bisphenol A (BPA), 143
Black beans, 18, 145, 221
Blood lipid levels. *See under* Cholesterol
Blood sugar levels, 7, 73–74, 226
Blueberries
  benefits, 128, 146, 221
  RDA information, 274–75
  shopping tips, 151
  subsidies for, 144
Blue cheese, 17
Blue dyes, 265
Blue foods, 150
Blue walls, appetite effects, 83
Body fat. *See also* Weight
  abdominal fat, 5, 215, 245–46
  vitamin D metabolism and, 245–47
Bok choy, 18, 55
Bone health, 54, 231, 262
Bowl size, 83
BPA (Bisphenol A), 143
Brain health, 230
Bran, wheat, 274–75
Bread/buns
  glycemic loads, 288
  RDA information, 274–75, 276–77, 278–79, 280–81
  recommendations regarding, 46, 188
  sodium in, 204
Bread crumbs, 176, 195

Breakfasts
  examples of (*see* Meal planning)
  protein in, 96
  recommendations regarding, 68, 71, 76, 100
  while traveling, tips for, 44–45
Brilliant blue (dye), 265
Broccoli, 146, 151, 221
Broccoli sprouts, 53
Broth, 177, 195
Brown rice syrup, 265
Brussels sprouts, 274–75
Buffalo, 54
Butter, 254
Button mushrooms, 152
Butylated hydroxyanisole/ hydroxytoluene, 265

C

Cabbage, 18, 145
Caffeine, 30, 62, 120, 132–33
Cake, 276–77
Calcitrol, 245
Calcium
  benefits, 263
  sodium and, 264
  sources of, 29, 50, 54, 55, 62, 113, 118, 146–47
  supplements, 215
  vitamin D and, 262
  weight loss and, 71
Calcium caseinate. *See* Casein
Calories
  about, 12–14
  in assessing food costs, 146
  counting of, 48, 69
  cutting of, 126
  fat as source of, 4, 12, 255
  liquid forms, 57–58
  in macronutrients, 12
  metabolism of, 13, 14
  in natural/health foods, 69
  on nutrition facts labels, 142
Cancer risk, 233, 265, 270
Candy, 276–77, 289
Cane juice/cane sugar, 266
Canned foods, 29, 177, 179, 190–91
Canola oil, 176, 195, 255
Cantaloupe, 137, 147, 276–77
Capsaicin, 44
Carbohydrates
  about, 7–8, 8
  activity levels and, 135
  benefits, 132

  calories in, 12
  in energy foods, 120
  fiber in, 241
  muscle-building role, 134, 135
  refined, 202
  simple vs. complex, 7–8, 200–201
Carmine, 266
Carnosine, 135
Carotenoids, 269
Carrageenan, 265
Carrots, 137, 276–77, 288
Casein, 10, 101, 215, 266
Cassis tea, 59
Catechins, 30, 233
Cauliflower, 276–77
CCK hormone, 240
Celery, 99, 276–77
Celiac disease, 8, 200
Cereal
  glycemic loads, 288–89
  packaged, recommendations, 188
  RDA information, 276–77
  as snack, 46, 107
Cheating, 79
Cheese
  lactose in, 217
  packaged, recommendations, 189
  RDA information, 276–77
  serving recommendations, 17
  as snack, 137
  sodium in, 204
  tips for using, 50
Cherries, 128, 276–77
Chia seeds, 118
Chicken
  organic, 251
  packaged, recommendations, 177, 189–90, 194
  RDA information, 276–77
  serving recommendations, 16
Chickpeas, 276–77
Children, snacks for, 79
Chili powder, 176
Chloride, 133
Chocolate
  cravings and, 75
  dark, benefits, 107, 147
  frozen yogurt, 128
  milk, 17, 137, 189
  packaged food recommendations, 193
  RDA information, 276–77

Cholesterol
  blood lipid levels
    fiber and, 240
    healthy fats and, 28, 54, 112, 136
    sugar and, 224
    supplements for, 231, 233, 261, 263
    trans fats and, 6
  dietary vs. serum, 28, 254
Choline, 260, _260_, 268
Cinnamon, 176
Citrus fruits, 128, _221_, _276–77_, _288_
Clams, 177, _276–77_
Cochineal extract, 266
Cocoa, _221_
Coconut milk, 218
Coenzyme Q-10, 231
Coffee
  about, 59–62
  benefits, 30
  cooking with, 60
  exercise and, 133
  flavored, 60, 62
  packaged food recommendations, 193, 194
  RDA information, _276–77_
  serving recommendations, 19
Cold cuts, 49, 143, 189, _204_, 266, _280–81_
Collard greens, _276–77_
Colon cancer, 241
Color, of food, 145, _147_, 150
Comfort foods, 106
Conjugated linoleic acid, 254
Cookies, 193, _276–77_, _278–79_, _288_
Cooking
  benefits of, 25, 94
  oils for, 176, 179, 195, 253–55
  pantry items, 175–77
  planning for, 77
  shortcuts for, 145
Copper, 263
Corn, 144, _221_, _276–77_, _288_
Corn oil, 24
Corn syrup, 224, 266, 267
Cortisol, 134, 261
Cost, of food, 144, 145, 146, 250–52
Cottage cheese, 101, 189, _276–77_
Counting, of calories, _48_, 69
Couscous, 176, _289_
Crabmeat, 177

Crackers, 192, _276–77_, _288_
Cranberries, 111, _137_, _276–77_
Crash dieting, 69
Cravings
  assessing, 77
  for chocolate, _75_
  for comfort foods, 106
  controlling, 25, 47, 73–79
  imagery and, 93–94
  saturated fat role, 91
C-reactive protein, 29
Cream cheese, 189, _278–79_
Creatine monohydrate supplements, 134–35
Cruciferous vegetables, _261_
Cucumbers, _278–79_
Cultured foods, 212
Cumin, 176
Cured meats, 49, 143, 189, _204_, 266, 271

D

Dairy foods
  benefits, 248, 262
  conjugated linoleic acid in, 251
  organic, 251
  packaged food recommendations, 189
  probiotics and, 212
  serving recommendations, 17
  subsidies for, 144
Dairy-free milks, 217–18
Dehydration, 46, 132, 134
Deli foods, 49–50, 189
Depression, 234
Dextrose, 266
Diabetes
  risk factors, 143, 205, 222, 224–26, 254, _262_
  supplement recommendations, 231–32
  travel and, 47
Dietary fat
  about, 4–6, 16
  as addictive food, 91
  calories in, 4, 12, 255
  cooking oils, 176, 179, 195, 253–55
  exercise/diet balance for, 136
  on nutrition facts labels, 142
  in snack foods, 74
  synthetic, 269
  taste adjustment for, 25
  timing of consumption, 99

"Diet" foods, 70
Diet pills, 236
Diet programs
  gluten-free, 199–202
  low-calorie, 14
  low-carb, 8, 71, 135
  low-fat, 4–5, 71
  low-salt, 203–7
  Paleo Diet, 8
  pitfalls of, 68–72
  visual cues and, 93
Diet soda, 63
Digestion/digestive process, 12–13, 232
Diglycerides, 268
Dining out
  calorie counts, _48_
  iodine levels and, 206
  labeling regulations and, _265_
  tips for, 44–50
Dinners
  examples of (see Meal planning)
  recommendations regarding, 100
  timing of, 68
Dips, 191
Distractions, in controlling cravings, _75_, 78
Dopamine, 90
Dragon Well tea, 59
Dried foods, 177, 179, 192, _278–79_
Drugs. See Medications
Duck, 194

E

Eating
  neurology and, 26, 90–94, 148, 266
  rules for, 23–26
  stress and, 92
  timing of, 68, 97
  variety in, _75_, 222
  while traveling, tips for, 44–50
  work habits and, 47, 78
Eating out. See Dining out
Ecological Food Manufacturers Association (EFMA), 25
Eczema, 210
Edamame, _137_
Eden Foods, 143
EFMA (Ecological Food Manufacturers Association), 25

EGCG, 233
Eggplant, 152, <u>278–79</u>
Eggs
   benefits, 28, 248
   as lecithin source, 268
   organic, 251
   packaged, recommendations, 189
   RDA information, <u>278–79</u>
   serving recommendations, 16, 222
   as snack, <u>137</u>
   yolk of, 28, <u>260</u>
80-20 eating strategy, 26
Elderberries, <u>221</u>
Elderly people, vitamin D deficiency in, 262
Electrolytes, 120, 133, 204
Emotional eating, 92, 106
Endorphins, 72, 91
Endurance, 132–33, 135, 232
Energy foods, 120–21, 133
Erectile dysfunction, 230–31, 264
Erythorbic acid, 266
Erythrosine, 270
Espresso, <u>61</u>
Evaporated cane juice, 266
Exercise
   food-reward response and, 94
   with friend, advantages of, 72
   metabolism and, 7–8, 9–10
   recovery, food/recipes for, 123–29
   rewards following, 72
   snacks for, 106, 108
   timing of, 106
Extra-virgin olive oil, 255

F

Fast foods, <u>48</u>, 92, <u>274–75</u>, <u>278–79</u>
Fat. *See* Body fat; Dietary fat
FDA, diet pill regulation, 236–37
Federal Trade Commission, 236
Fermented foods, 212
Fiber
   about, 239–41
   benefits, 7, 273
   digestion of, 13
   exercise and, 132
   "functional," as food additive, 240
   insoluble vs. soluble, 212, 240
   lack of, 202

   on nutrition facts labels, 142
   sources of, 55, 110, 115, 118, 146–47, 241, <u>241</u>
Figs, 55
Fish and seafood
   benefits, 248, 261, 262
   packaged, recommendations, 190
   for pantry, 177
   serving recommendations, 16
Fish oil, 231
5-Day Meal Plan, 32–41
Flavor
   vs. added sodium, 49
   artificial flavorings, 264–65
   enhancement of, 25
   of side dishes, styles of, 87
Flaxseed oil, <u>232</u>
Flour, whole-wheat, 176, 188
Folate/folic acid
   benefits, 261
   sources of, 29, 55, 115, 147, <u>261</u>
Foo, Susan, 86
Food additives, list of, 264–69
Food diaries, 68, 78
Food porn, 92–93
Food rating systems, 25, 148
Food safety issues, 49, 178, 215
Food storage, 176, 178–79
Formula 47 cooking oil, 253
Free radicals, 220–22
Freezing/frozen foods
   benefits, 24
   coffee, 62
   frozen yogurt, 70, 106, 124, 128
   packaged food recommendations, 189–90
   as pantry item, 177–79
Fructose, 224, 227
Fruit
   benefits, 143, 212
   dried, 192, <u>278–79</u>
   vs. juices, 62–63
   organic, 251
   packaged, recommendations, 190
   for pantry, 177
   serving recommendations, 17, 222
   shopping tips, 151–54, 251
   as snack, 46
   subsidies for, 144

Fruit juice
   exercise and, 133
   glycemic load, <u>288</u>
   RDA information, <u>278–79</u>
   recommendations regarding, <u>147</u>, 193
   for smoothies, 128
   vs. whole fruit, 62–63
Fully hydrogenated vegetable oil, 266–67
"Functional" fiber, 240

G

Game meats, 17
Garlic, <u>221</u>, <u>278–79</u>
"Gateway" foods, 89
Gatorade, 134
Genetically modified ingredients, <u>250</u>, 268
Genmaicha tea, 58
Ghrelin, 68, 91, 231
Ginkgo biloba, <u>232</u>
Ginseng, 230–31
Glassware, size of, 83
Glucosamine, 233
Glucose, 7, 13, 132
Glucosinolate, 55
Gluten-free diets, 199–202
Gluten sensitivity, 8, 200, <u>201</u>
Glycemic loads, <u>288–89</u>
Glycogen, 132, 134, 224
Goals/goal-setting, 74, 92
Grains
   gluten-free varieties, 202
   packaged, recommendations, 188
   for pantry, 176
   refined, 220
   whole vs. processed, 17, 200–201, 241
Granola, 45, 188
Granola bars, <u>137</u>, <u>278–79</u>
Grapefruit, 115, <u>288</u>
Grapes, 152, <u>288</u>
Grapeseed oil, 16, 255
Grass-fed meats, 28–29
Grazing, pitfalls of, 68
Green beans, 152
Green foods, 145, 150
Guacamole, 191
Guarana, 120
Guar gum, 267
Guiding Starts rating system, 148
Gunpowder tea, 59

H

Ham, 278–79
Hand, as gauge for portion sizes, 82–83
HDL. *See* Cholesterol, blood lipid levels
Headaches, 231, 263
Healthy eating habits, 70
Heart disease, 231
Heavy metals, in salmon feed, 52
Hemp milk, 217–18
Herbs, 25, 176, 179
HFCS (high-fructose corn syrup), 224, 267
High blood pressure, 203, 205, 231, 264
High-fructose corn syrup (HFCS), 224, 267
High Mountain Oolong, 59
Hojicha tea, 59
Homocysteine, 260, 260, 261
Honey, 288
Honey Phoenix tea, 59
Hormel Natural Choice, 143
Hormones, in animal products, 214, 250, 251
Hot dogs, 194
Hotels, eating tips for, 47
Hot sauce, 44, 195
Hummus, 137, 177, 191
Hunger, assessing, 77
Huynh, Michael "Bao," 85
Hydrogenated fats, 6, 254, 266–67
Hydrolyzed protein, 143, 267
Hydroxycut, 231
Hyperglycemia, 226
Hypertension. *See* High blood pressure
Hypoglycemia, 226

I

Ice, in smoothies, 128
Ice cream, 190, 278–79
Imagery, appetite and, 47–48, 75, 93–94
Immune system health, 210
Impulse buying, avoiding, 144
Indigotine, 265
Indole, 55
Indulgences, 79, 176

Inflammation
 dietary causes, 232
 in muscles/joints, 133, 233
 omega fatty acids and, 28, 231, 254
Ingredients lists, 143
Injury healing support, 126, 233
Inositol, 268
Insoluble fiber, 212, 240
Insulin
 production of, 68, 74, 90
 protein breakdown role, 9–10
 simple carbs and, 7
Insulin resistance, 245
Insulin sensitivity, 205, 222, 262
Interesterified fat, 267
Intestinal bacteria. *See* Probiotics
Inulin, 55, 240–41, 267
Iodine, 204, 205–6, 207, 269
Iron
 absorption of, 266
 benefits, 263
 gluten-free diets and, 202
 sources of, 28, 54, 55, 114, 126, 146–47

J

Jams, 191, 278–79
Jarred foods. *See* Canned foods
Jerky, 46, 99, 137, 143, 192
Jerusalem artichokes, 55–56
Jicama, 117
Joint pain, 233
Juice. *See* Fruit juice; Vegetable juice

K

Kale, 113, 278–79
Kefir, 116, 217
Ketchup, 191, 278–79
Kids' foods, 79
Kitchen. *See* Cooking; Pantry, stocking of
Kiwifruit, 152, 278–79, 288
Korean red panax ginseng, 230–31
Kosher salt, 205
Kukicha tea, 59

L

Labels/labeling
 additives, list of, 264–69
 of "diet" foods, 70

food without, 58, 143
 "natural"/"organic," 250
 nutrition facts, 24–25, 58, 142, 148
 of probiotics, 211
 regulation of, 265
 in rules for healthy eating, 24
Lactose intolerance, 216–17
Lamb, 17
Lasagna, 278–79
LDL. *See* Cholesterol, blood lipid levels
Lecithin, 268
Leftovers, storage of, 176, 178
Legumes, 18, 177
Lentils, 114, 221, 278–79
Leptin, 245, 267
Lettuce, 147, 153, 278–79
Leucine, 10, 134, 248
Lifestyle factors, 48, 72, 79
Lignans, 119
Liquid calories, 58
Liver, 278–79
Low-carb diets, 8, 71, 135
Low-fat diets, 4–5, 71
Low-salt diets, 203–7
Lunches
 examples of (*see* Meal planning)
 planning for, 78
 recommendations regarding, 100
Lutein, 56
Lycopene, 115, 230, 233

M

Macadamia nuts, 28
Mackerel, 28, 248
Macronutrients, 4–10, 12. *See also* Carbohydrates; Dietary fat; Protein
Magnesium
 benefits, 45, 133, 231, 263
 daily recommendations, 29
 sources of, 29, 54
Maltodextrin, 268
Maltose/malt sugar, 268
Manganese, 55, 263
Mangoes, 128
Mannitol, 268
Maple syrup, 147, 192
Margarine, 254
Marinades, 176–77, 191
Marketing, 47–48, 74, 93, 141, 236

Index **295**

Matcha tea, 58–59
Mayonnaise, 192
Meal planning
  exercise recovery, 123–29
  5-Day Meal Plan, 32–41
  timing considerations, 68, 78, 96–101
Meat
  as condiment, 24
  cured/processed, 49, 143, 189, 204, 266, 271
  grass-fed, 28–29
  organic, 251
  sodium in, 204
  storage of, 178
Meat loaf, 280–81
Medications
  prescription diet pills, 236
  supplement interactions, 231, 232, 261, 263
Mediterranean diets, 24, 254
Mediterranean flavors, for side dishes, 87
MedWatch program, 237
Mega-T, 231
Melatonin, 147
Melon, 147, 280–81
Memory
  as aid in appetite control, 266
  nutritional boosters for, 232–33, 260, 261
  sugar and, 91
Menus, tips for navigating, 47–48
Metabolism
  basal, 14
  of calories, 13, 14
  crash diets and, 69
  of macronutrients, 12–13
  undereating effects on, 71
Migraines, 231, 263
Milk. *See also* Whey protein
  allergies to, 266
  alternatives, 217–18
  brand recommendations, 189
  flavored, 17, 62, 137
  glycemic load, 288
  health assessments of, 213–17
  as muscle-building food, 215
  1%, 29, 128
  raw, 215
  RDA information, 280–81
  serving recommendations, 62
  skim, 134, 189, 248
  in smoothies, 128
  as snack, 107, 137

2%, 189
  weight loss and, 215
Mindful eating, 26, 68, 78, 92, 202
Minerals
  about, 263–64
  absorption of, 210
Mistakes, moving on after, 79
Modified food starch, 268
Monoglycerides, 268
Monosodium glutamate (MSG), 143, 267, 269
Monounsaturated fats, 5, 28, 254
Monterey Mushrooms, 247
Motivation, 75
Mozzarella, 50
MSG (monosodium glutamate), 143, 267, 269
Muffins, 188, 280–81
Mullen, Seamus, 84
Multivitamins, 207, 229–30, 273
Muscle
  building of, 28–30, 126–27, 133–34
  loss of, 69
  preserving, 264
Mushrooms, 147, 152, 247, 248, 280–81
Mustard, 192
Myelin, 261

N

Nachos, 280–81
Natural food stores, 148
"Natural" labeling, 250
Navy beans, 29, 221
NEAT (non-exercise activity thermogenesis), 14
Nectarines, 280–81
Neotame, 269
Neoxanthin, 29
Neurology, eating and, 90–91, 266
Niacin, 119, 261
Nighttime eating, 68
Nitrates/nitrites, 49, 143, 266, 271
Nitric oxide supplements, 134
Non-exercise activity thermogenesis (NEAT), 14
Nut butters, 46, 54, 177
Nutrition
  in assessing food costs, 146
  daily consumption recommendations, 15–19
  exercise and, 132–36
  RDA in common foods, 273–85

Nutritional deficiencies, 75, 201–2, 244, 262
Nutritional Labeling and Education Act of 1990, 265
Nutrition facts labels, 24–25, 58, 142, 148
Nuts
  benefits, 45
  packaged, recommendations, 192
  for pantry, 177
  serving recommendations, 16
NuVal food rating system, 25, 145, 148

O

Oats/oatmeal
  benefits, 29, 146
  glycemic loads, 288–89
  packaged, recommendations, 188
  RDA information, 280–81
  subsidies for, 144
Obesity/overweight
  HFCS link, 267
  sugar and, 224, 225
  vitamin D requirements and, 244, 244, 247
OGTT (oral glucose tolerance test), 224, 226
Oh Boy! Oberto, 143
Oils, for cooking, 176, 179, 195, 253–55
Olestra, 269
Oligofructose. *See* Inulin
Olive oil, 28, 176, 195, 255
Olives, 191, 280–81
Omega-3 fatty acids
  about, 6
  ratio to omega-6, 28, 136, 254
  sources of, 52, 112, 118, 218, 232, 248
  from supplements, 231
Omega-6 fatty acids, 6, 28, 136, 254
Onion rings, 280–81
Oral glucose tolerance test (OGTT), 224, 226
Orange foods, 145, 150
Orange juice, 248, 288
Oranges, 128, 221, 288
Oregano, 176
Organic foods, 121, 188–95, 250–52
"Organic" labeling, 250

Oringer, Ken, 86
Oryzanol, 255
Overeating, 90–91, 225
Overweight. *See* Obesity/overweight
Oxidation/oxidative stress, 220–22
Oysters, <u>280–81</u>

P

Packaged food recommendations, 187–95
Packaging. *See* Labels/labeling
Paleo Diet, 8
Panko bread crumbs, 176, 195
Pantothenic acid, 261
Pantry, stocking of, 76, 175–77, 179, 182, 195
Papayas, 152
Paprika, 176, 195
Parathyroid hormone (PTH), 245
Parsnips, 55
Partially hydrogenated fats, 6, 267, 270
Pasta
  glycemic loads, <u>288–89</u>
  packaged, recommendations, 188, 190
  RDA information, <u>280–81</u>, <u>282–83</u>
  sodium in, <u>204</u>
  whole wheat, 176
Peaches, 153, <u>280–81</u>, <u>288</u>
Peanut butter, 99, 128, 177, 192, <u>280–81</u>
Peanuts, 107, <u>137</u>, <u>280–81</u>, <u>288</u>
Pears, 153, <u>280–81</u>, <u>288</u>
Peas, 18, 193, <u>288</u>
Pectin, 270
Pepper, 195
Peppers, bell, 151, <u>280–81</u>
Pesticide residue, on foods, 250–51
Phosphorus, 29, 54, 262, 263
Phytochemicals, 273
Pickles, 191, 212
Pineapple, 153, <u>288</u>
Pineapple-orange juice, 128
Pistachios, <u>137</u>
Pita, 188
Pizza, 188, 190, <u>204</u>, <u>280–81</u>
Plates
  portioning of food on, 124
  size of, 83, 84

Pleasure response, to food, 26, 90, 94, 148
Plums, <u>280–81</u>, <u>288</u>
Polydextrose, 240–41
Polysorbates, 270
Polyunsaturated fats, 5, 254
Pomegranate juice, <u>147</u>
Popcorn
  brand recommendations, 192
  glycemic load, <u>288</u>
  RDA information, <u>280–81</u>
  as snack, 79, 106
  as whole grain, 17
Pork, 16, 28, 194, <u>274–75</u>, <u>280–81</u>
Portion control. *See also* Serving sizes
  of dietary fats, 6
  vs. "diet" foods, 70
  of snacks, 105, 106
  tips for, 82–83
  while dining out, 48
Potassium
  benefits, 133, 205, 263, <u>264</u>
  sources of, 29, 55, 115, 147
Potassium iodide, 207
Potato chips, 193
Potatoes, 144, <u>147</u>, <u>280–81</u>, <u>288–89</u>
Poultry, 16, 177, <u>204</u>
Prebiotics, 212
Prediabetes, 226
Pretzels, <u>137</u>, 192, <u>282–83</u>
Probiotics, 45, 116, 209–12, 232
Processed foods
  additives in, 264–69
  avoiding, 24, 49, 200–201, 202
  fructose in, 224
  "functional" fiber in, 240
  labels of, 58
  pitfalls of, 212
  sodium in, 204, 206
  vs. whole foods, 222
Propyl gallate, 270
Prostate health, 233, 234, 263
Protein
  about, 9–10, 142
  in breakfasts, 96
  calories in, 12
  for muscle-building, 127, 133–34
  on nutrition facts labels, 142
  in snack foods, 101
  sources of, 9–10, 52, 62, 97, 101, 126
  in weight loss regimens, 135–36

Protein bars, 45, 99, 120
Protein powder. *See* Whey protein
Protein synthesis, 9, 10
Psyllium husk, 231–32
PTH (parathyroid hormone), 245
Pu-Erh Tuocha tea, 59
Pumpkin seeds, 192
Purple foods, 145, 150
Pycnogenol, 232–33

Q

Quinoa, 17, 52

R

Raisins, <u>282–83</u>, <u>289</u>
Raspberries, 29, 128, <u>137</u>, 153, <u>282–83</u>
Raw foods, 215
RBGH (recombinant bovine growth hormone), 214
RDA, of common foods, <u>273–85</u>
Recovery, from exercise, 123–29, 134, 194
Red dyes, 270
Red foods, 150
Red-pepper flakes, 176
Red wine, 30, <u>147</u>, 194, <u>284–85</u>
Red yeast rice, 233
Refrigerator storage tips, 178, 179
Relationships, 48, 72, 79
Restaurants. *See* Dining out
Resveratrol, 30, 152, 233
Reward-seeking behavior, 26, 90, 94, 148
Riboflavin, 261
Rice, 17, <u>147</u>, 176, 188, <u>282–83</u>, <u>289</u>
Rice bran oil, 255
Rice milk, 218
Ricotta cheese, <u>282–83</u>
Roasting, of coffee beans, 60
Robusta coffee, 60
Romaine lettuce, 153, <u>278–79</u>
Rosemary, 176
Rules to eat by, 23–26

S

Saccharin, 226, 270
St. John's Wort, <u>232</u>
Salad dressing, <u>48</u>, 192, <u>282–83</u>
Salads, 46, <u>48</u>, 87, <u>276–77</u>, <u>282–83</u>

Index **297**

Salmon
  benefits, 247, 248
  canned, 177, 191
  packaged, recommendations, 190
  RDA information, 282–83
  serving recommendations, 16
  wild vs. farm-raised, 248
Salsa, 177, 192, 282–83
Salt, brand recommendation, 195. *See also* Sodium
SAMe, 234
Sandwiches, 49, 190, 204, 278–79, 282–83
Santos, Chris, 85
Sardines, 16, 248
Sashimi, 137
Satiety, beverages and, 58. *See also* Appetite
Saturated fats, 5, 91, 254
Sauces, prepared, 176–77, 191–92
Sauerkraut, 212, 282–83
Sausage, 194, 282–83
Saw palmetto, 234
Seafood. *See* Fish and seafood
Sea salt, 205
Selenium, 29, 147, 262, 263
Sencha tea, 59
Serotonin, 46, 129, 231
Serving dishes, size of, 83
Serving sizes, 24–25, 142. *See also* Portion control
Shakes, protein, 136. *See also* Smoothies
Shopping tips
  food rating systems, 25, 148
  impulse buying, avoiding, 144
  for produce, 151–54
  sample list, 182
  supermarket strategies, 24
Shrimp, 16, 137, 282–83
Skin cancer, 246, 255
Skirt steak, 17
Sleep/sleep issues, 47, 94
Smell, as distraction, 75
Smoked paprika, 195
Smoke point, of cooking oils, 255
Smoothies
  prepared, 193
  tips for, 128, 136
  as travel food, 44–45
Snack bars, 45, 99, 120, 193
Snacks
  availability of, 76, 92, 176
  benefits, 25, 105
  examples of, 137 (*see also* Meal planning)
  family-friendly, 79
  mindfulness and, 266
  packaged, recommendations, 192–93
  pre-/postworkout, 106, 137
  protein in, 97, 101
  sodium in, 204
  timing of, 78
  tips for, 97, 99, 101, 106, 108
  while traveling, 45, 46
Social relationships, 48, 72, 79
Soda, 24, 57–58, 63, 282–83
Sodium
  about, 263–64
  benefits, 204
  exercise and, 133
  low-salt diets, 203–7
  on nutrition facts labels, 142
  potassium and, 205
  reducing, with flavor enhancement, 49
  sources of, 46, 204
  taste adjustment for, 25
Sodium ascorbate, 265
Sodium caseinate. *See* Casein
Sodium nitrate/sodium nitrite. *See* Nitrates/nitrites
Soluble fiber, 240
Sorbitol, 271
Sorghum, 144
Soup
  canned, 177, 190, 204
  glycemic loads, 288
  pitfalls of, 48
  RDA information, 282–83
  as travel meal, 46
Sour cream, 17
Soy
  as food additive, 267, 268
  as protein source, 126
Soybean oil, 136
Soybeans, 137, 144, 282–83
Soy milk, 218, 280–81, 288
Soy sauce, 177, 195
Spices
  brand recommendations, 195
  for flavor enhancement, 25
  as pantry item, 176
  storage of, 179
Spinach, 29, 147, 221, 282–83
Spirits, 19
Spoon size, 83
Sports drinks, 133, 194
Sports nutrition, 132–36
Spreads, 176–77, 192
Starches, 13, 268
Starchy vegetables, 18
Steak sauce, 192
Stevia, 226
Stock, 177
Storage, of food, 178–79
Strawberries
  RDA information, 282–83
  serving recommendations, 17, 146
  shopping tips, 153
  as snack, 101, 137
Strength training, 133–34
Stress, 92, 106, 134
Strip steak, 28–29, 194
Subsidies, 144
Sucralose, 14, 227, 271
Sugar
  about, 224–26
  added, 24, 62, 74
  as addictive food, 91
  craving role, 76
  in energy foods, 120–21
  memory and, 91
  on nutrition facts labels, 142
  in snack foods, 74
  in soda/drinks, 57–58
  subsidies for, 147
  substitutes for, 226–27, 264, 265, 266, 268, 271
  in teas, 58
Sugar alcohols, 271
Sulforaphane, 53
Sunchokes, 55–56
Sunflower oil, 136
Sunflower seeds, 137, 177, 282–83
Sunlight, vitamin D production and, 134, 244–46, 244
Sunset yellow (dye), 271
Supermarket rating systems, 25, 148
Supernormal stimuli, 93
Supplements
  discredited, 232
  drug interactions, 230, 232, 261, 263
  multivitamins, 207, 229–30, 273
  for muscle-building, 134–35
  recommendations regarding, 230–34
  vitamin D, 246
  for weight loss, cautions regarding, 231

298 Index

Sur le Nil tea, 59
Sweet potatoes, 18, <u>146</u>, <u>147</u>, <u>282–83</u>, <u>289</u>
Swiss chard, 56
Swiss cheese, 50
Syrup, 192

T

Table-setting, tips for, 83
Tartrazine, 271
Taste
   adjustment of, 25
   of cooking oils, 255
   of organic vs. conventionally-raised foods, 251
   sweetness, preference for, 63
Tea
   bottled, 193
   green, 19, 30, 233
   recommendations regarding, 58–60, 193, 194
Teriyaki sauce, 177, 195
Testosterone, 134
Theobromine, 121
Theophylline, 121
Thiamin, 261
Thyme, 176
Time management, 77
Timing, of meals/snacks, 68, 78, 96–101
Tobacco subsidies, 144
Tocopherol, 255
Tocotrienol, 255
Tofu, <u>282–83</u>
Tomatoes, <u>137</u>, <u>146</u>, 154, 191, <u>282–83</u>
Tomato sauce, 177, 192
Tortilla chips, 192
Tortillas, 176, 188
Trail mix, 107, 193
Trans fats, 6, 254–55, 266–67, 270
Travel, eating tips for, 44–50
Triggers, 92
Triglyceride levels, 224, 225
Tuna, <u>137</u>, 177, 191, 248, <u>282–83</u>
Turkey, 16, 46, <u>137</u>, 194, <u>284–85</u>
25-hydroxy vitamin D test, <u>244</u>

U

UIC (urinary iodine concentration test), 206
Undereating, effects of, 71
Unpasteurized milk, 215
UPC codes, food without, 143
Urinary iodine concentration test (UIC), 206
Urinary tract infections, 210
Urine, in assessing water intake, 132

V

Valerian, <u>232</u>
Vanilla Rooibos tea, 59
Variety, in diet, <u>75</u>, 222
Vegan diets, 261
Vegetable juice, <u>137</u>, 194, <u>284–85</u>
Vegetable oils, 254
Vegetables
   benefits, 24, 49, 143, 212
   cruciferous, <u>261</u>
   dining out, tips for, 47–48, 50
   organic, 251
   packaged, recommendations, 190
   for pantry, 177
   preparation tips, 87
   serving recommendations, 18, 222
   shopping tips, 151–54, 251
   as snacks, 106
   starchy, 18
   subsidies for, 144
Vegetable shortening. *See* Partially hydrogenated fats
Vegetarian diets
   eating plan for, 126
   food additive considerations, 266
   packaged food recommendations, 190
   protein sources, 9, 52
   travel and, 46
Venison, 17
Vinegars, 176, 195
Visual cues, appetite and, 47–48, <u>75</u>, 93–94
Vitamin A
   benefits, 260
   sources of, 28, 29, 56, 113, 115, 146–47
Vitamin B complex
   benefits, 261
   gluten-free diets and, 202
   sources of, 28, 115, 126, 147
Vitamin C
   benefits, 233, 262
   sources of, 29, 55, 110, 111, 113, 117, 146–47, 265
   weight loss and, 71
Vitamin D
   about, 243–47
   benefits, 231, 262
   deficiency, <u>244</u>
   exercise and, 134
   sources of, 28, 248
   supplements for, 246
Vitamin E, 28, 217, 262, 264
Vitamin K
   benefits, 262, <u>262</u>
   sources of, 29, 55, 56, 113, 146–47
Vitamins
   fat-soluble, 4, 269
   intestinal microbe production of, 210
   overview of, 260–62

W

Wall color, appetite effects, 83
Walnuts, 16, 45, 112, 177, <u>284–85</u>
Water
   bottled, 193
   consumption recommendations, 57–58, 128, 132, 134
   flavored, 193
   pollution of, 251
Watermelon, 154, <u>284–85</u>, <u>288</u>
Web sites
   food/nutrition resources, 25, 52, 60, 133, 255
   as food porn, 93–94
   supplement regulations, 237
Weight
   calorie intake and, 225
   fluctuations in, 71
   gain, 201 (*see also* Obesity/overweight)
   loss
      eating plan for, 126
      exercise/diet balance in, 135–36
      goals for, 70
      healthy rate of, 69
      nutritional support of, 222, 233
      supplements for, <u>231</u>, 235–37
   maintenance of, 70

Wheat
  bran, 274–75
  germ, 284–85
  gluten in, 8, 200
  subsidies for, 144
Whey protein
  benefits, 10
  exercise and, 134, 135
  in milk, 215
  packaged food recommendations, 195
  RDA information, 284–85
  in smoothies, 128
"Whole cuts," 49
Whole foods, 222
Wine, 19, 30, 147, 194, 284–85
Wood Dragon Oolong tea, 59
Work environment/habits, 47, 78
Workouts. *See* Exercise
Wraps, 44, 46

X

Xanthan gum, 271
Xylitol, 271

Y

Yellow dyes, 271
Yellow foods, 145, 150
Yellow walls, appetite effects, 83
Yerba maté, 121

Yogurt
  frozen, 70, 106, 124, 128, 137, 190
  glycemic load, 288
  lactose in, 217
  packaged food recommendations, 189
  probiotics and, 211
  RDA information, 284–85
  in smoothies, 45, 128
  as snack, 45, 137
  vitamin D-fortified, 247, 248

Z

Zeaxanthin, 56
Zinc, 28, 126, 147, 264

Recipe Index

An asterisk (*) indicates that recipe photos are shown in the color insert pages.

A

Almonds
  Almond-Blueberry Oatmeal, 159
  Cran-Almond Muffins, 111
Apples
  Apple-Sausage Sauté, 110
Arctic char
  Seared Arctic Char with Citrus-Fennel Salsa, 53
Artichokes
  Artichoke Hummus,* 155
Arugula
  Grilled Mustard-Garlic Skirt Steak with Arugula, 185
Asparagus
  Asparagus Stir-Fry,* 156
  roasted, 87
  Shrimp Stir-Fry, 145
Avocado
  Green Goddess Smoothie,* 116
  Tropical Guac, 169
  Turkey and Avocado Sandwich with Slaw,* 157

B

Bacon
  Watermelon, Spinach, and Bacon Salad, 174
Bananas
  Heart Helper smoothie, 129
  Muscle Builder smoothie, 129
  Strawberry and Banana Workout Shake, 96
Barley
  Spinach Barley Salad,* 119
Beans
  canned
    Artichoke Hummus, 155
    Chickpeas with Chorizo, 86
    Escarole Soup with Fennel, Navy Beans, and Mini Meatballs, 36–37
    Pan-Fried Salmon with Broccoli and Beans, 100
    Pork Braised in Kiwi-Coconut Sauce with White Beans,* 165
    Quick Chicken Adobo and Black Bean Tacos, 184
    Quinoa Salad with Black Beans and Sweet Potatoes, 52
  green
    Lemony Green Beans, 164
Beef
  Grilled Mustard-Garlic Skirt Steak with Arugula, 185
  Mini Blue-Cheese Steaks on Salad, 85
  Steak Quesadilla,* 38
Beverages. *See also* Smoothies and shakes
  Golden Gazpacho, 166
  Pear-Thyme Bellini,* 168
  Pomegranate-Cranberry Soda, 163
Black beans
  Quick Chicken Adobo and Black Bean Tacos, 184
  Quinoa Salad with Black Beans and Sweet Potatoes, 52
Blueberries
  Almond-Blueberry Oatmeal, 159
  Brain Booster smoothie, 129
  Mood Maker smoothie, 129

Blue cheese
  Mini Blue-Cheese Steaks on Salad, 85
Breads
  Breakfast Stuffins,* 34–35
  Green Tea French Toast, 40
Broccoli
  Chicken with Cheesy Broccoli Soup, 160
  Pan-Fried Salmon with Broccoli and Beans, 100
Broccoli rabe
  Spicy Sausage Bolognese with Fettuccine and Broccoli Rabe, 184–85
Broccoli sprouts
  Shrimp and Sprout Lettuce Wraps, 53
Buffalo
  Buffalo Burgers in Pita with Mint-Yogurt Dressing, 54–55

C

Cabbage
  Chicken with Slaw, 145
  Turkey and Avocado Sandwich with Slaw,* 157
  Vietnamese Pork Salad,* 32–33
Cannellini beans
  Pork Braised in Kiwi-Coconut Sauce with White Beans,* 165
Cantaloupe
  Tropical Guac, 169
Carrots, roasted, 87
Cheese
  Baby Spinach Salad with Goat Cheese and Toasted Pistachios, 40
  Chicken with Cheesy Broccoli Soup, 160
  Heirloom Tomato and Eggplant Stacks,* 162
  Italian Frittata,* 173
  Mini Blue-Cheese Steaks on Salad, 85
  Steak Quesadilla,* 38
Cherries
  Smooth Operator smoothie, 129
Chia seeds
  Mango-Coconut Chia Pudding, 118

Chicken
  Apple-Sausage Sauté, 110
  Chicken Fajitas, 125
  Chicken with Cheesy Broccoli Soup, 160
  Chicken with Grapefruit,* 115
  Chicken with Roasted Onions, Peppers, and Tomatoes, 183
  Chicken with Slaw, 145
  Garden Chicken Burger with Strawberry Sauce,* 172
  Italian-Style Chicken and Mushrooms,* 33
  Quick Chicken Adobo and Black Bean Tacos, 184
  Vietnamese Chicken Skewers, 85
Chickpeas
  Artichoke Hummus,* 155
  Chickpeas with Chorizo, 86
Chili
  Lean Turkey Chili, 161
Chocolate
  Muscle Builder smoothie, 129
  Protein Pudding, 101
  Rich Chocolate Pudding, 37
Coconut milk
  Kiwi-Coconut Sauce, 165
  Mango-Coconut Chia Pudding, 118
Cod
  Roast Cod with Pomegranate-Walnut Sauce,* 40
Coffee
  Raspberry Java Smoothie, 38
  Thai Iced Coffee Pop, 35
Coleslaw
  Chicken with Slaw, 145
  Vietnamese Pork Salad,* 32–33
Cookies
  Butterscotch Chip Macadamia Cookies, 33
Cranberries
  Cran-Almond Muffins, 111
  Pomegranate-Cranberry Soda, 163
Cucumbers
  Golden Gazpacho, 166
  Green Goddess Smoothie,* 116
  Shrimp Ceviche,* 117

D

Desserts
  Butterscotch Chip Macadamia Cookies, 33
  Mango-Coconut Chia Pudding, 118
  Protein Pudding, 101
  Rich Chocolate Pudding, 37
  Rum Berry Sherbet, 170
  Thai Iced Coffee Pop, 35
Dill
  Dill-Yogurt Sauce, 247
Dips. See Sauces and dips
Dressings
  Mint-Yogurt Dressing, 54–55

E

Eggplant
  Baked Eggplant with Tomato Chutney, 39
  Heirloom Tomato and Eggplant Stacks,* 162
Eggs
  Breakfast Stuffins,* 34–35
  Chef's Salad, 98
  Eggs and Salsa, 145
  Italian Frittata,* 173
  Spicy Omelet, 96
Escarole
  Escarole Soup with Fennel, Navy Beans, and Mini Meatballs, 36–37

F

Fennel
  Citrus-Fennel Salsa, 53
  Escarole Soup with Fennel, Navy Beans, and Mini Meatballs, 36–37
Fish and seafood
  Braised Salmon with Soy and Ginger, 86
  Grilled Salmon with Peach Salsa, 167
  Grilled Wild Salmon, 247
  Mexi-Tuna, 97
  Pan-Fried Salmon with Broccoli and Beans, 100
  Perfect Grilled Mackerel,* 35
  Roast Cod with Pomegranate-Walnut Sauce,* 40

Seared Arctic Char with
    Citrus-Fennel Salsa, 53
Shrimp and Sprout Lettuce
    Wraps, 53
Shrimp Ceviche,* 117
Shrimp Stir-Fry, 145
Spicy Garlic Shrimp, 84
French toast
    Green Tea French Toast, 40

G

Ginger
    Braised Salmon with Soy and
        Ginger, 86
Goat cheese
    Baby Spinach Salad with Goat
        Cheese and Toasted
        Pistachios, 40
    Heirloom Tomato and
        Eggplant Stacks,* 162
Grains
    Lentil Quinoa Burgers,* 114
    Quinoa Salad with Black Beans
        and Sweet Potatoes, 52
    Spinach Barley Salad,* 119
Grapefruit
    Chicken with Grapefruit,* 115
    Citrus-Fennel Salsa, 53
Greens. See also Salads; Spinach
    Grilled Mustard-Garlic Skirt
        Steak with Arugula, 185
    preparation tips, 55
    Smoky Paprika Kale Chips,* 113

H

Hummus
    Artichoke Hummus,* 155

J

Jicama
    Shrimp Ceviche,* 117

K

Kale
    Smoky Paprika Kale Chips,* 113
Kefir
    Green Goddess Smoothie,* 116

Kidney beans
    Pan-Fried Salmon with
        Broccoli and Beans, 100
Kiwifruits
    Kiwi-Coconut Sauce, 165

L

Legumes. See Beans; Lentils
Lemon
    Lemony Green Beans, 164
Lentils
    Lentil Quinoa Burgers,* 114
Lettuce. See also Salads
    Shrimp and Sprout Lettuce
        Wraps, 53

M

Macadamia nuts
    Butterscotch Chip Macadamia
        Cookies, 33
Mackerel
    Perfect Grilled Mackerel,* 35
Mangoes
    Golden Gazpacho, 166
    Mango-Coconut Chia Pudding, 118
    Mood Maker smoothie, 129
    Shrimp Ceviche,* 117
    Smooth Operator smoothie, 129
    Tropical Guac, 169
Matcha powder
    Green Tea French Toast, 40
Melon
    Golden Gazpacho, 166
Mint
    Mint-Yogurt Dressing, 54–55
Muffins
    Breakfast Stuffins,* 34–35
    Cran-Almond Muffins, 111
Mushrooms
    Balsamic-Glazed Mushrooms
        and Onions, 247
    Italian-Style Chicken and
        Mushrooms,* 33
    Mushroom and Dumpling
        Soup, 145

N

Navy beans
    Escarole Soup with Fennel,
        Navy Beans, and Mini
        Meatballs, 36–37

Nuts
    Baby Spinach Salad with Goat
        Cheese and Toasted
        Pistachios, 40
    Butterscotch Chip Macadamia
        Cookies, 33
    Linguine with Walnut-Tomato
        Pesto,* 112
    Pomegranate-Walnut Sauce,* 40

O

Oatmeal
    Almond-Blueberry Oatmeal, 159
    Maple-Bacon Oatmeal, 36
    Protein-Packed Oatmeal, 96
Omelets
    Spicy Omelet, 96
Onions
    Balsamic-Glazed Mushrooms
        and Onions, 247
    Chicken with Roasted Onions,
        Peppers, and Tomatoes, 183
    roasted, 87
Orange juice
    Golden Gazpacho, 166

P

Papaya
    Golden Gazpacho, 166
Parsnips
    Chicken with Cheesy Broccoli
        Soup, 160
    Parsnip Cakes, 55
Pasta dishes
    Linguine with Walnut-Tomato
        Pesto, 112
    Pasta Dinner, 145
    Spaghetti with Roasted Red
        Pepper Sauce, 158
    Spicy Sausage Bolognese with
        Fettuccine and Broccoli
        Rabe, 184–85
Peaches
    Peach Salsa, 167
Peanut butter
    Heart Helper smoothie, 129
    Muscle Builder smoothie, 129
Pears
    Pear-Thyme Bellini,* 168

Peppers
    Breakfast Stuffins,* 34–35
    Chicken with Roasted Onions, Peppers, and Tomatoes, 183
    Spaghetti with Roasted Red Pepper Sauce, 158

Pineapple
    Golden Gazpacho, 166
    Tropical Guac, 169

Pineapple-orange juice
    Brain Booster smoothie, 129
    Mood Maker smoothie, 129

Pistachios
    Baby Spinach Salad with Goat Cheese and Toasted Pistachios, 40

Pomegranates
    Pomegranate-Cranberry Soda, 163

Pork
    Apple-Sausage Sauté, 110
    Chickpeas with Chorizo, 86
    Escarole Soup with Fennel, Navy Beans, and Mini Meatballs, 36–37
    Italian Frittata,* 173
    Pork Braised in Kiwi-Coconut Sauce with White Beans,* 165
    Spicy Sausage Bolognese with Fettuccine and Broccoli Rabe, 184–85
    Vietnamese Pork Salad,* 32–33
    Watermelon, Spinach, and Bacon Salad, 174

Puddings
    Mango-Coconut Chia Pudding, 118
    Protein Pudding, 101
    Rich Chocolate Pudding, 37

Q

Quinoa
    Lentil Quinoa Burgers,* 114
    Quinoa Salad with Black Beans and Sweet Potatoes, 52
    Spaghetti with Roasted Red Pepper Sauce, 158

R

Raspberries
    Brain Booster smoothie, 129
    Heart Helper smoothie, 129
    Raspberry Java Smoothie, 38
    Rum Berry Sherbet, 170

Romaine lettuce
    Tuna Niçoise Salad,* 171

S

Salads
    Baby Spinach Salad with Goat Cheese and Toasted Pistachios, 40
    Chef's Salad, 98
    Mini Blue-Cheese Steaks on Salad, 85
    preparation tips, 87
    Quinoa Salad with Black Beans and Sweet Potatoes, 52
    Spinach Barley Salad,* 119
    Tuna Niçoise Salad,* 171
    Vietnamese Pork Salad,* 32–33
    Watermelon, Spinach, and Bacon Salad, 174

Salmon
    Braised Salmon with Soy and Ginger, 86
    Grilled Salmon with Peach Salsa, 167
    Grilled Wild Salmon, 247
    Pan-Fried Salmon with Broccoli and Beans, 100

Salsas. *See also* Sauces and dips
    Citrus-Fennel Salsa, 53
    Peach Salsa, 167

Sandwiches and wraps
    Buffalo Burgers in Pita with Mint-Yogurt Dressing, 54–55
    Garden Chicken Burger with Strawberry Sauce,* 172
    Lentil Quinoa Burgers,* 114
    Shrimp and Sprout Lettuce Wraps, 53
    Smoky & Spicy Sausage Heroes, 183
    Steak Quesadilla,* 38
    Tuna Sandwich, 98
    Turkey and Avocado Sandwich with Slaw,* 157

Sauces and dips. *See also* Salsas
    Adobo, 184
    Artichoke Hummus,* 155
    Dill-Yogurt Sauce, 247
    Kiwi-Coconut Sauce, 165
    Pomegranate-Walnut Sauce,* 40
    Roasted Red Pepper Sauce, 158
    Spicy Sausage Bolognese, 184–85
    Spinach Dip,* 39
    Strawberry Sauce, 172
    Tropical Guac, 169
    Walnut-Tomato Pesto, 112

Seafood. *See* Fish and seafood
Shakes. *See* Smoothies and shakes

Shitake mushrooms
    Mushroom and Dumpling Soup, 145

Shrimp
    Shrimp and Sprout Lettuce Wraps, 53
    Shrimp Ceviche,* 117
    Shrimp Stir-Fry, 145
    Spicy Garlic Shrimp, 84

Smoothies and shakes
    Berry Smoothie, 247
    Brain Booster, 129
    Green Goddess Smoothie,* 116
    Heart Helper, 129
    Mood Maker, 129
    Muscle Builder, 129
    Raspberry Java Smoothie, 38
    Smooth Operator, 129
    Strawberry and Banana Workout Shake, 96

Sodas
    Pomegranate-Cranberry Soda, 163

Soups and stews
    Chicken with Cheesy Broccoli Soup, 160
    Escarole Soup with Fennel, Navy Beans, and Mini Meatballs, 36–37
    Golden Gazpacho, 166
    Hearty Minestrone Soup,* 35
    Lean Turkey Chili, 161
    Mushroom and Dumpling Soup, 145

Spinach
    Baby Spinach Salad with Goat Cheese and Toasted Pistachios, 40
    Breakfast Stuffins,* 34–35
    Green Goddess Smoothie,* 116
    Mushroom and Dumpling Soup, 145
    Spinach Barley Salad,* 119
    Spinach Dip,* 39
    Watermelon, Spinach, and Bacon Salad, 174

Stews. *See* Soups and stews
Stir-fries
  Asparagus Stir-Fry,* 156
  Shrimp Stir-Fry, 145
Strawberries
  Strawberry and Banana Workout Shake, 96
  Strawberry Sauce, 172
Sweet potatoes
  Quinoa Salad with Black Beans and Sweet Potatoes, 52

T
Tacos
  Quick Chicken Adobo and Black Bean Tacos, 184
Tomatoes
  Baked Eggplant with Tomato Chutney, 39
  Chicken with Roasted Onions, Peppers, and Tomatoes, 183
  Heirloom Tomato and Eggplant Stacks,* 162
  Linguine with Walnut-Tomato Pesto,* 112
Tortillas
  Chicken Fajitas, 125
  Quick Chicken Adobo and Black Bean Tacos, 184
  roasted, 87
  Steak Quesadilla,* 38

Tuna
  Mexi-Tuna, 97
  Pasta Dinner, 145
  Tuna Niçoise Salad,* 171
  Tuna Sandwich, 98
Turkey
  Lean Turkey Chili, 161
  Smoky & Spicy Sausage Heroes, 183
  Turkey and Avocado Sandwich with Slaw,* 157

V
Vegetables
  Balsamic-Glazed Mushrooms and Onions, 247
  Green Goddess Smoothie,* 116
  Heirloom Tomato and Eggplant Stacks,* 162
  Lemony Green Beans, 164
  roasted, 87
  Smoky Paprika Kale Chips,* 113
Vegetarian main dishes
  Asparagus Stir-Fry,* 156
  Baked Eggplant with Tomato Chutney, 39
  Hearty Minestrone Soup,* 35
  Lentil Quinoa Burgers,* 114
  Spaghetti with Roasted Red Pepper Sauce, 158

W
Walnuts
  Linguine with Walnut-Tomato Pesto,* 112
  Pomegranate-Walnut Sauce,* 40
Watermelon
  Watermelon, Spinach, and Bacon Salad, 174
Whey protein powder
  Muscle Builder smoothie, 129
  Protein-Packed Oatmeal, 96
  Strawberry and Banana Workout Shake, 96
Wine, sparkling
  Pear-Thyme Bellini,* 168
Wraps. *See* Sandwiches and wraps; Tortillas

Y
Yogurt
  Berry Smoothie, 247
  Brain Booster smoothie, 129
  Dill-Yogurt Sauce, 247
  Green Goddess Smoothie,* 116
  Heart Helper smoothie, 129
  Mint-Yogurt Dressing, 54–55
  Spinach Dip,* 39